AF577325

LYMPHOID MALIGNANCY

Immunocytology and Cytogenetics

International Colloquium on Lymphoid Malignancy
August 27–September 1, 1987
Kyoto International Conference Hall, Kyoto, Japan

Organizers

Masao Hanaoka (Kyoto)
Masahiro Kikuchi (Fukuoka)
Taizan Suchi (Nagoya)

Honorary Advisor

Mizu Kojima (Mito)

Members of Executive Committee

Yutaka Imai (Yamagata)
Atsuo Mikata (Chiba)
Noboru Mohri (Tokyo)
Naoyoshi Mori (Tsukuba)
Shigeo Mori (Tokyo)
Makoto Motoi (Okayama)
Koji Nanba (Hiroshima)
Mikihiro Shamoto (Nagoya)
Keizo Takagi (Tokyo)
Haruki Wakasa (Fukushima)
Shaw Watanabe (Tokyo)
Hirohiko Yamabe (Kyoto)

LYMPHOID MALIGNANCY

Immunocytology and Cytogenetics

Edited by

Masao Hanaoka, M.D.
Department of Pathology
Institute for Virus Research
Kyoto College of Medical Technology
Kyoto, Japan

Marshall E. Kadin, M.D.
Department of Pathology and Charles A. Dana Research Institute
Beth Israel Hospital and Harvard Medical School
Boston, Massachusetts, U.S.A.

Atsuo Mikata, M.D.
First Department of Pathology
School of Medicine
Chiba University
Chiba, Japan

Shaw Watanabe, M.D.
Epidemiology Division
National Cancer Center Research Institute
Tokyo, Japan

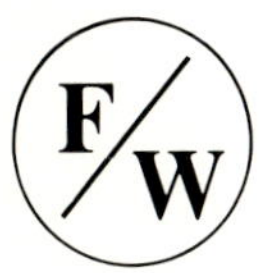

FIELD & WOOD
Medical Publishers, Inc.

Distributed by W. W. Norton & Company, Inc.

500 Fifth Avenue, New York, NY 10110

Distributed by:

W. W. Norton & Company, Inc.
500 Fifth Avenue
New York, New York 10110

Library of Congress Catalog Card Number: 89–080874

ISBN 0–938607–24–3

Printed in the United States of America

Printing: 1 2 3 4 5 6 7 8 9 10

Contents

Contributors

Masafumi Abe, M.D.
First Department of Pathology
Fukushima Medical College
Fukushima, Japan

Ryuichi Amakawa, M.D.
Department of Internal Medicine and
Anatomical Pathology
Kyoto University
Kyoto, Japan

Yuu Arita, M.D.
The First Division of Internal Medicine
Kyoto University
Kyoto, Japan

Shigeyuki Asano, M.D.
First Department of Pathology
Fukushima Medical College
Fukushima, Japan

Raul C. Braylan, M.D.
Department of Pathology
University of Florida Medical College
Gainesville, Florida, U.S.A.

V. Brito-Babapulle, M.D.
MRC Leukaemia Unit
Department of Haematology
Royal Postgraduate Medical School
London, U.K.

Daniel Catovsky, M.D.
MRC Leukaemia Unit
Royal Postgraduate Medical School
London, U.K.

Carlo M. Croce, Ph.D.
The Wistar Institute of Anatomy and Biology
Philadelphia, Pennsylvania, U.S.A.

J. Davis, M.D.
The Departments of Pathology and Microbiology
and Pediatrics, and the Eppley Institute for
Research in Cancer and Allied Diseases
University of Nebraska Medical Center
Omaha, Nebraska, U.S.A.

C. Dearden, M.D.
MRC Leukaemia Unit
Department of Haematology
Royal Postgraduate Medical School
London, U.K.

C. De Wolf-Peeters, M.D.
Pathologische
Ontleedkunde II
Universitaire Ziekenhuizen
Leuven, Belgium

Shoichi Doi, M.D.
First Department of Internal Medicine
Kyoto University
Kyoto, Japan

Ronald F. Dorfman, M.D.
Co-Director, Surgical Pathology
Stanford University Medical Center
Stanford, California, U.S.A.

Tadaaki Eimoto, M.D.
First Department of Pathology
School of Medicine
Fukuoka University
Fukuoka, Japan

Lawrence Fagan, M.D., Ph.D.
Stanford University School of Medicine
Medical Computer Science Group
Stanford, California, U.S.A.

L. Foroni
Laboratory of Molecular Genetics
Department of Haematology
Royal Postgraduate Medical School
London, U.K.

Glauco Frizzera, M.D.
Department of Laboratory Medicine and Pathology
University of Minnesota Medical School
Minneapolis, Minnesota, U.S.A.

Junichiro Fujimoto, M.D.
Department of Pathology
National Children's Medical Research Center
Tokyo, Japan

Shirou Fukuhara, M.D.
First Department of Internal Medicine
Kyoto University
Kyoto, Japan

A. Gates
MRC Leukaemia Unit
Department of Haematology
Royal Postgraduate Medical School
London, U.K.

H. Grierson, M.D.
The Departments of Pathology and Microbiology and Pediatrics, and the Eppley Institute for Research in Cancer and Allied Diseases
University of Nebraska Medical Center
Omaha, Nebraska, U.S.A.

Shuichi Hanada, M.D.
Second Department of Internal Medicine
Kagoshima University
Kagoshima, Japan

Masao Hanaoka, M.D.
Department of Pathology
Institute for Virus Research
Kyoto College of Medical Technology
Kyoto, Japan

Akira Hasegawa, M.D.
Fundamental Research Laboratory
Toa Nenryo Kogyo Co., Ltd.
Saitama, Japan

Kazuhisa Hasui, M.D.
Second Department of Pathology
Kagoshima University
Kagoshima, Japan

Jun-ichi Hata, M.D.
Department of Pathology
National Children's Hospital, Medical Research Center
Taishido, Setagaya-ku
Tokyo, Japan

Toshio Hattori, M.D.
Second Department of Internal Medicine
Kumamoto University School of Medicine
Kumamoto, Japan

David Heckerman, Ph.D.
Stanford University Medical Center
Medical Computer Science Group
Stanford, California, U.S.A.

Hiroshi Hojo, M.D.
First Department of Pathology
Fukushima Medical College
Fukushima, Japan

Hiroshi Horie, M.D.
First Department of Pathology
School of Medicine
Chiba University
Chiba, Japan

Eric Horvitz, Ph.D.
Stanford University Medical Center
Medical Computer Science Group
Stanford, California, U.S.A.

Yutaka Imai, M.D.
Department of Pathology
Yamagata University School of Medicine
Yamagata, Japan

Hiroshi Iwasaki, M.D.
First Department of Pathology
School of Medicine
Fukuoka University
Fukuoka, Japan

Elaine S. Jaffe, M.D.
Hematopathology Section
Laboratory of Pathology
National Cancer Institute
National Institutes of Health
Bethesda, Maryland, U.S.A.

Marshall E. Kadin, M.D.
Department of Pathology and Charles A. Dana Research Institute
Beth Israel Hospital and Harvard Medical School
Boston, Massachusetts, U.S.A.

Nanao Kamada, M.D.
Research Institute of Nuclear Medicine and Biology
Hiroshima University
Hiroshima, Japan

Yasuhiko Kaneko, M.D.
Department of Laboratory Medicine
Saitama Cancer Center
Saitama, Japan

Kokichi Kikuchi, M.D.
Department of Pathology
Sapporo Medical College
Sapporo, Japan

Masahiro Kikuchi, M.D.
First Department of Pathology
School of Medicine
Fukuoka University
Fukuoka, Japan

Kenkichi Kita, M.D.
Department of Internal Medicine
Mie University Medical School
Mie, Japan

Michiaki Kohno, M.D.
Faculty of Liberal Arts
Gifu Pharmaceutical School
Gifu City, Japan

Tseng-Tong Kuo, M.D.
Department of Pathology
Chang Gung Medical College and Chang Gung Memorial Hospital
Taipei, Taiwan

Kunihiko Maeda, M.D.
Department of Pathology
Yamagata University School of Medicine
Yamagata, Japan

Yoshiaki Maeda, M.D.
Fukuoka Red Cross Blood Center
Fukuoka, Japan

Nobuo Maseki, M.D.
Hematology Clinic
Saitama Cancer Center
Saitama, Japan

Atsuko Masunaga, M.D.
Department of Pathology
Yamagata University School of Medicine
Yamagata, Japan

Mikio Matsuda, M.D.
Department of Pathology
Yamagata University School of Medicine
Yamagata, Japan

Masao Matsuoka, M.D.
Second Department of Internal Medicine
Kumamoto University Medical School
Kumamoto, Japan

E. Matutes, M.D.
MRC Leukaemia Unit
Department of Haematology
Royal Postgraduate Medical School
London, U.K.

Atsuo Mikata, M.D.
First Department of Pathology
School of Medicine
Chiba University
Chiba, Japan

Youichi Minamishima, M.D.
Department of Microbiology
Miyazaki Medical College
Miyazaki, Japan

Hiroshi Miwa, M.D.
Department of Internal Medicine
Mie University Medical School
Mie, Japan

Tenjun Mizukami, M.D.
First Department of Pathology
School of Medicine
Chiba University
Chiba, Japan

Shigeo Mori, M.D.
Department of Pathology
Institute of Medical Science
University of Tokyo
Tokyo, Japan

Kiyoshi Mukai, M.D.
Pathology Division
National Cancer Center Research Institute and Hospital
Tokyo, Japan

Yujiro Namba, M.D.
Institute for Virus Research
Kyoto University
Kyoto, Japan

Reiko Namikawa, M.D.
The First Department of Pathology
Aichi Medical University
Nagoya, Japan

Kohji Nanba, M.D.
Department of Health Science
Faculty of Integrated Arts and Sciences
Hiroshima University
Hiroshima, Japan

Masaru Narabayashi, M.D.
Department of Pathology
Yamagata University School of Medicine
Yamagata, Japan

Kaori Nasu, M.D.
Department of Internal Medicine
Osaka Red Cross Hospital
Osaka, Japan

Bharat N. Nathwani, M.D.
Professor of Pathology
Chief of Hematopathology
University of Southern California School of Medicine
Los Angeles, California, U.S.A.

Tetsuya Nosaka, M.D.
Department of Serology and Immunology
Institute of Virus Research
Kyoto University
Kyoto, Japan

Yoshihiro Nozawa, M.D.
First Department of Pathology
Fukushima Medical College
Fukushima, Japan

Yuichi Obata, M.D.
Laboratory of Immunology
Aichi Cancer Center
Nagoya, Japan

Hisako Ochi, Ph.D.
Epidemiology Division
National Cancer Center Research Institute and Hospital
Tokyo, Japan

Toshiyuki Ohno, M.D.
First Department of Internal Medicine
Kyoto University
Kyoto, Japan

Akitsugu Ojima, M.D.
Department of Pathology
Gifu University School of Medicine
Gifu City, Japan

M. Okano, M.D.
The Departments of Pathology and Microbiology and Pediatrics, and the Eppley Institute for Research in Cancer and Allied Diseases
University of Nebraska Medical Center
Omaha, Nebraska, U.S.A.

T. Perrone, M.D.
Department of Laboratory Medicine and Pathology
University of Minnesota Medical School
Minneapolis, Minnesota, U.S.A

D.T. Purtilo, M.D.
The Department of Pathology and Microbiology and Pediatrics, and the Eppley Institute for Research in Cancer and Allied Diseases
University of Nebraska Medical Center
Omaha, Nebraska, U.S.A.

Chen-Feng Qi, M.D.
Department of Pathology
Gifu University School of Medicine
Gifu City, Japan

Hitoshi Sakano, M.D.
Department of Microbiology
University of California
Berkeley, California, U.S.A.

Keiko Sakatani, M.D.
Department of Hematology
Research Institute for Nuclear Medicine and Biology
Hiroshima University
Hiroshima, Japan

Masaharu Sakurai, M.D.
Department of Internal Medicine
Saitama Cancer Center
Saitama, Japan

Naomi Sasaki, M.D.
Department of Pathology
Kure Mutual Aid Hospital
Hiroshima, Japan

Eiichi Sato, M.D.
The Second Department of Pathology
Faculty of Medicine
Kagoshima University
Kagoshima, Japan

Mikihiro Shamoto, M.D.
Department of Pathology
Fujita-Gakuen Health University
School of Medicine
Toyoake City, Japan

Lee-Yung Shih, M.D.
Division of Hematology
Department of Internal Medicine
Chang Gung Medical College and Chang Gung Memorial Hospital
Taipei, Taiwan

Masanori Shimoyama, M.D.
Drug Therapy Division
National Cancer Center Research Institute and Hospital
Tokyo, Japan

Shigeru Shirakawa, M.D.
Department of Internal Medicine
Mie University Medical School
Mie, Japan

Jeffrey Sklar, M.D.
Department of Pathology
Stanford University Medical Center
Stanford, California, U.S.A.

Taizan Suchi, M.D.
Department of Pathology and Clinical Laboratories
Aichi Cancer Center Hospital
Nagoya, Japan

Haruo Sugiyama, M.D.
Third Department of Internal Medicine
University of Osaka
Osaka, Japan

Hirotaka Suzuki, M.D.
The First Department of Internal Medicine
Nagoya University School of Medicine
Nagoya, Japan

Toshitada Takahashi, M.D.
Laboratory of Immunology
Aichi Cancer Center
Nagoya, Japan

Tsuyoshi Tamaki, M.D.
Department of Pathology
Gifu University School of Medicine
Gifu City, Japan

Kiyoshi Takatsuki, M.D.
Second Department of Internal Medicine
Kumamoto University Medical School
Kumamoto, Japan

Morishige Takeshita, M.D.
First Department of Pathology
School of Medicine
Fukuoka University
Fukuoka, Japan

Kimio Tanaka, M.D.
Department of Hematology
Research Institute for Nuclear Medicine and Biology
Hiroshima University
Hiroshima, Japan

G. Thiele, Ph.D.
The Departments of Pathology and Microbiology and Pediatrics, and the Eppley Institute for Research in Cancer and Allied Diseases
University of Nebraska Medical Center
Omaha, Nebraska, U.S.A.

Kennsei Tobinai, M.D.
Drug Therapy Division
National Cancer Center Research Institute and Hospital
Tokyo, Japan

Takahiro Tokudome, M.D.
Department of Pathology
Kagoshima Municipal Hospital
Kagoshima, Japan

Masayoshi Tokunaga, M.D.
Department of Pathology
Kagoshima Municipal Hospital
Kagoshima, Japan

Kunihiko Tominaga, M.D.
First Department of Pathology
Fukushima Medical College
Fukushima, Japan

Fumiyo Tsubai, M.D.
Department of Pathology
Institute for Virus Research
Kyoto College of Medical Technology
Kyoto, Japan

Yoshihide Tsujimoto, M.D.
The Wistar Institute of Anatomy and Biology
Philadelphia, Pennsylvania, U.S.A.

Haruto Uchino, M.D.
First Department of Internal Medicine
Kyoto University
Kyoto, Japan

Ryuzo Ueda, M.D.
Laboratory of Chemotherapy
Aichi Cancer Center Research Institute
Nagoya, Japan

Haruki Wakasa, M.D.
First Department of Pathology
Fukushima Medical College
Fukushima, Japan

Yuji Wano, M.D.
Department of Internal Medicine
Howard Hughes Medical Institute
Duke University
Durham, North Carolina, U.S.A.

Shaw Watanabe, M.D.
Epidemiology Division
National Cancer Center Research Institute
and Hospital
Tokyo, Japan

Kazuyoshi Yamaguchi, M.D.
MRC Leukaemia Unit
Royal Postgraduate Medical School
London, U.K.

Seiko Yamamoto, M.D.
Second Department of Internal Medicine
Kumamoto University Medical School
Kumamoto, Japan

You-Li Zu, M.D.
Department of Pathology
Institute for Virus Research
Kyoto University
Kyoto, Japan

Preface

This monograph presents the Proceedings of the International Colloquium on Lymphoid Malignancy, which was held from August 27 to September 1, 1987 in Kyoto Japan, in memory of Dr. Kenji Kiyono and Dr. Shigeyasu Amano who promoted the study of hematopathology.

Kyoto is not only a place of historic interest, but it also has taken the lead in the development of civilization in each age for 1,000 years. In the past 100 years, achievements in scientific fields have been produced in Kyoto. In the field connected with this meeting, excellent research has been presented by pioneers. Dr. Akira Fujinami, the first professor in the Department of Pathology, Kyoto University, is one of those pioneers. About 80 years ago, a poultryman in Nagoya, a center of poultry in Japan, carried a dead chicken with abdominal inflation to Fujinami's laboratory for the purpose of knowing how to prevent the spread of the disease. At autopsy, white-grey tubercles were found in the peritoneal cavity; Dr. Fujinami thought the chicken died of tuberculosis. However, frozen sections showed a histologically neoplastic pattern. Dr. Fujinami was surprised and glad to get such material. He then asked the poultryman to bring similar chickens and began his research on transplantable avian sarcoma. The results were reported in 1909, and he believed this tumor was the only example of animal neoplasia. However, he later learned that Dr. Rous at the Rockefeller Institute reported a histologically similar sarcoma in chickens in 1910. In fact, the first case of avian sarcoma was reported by Ellenman-Bang in 1908. Dr. Fujinami and Dr. Rous began their research on cell-free transmission of the sarcoma. This was the dawn of the study of oncovirology of avian sarcoma-leukosis and oncogenes, fps, and src.

In 1909 when Dr. Fujinami reported the avian sarcoma, a freshman, Dr. Kenji Kiyono entered Dr. Fujinami's laboratory. During a one year period of research, Dr. Kiyono questioned why tissues were fixed for staining. He thought living cells should be stained in a living state. Accordingly, Dr. Kiyono tried and succeeded in staining living cells in rabbits repeatedly injected with lithion-carmin. One day, he found a small abcess in the neck of a rabbit, where he injected carmin repeatedly. After the vital staining, the tissue surrounding the abscess became red, and histologically, many cells containing red granules accumulated there. Dr. Kiyono could not identify what kind of cells were stained, at that time. It was his first encounter with histiocytes, later named by him. In 1912, Dr. Kiyono visited Dr. Ashoff in Freiburg and showed the section of the vitally stained abscess tissue. After observation of the section under a microscope by the window, Dr. Ashoff said to him "you should study hematology here." For 2 years until the outbreak of the First World War, Dr. Kiyono had observed cells selectively taking up carmin particles in the liver and hematopoietic organs, and published the results in a monograph entitled *Vitale Karmin Speicherung* in which he proposed the name histiocyte. Six years after coming back to Kyoto, he formulated the idea of the histiocytic system. This concept later evolved into the Reticulendothelial system as described by Ashoff and Kiyono.

In 1929, Dr. Shigeyasu Amano, my teacher, entered Dr. Kiyono's laboratory. His early research concerned physicochemical and cytochemical studies of hematopoietic cells, particularly on monocytes. Since 1945, his project has focused on two fields. One is the proliferation and function of lymphocytes and plasma cells. Already in 1945, he proposed antibody formation by plasma cells. The project of lymphocyte proliferation is being continued by us as our research on the intracellular mechanism of proliferating T cells and their neoplastic cells. The second project was the viral origin of leukemia.

When Dr. Amano moved to the Institute for Virus Research, Kyoto University, in 1956 he participated in the 6th International Congress of Hematology held in Boston. On that occasion, he was invited to Dr. Furth's residence with Dr. Beard and others. On discussion with them he found that no one had yet succeeded in directly observing virus particles in leukemia cells of experimental animals by electron microscopy. After coming back to Kyoto, he began his second project immediately, using SL mice that spontaneously developed lymphoid leukemia and had already been bred in our laboratory. Later, in 1957, Dr. Ichikawa found C-particles on the surface of leukemia cells of SL mice.

The traditional studies of hematology and oncovirology at Kyoto University formed the foundation of the discovery of adult T-cell leukemia by Dr. Takatsuki and others in Kyoto. When I observed histologically the first autopsy case of ATL reported in 1977, I was shocked, because the neoplastic tissues showed the pattern of reticulum cell sarcoma. This resulted in a new classification of lymphoma including diffuse lymphoma, pleomorphic type, by our lymphoma study group. Rapid progress in virological research on ATL followed thereafter as is well known.

In the last decade, lymphoma studies and diagnosis have experienced a dynamic development using immunocytologic and molecular genetic techniques, especially in situ. On this occasion, it was significant to hold the Colloquium on Lymphoid Malignancies from histologic and molecular aspects.

Finally, I thank for Dr. Kiyono's and Dr. Amano's Foundation on Hematopathological Studies for making it possible to invite guests from overseas and for the publication of these proceedings. I also wish to thank the Ministry of Education, Culture and Science, and the Prime Minister Nakasone's 10 Years Strategies for the Aid of Cancer Research for practical support and invitation of the guests.

Masao Hanaoka

Part I

Modern Techniques in the Diagnosis of Lymphoma-Leukemia

1

Molecular Genetic Analysis of Lymphoid Malignancies

Kenkichi Kita
Hiroshi Miwa
Tetsuya Nosaka
Toshiyuki Ohno
Kaori Nasu
Kohji Nanba
Shigeru Shirakawa

Molecular genetic analysis of immunoglobulin (Ig) and T-cell antigen receptor (TcR) genes have greatly contributed to elucidating the cellular origin and monoclonality of hematopoietic disorders, especially of lymphoproliferative disorders (LPD)[1–4] Ig heavy chain (IgH) gene is recombined to produce IgH molecules, followed by Ig kappa (Igκ) and lambda (Igλ) chain gene recombination and expression during successful B-cell differentiation process.[1,5,6] TcRα, TcRβ and TcRγ chain genes which were already isolated, are also rearranged in the early stage of intrathymic T-cell differentiation[7,8] and gene rearrangements of TcRγ and TcRβ are thought to occur prior to those of TcRα.[2,4–7]

The cytochemical and immunophenotypical methods are powerful tools to clarify the clinical manifestations in relation to the nature of tumor cells.[9–11] Nevertheless, the precise cellular origin of tumor cells or the neoplastic nature of some LPD (i.e., non-T non-B acute lymphoblastic leukemia, [ALL] angioimmunoblastic lymphadenopathy with dysproteinemia [AILD], and Hodgkin's disease [HD], are still undetermined even by using these techniques.[12–18] Introduction of molecular study in the field of hematopoietic disorders, especially of LPD, is therefore expected to work out such problems and to make an insight into hematopoietic cell differentiation.

In this report, Kita et al present the results of 165 LPD cases, analyzed for Ig and TcR genes with immunophenotyping, and two points are discussed as follows: (1) Is it possible to determine the precise cellular origin of leukemic cells in relation to immature hematopoietic differentiation; and (2) is this new technique useful for confirming the clonality of cells in the mature type of LPD, especially AILD and HD?

MORPHOLOGIC AND PHENOTYPICAL DIAGNOSIS

The diagnosis was made by the cytologic and histologic stainings of peripheral blood, bone marrow, or tissue sections, and was followed by FAB classification with cytochemical stainings for acute leukemias, Working Formulation (WF) or Japanese LSG classification for non-Hodgkin's lymphoma (NHL), and Rye classification for HD. The diagnosis of AILD was made according to the definition in the first report by Frizzera et al.[13] Nevertheless, occasionally the existence of cells with atypia in lymph nodes with AILD lesions occurs. Indeed, when the cellular atypia was focused upon, some AILD cases were diagnosed as malignant lymphoma, an immunoblastic clear cell type according to WF. In this study, cases with the cellular atypia were regarded as AILD unless such cells could be definitively recognized as taking a main role for the diffuse destruction of lymph nodes. Here, note that the histologic diagnoses of malignant lymphoma was made independently of other diagnostic methods.

Phenotypical diagnosis of leukemia and lymphoma cells were made by a panel of monoclonal antibodies. Cell suspension and the frozen sections of lymph nodes or tissues were stained by immunofluorescence and an avidin-biotin complex method, respectively. Fifty-five cases with ALL, 42 with NHL, 9 with adult T-cell leukemia/lymphoma (ATL), 29 with chronic lymphocytic leukemia (CLL) and related disorders, 10 with HD, and 20 with AILD were examined in this study.

MOLECULAR GENETIC EXAMINATIONS

High-molecular weight DNAs were obtained from cells or tissues. DNAs completely digested with EcoRI or BamHI, separated by 0.6% agarose gel, and transferred to nitrocellulose membrane.[19] Total cellular RNA was extracted by the guanidine isothiocyanate technique, and the poly(A)-containing fraction was purified by oligodeoxythymidylic acid cellulose chromatography, then 2μg of poly(A)+ RNAs were denaturated.[20] After electrophoresis through 1% agarose with 6% formaldehyde, the DNAs were transferred to the gene screen by Northern blotting. The membranes both of Southern blot and Northern blot were hybridized to Nick-translated ^{32}P-labeled DNA probe, and autoradiographed.

DNA probes used for the determination of gene structures of Ig and TcR were as follows with sizes of the germline genes and used restriction enzymes; JH for joining(J) region genes of IgH(19kb by BamHI). Jκ for J region genes of Igκ (10kb by BamHI), Cβ1 for constant (C) region genes of TcRβ (23kb by BamHI, and 10.5kb and 4kb by EcoRI), and Jγ1 for J region genes of TcRγ (15kb and 12.5kb by BamHI, and 3.3kb and 1.8kb by EcoRI). Probe Cμ for Cμ region of IgH was used for Northern blot study.

Sensitivity of Southern-Blotting Analysis

The results clearly showed the utility of DNA study for LPD to clarify the cellular origin and the clonality of tumor cells, and were able to give a new explanation for the relationship between the LPD and lymphocyte differentiation process. The genomic study using the Southern method did not show higher sensitivity than the histologic study with the high-resolution immunologic methods in order to identify the existence of neoplastic components in specimen, especially in lymph node samples. Indeed, in comparison with the study using cell lines, over 5% of monoclonal populations in fresh samples are necessary in the Southern-blotting assay using immune genes. The definite band(s) on films can be regarded as an evidence of the existence of the clonally proliferative cells, and there is a possibility that the clonal cells below the sensitivity of Southern method may exist.

In the analysis for TcRγ genes, cells from peripheral blood and lymph nodes in non-neoplastic individuals occasionally demonstrated several non-germ line bands by using EcoRI digested DNA. These bands can not be regarded as clonal ones because of the limited rearranged pattern of TcRγ genes, as previously described.[21] Therefore, the analysis of TcRβ genes is superior to that of TcRγ genes in identifying the clonality of cells, especially in lymphoid tissue with heterogenous populations. In addition, take notice of the fact that the disordered rearrangements of the immune genes may occur, for example in consequence of chromosomal rearrangements.[22] Despite such limitations, the present genomic findings are thought enough evidence to represent pathogenesis of LPD closely relating to the cellular origin of tumor cells.

IMMATURE LYMPHOID NEOPLASMS

Relation Between Genotypes and Phenotypes in ALL Cells

Subtypes and numbers of immature type lymphoid neoplasms examined are listed in Table 1-1. Here, acute unclassified (or undifferentiated) leukemia (AUL) was defined as follows: (1) there are no morphological or cytochemical properties of myeloid cells such as POX; (2) there are no immunologic features corresponding to the typical T-cell ALL (T-ALL), B-cell ALL (B-ALL), and common-ALL (c-ALL); and (3) coexpression of different lineage-associated antigens exist. Lymphoblastic lymphoma (LBL) was taken together with T-ALL, because it was not easy to distinguish LBL from T-ALL, not only phenotypically, but also clinically. On the basis of phenotypes, 20 cases were diagnosed as AUL, 18 as c-ALL, 2 as B-ALL, and 26 as T-ALL/LBL.

According to genotypes of Ig and TcR genes, ALL was subclassified to 4 groups: (1) the germ line, (2) the IgH rearranged, (3) the TcR rearranged, and (4) the dual-genotype (with simultaneous rearrangements of Ig and TcR genes) groups. the rearranged bands of Ig and TcR genes were one or two on both regular- and long-exposed films of all ALL cases tested, indicating monoclonal origin of leukemic cells, found in either phenotype-genotype or genotype-genotype discordant cases.

The relationship between genotypes and phenotypes in AUL cells was very complex. Nine AUL cases were positive for one or more of anti-myeloid cell antibodies, even though they were completely negative for the myeloid-specific cytochemical stainings including ultrastructural peroxidase. Four myeloid antigen positive AUL had the IgH rearranged genotype, and one of them also had the Igκ rearranged one. The simultaneously rearranged Ig and TcR genes were demonstrated in 2 cases: one had the rearranged IgH and TcRβ genes, and the other the rearranged IgH, TcRγ and TcRβ genes. Since no lymphocyte-associated antigens were found on these leukemic cells, there is the

TABLE 1-1
Genotypes of Acute Leukemia

		IgH	Igκ	TcRγ	TcRβ
AUL:	null	2*/ 3	1 / 3	1 / 3	2 / 3
	My-Ag(+)	2*/ 9	1 / 9	1 / 9	2 / 9
	CD19(+)	6 / 8	1 / 8	1†/ 8	0 / 8
c-ALL:	CD20(−)	7 / 7	2 / 7	1 / 7	1 / 7
	CD20(+)	11 / 11	2 / 11	7 / 11	4 /11
B-ALL		2 / 2	2 / 2	0 / 2	0 / 2
T-ALL/LBL:	stage I	0 / 11		4 / 11	3 / 11
	II	2 / 9		7 / 8	8 / 9
	III	0 / 3		3 / 3	3 / 3
	undetermined	0 / 3		2 / 3	2 / 3

Cases with clonal gene rearrangements / cases examined
*: with simulaneous rearrangement of TcR genes
†: without Ig gene rearrangements

possibility that these IgH gene rearrangements correspond to the abortive IgH gene rearrangements reported in some acute myeloblastic leukemia and T-ALL.[23,24] Such AUL cells called into doubt the variety of genomic studies as a tool for simple lineage-determination of AUL cells. In myeloid antigen negative AUL, 8 cases had the IgH rearranged-genotype, and 2 of them were dual genotypic. In this group, 8 cases were positive for CD19, which reacts with the earliest B-cell progenitor cells,[25] and were discussed together with c-ALL cases.

On the basis of expression of CD19, CD10, and CD20 antigens,[25] B-cell progenitor cell leukemia can be divided into 3 groups: (1) CD19(+), CD10(−), and CD20(−); (2) CD19(+), CD10(+), and CD20(−); and (3) CD19(+), CD10(+), and CD20(+). The first group is diagnosed as CD19(+)AUL shown in Table 1-1, and the second and third groups as c-ALL, generally. Most of these cases had the clonally rearranged IgH genes (Table 1-1 and Fig. 1-1), and Cμ mRNA were demonstrated by Northern-blot analysis using RNAs of CD19-positive AUL and c-ALL cells (Fig. 1-2). Thus, these finding strongly suggested a B-cell progenitor cell origin of these leukemias. Nevertheless, 8 c-ALL cases had the clonally rearranged TcRγ genes, and 5 of them also had the rearranged TcRβ genes. More interestingly, most of such dual-genotypic c-ALL cases were positive for CD20 (Fig. 1-1).

In T-ALL and LBL cases, a good relation between gene rearrangements of TcR and expression of T-cell differentiation antigens were found,[26] and there were only 2 dual-genotype T-ALL/LBL cases. Note here the two findings: 4 of 11 cases corresponding to the earliest stage of T-cell ontogeny had the rearranged TcR genes, and each of 2 dual-genotype cases had phenotypes of stage II of intrathymic differentiation.

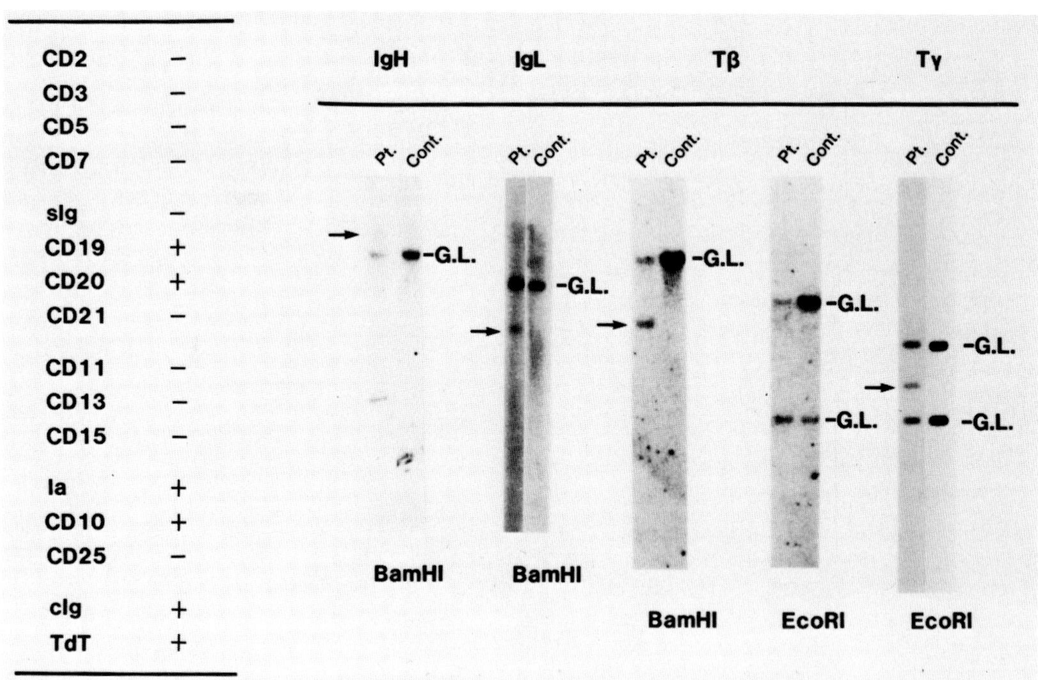

Fig. 1-1. CD20-positive c-ALL with the dual-genotype. Phenotypes of leukemic cells corresponded to those of the most mature B-cell progenitor cells. Rearrangements of TcR genes in this case were caused in consequence of those of IgH genes by putative common recombinase. Indeed, only Ig genes were transcribed as shown in lane 6 of Cμ in Figure 1-4.

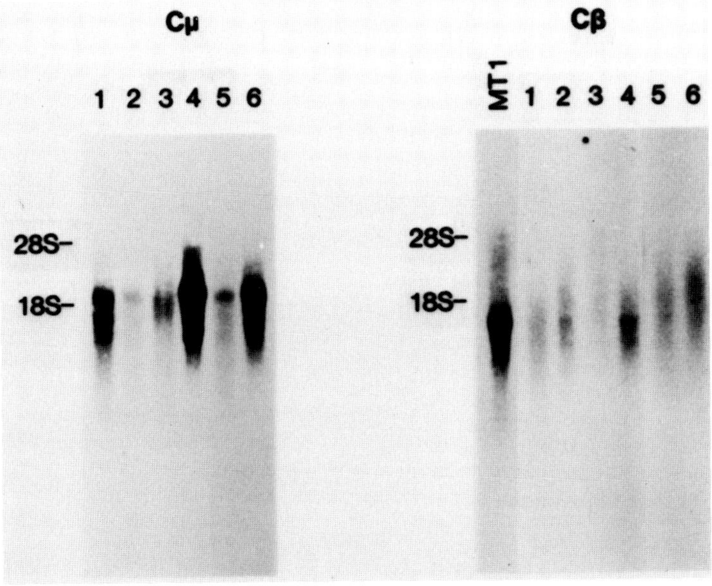

Fig. 1-2. Northern-blot of Cμ and Cβ genes. Lanes 1–3 are CD19(+)CD20(−) ALL, lane 4 CD20(−) c-ALL, and lanes 5 and 6 CD20(+) c-ALL. Cμ gene transcripts were found in 5 of 6 examined cases, but no Cβ transcripts were found in any cases. Here, faint bands of Cβ were observed in lanes 2 and 4, but might be considered as Cβ transcripts of contaminated normal T-cells.

Simultaneous Rearrangements of Ig and TcR Genes in ALL Cells

Simultaneous rearrangements of Ig and TcR genes were often observed in the IgH rearranged-genotypic AUL and c-ALL, while such genotypes were rare in T-ALL/LBL and mature LPD. This suggests that such gene rearrangements occurred in the different develomental stages of early immature hematopoiesis. In the dual-genotypic AUL cases, most of which expressed myeloid antigen(s), there was no significant relation between genotypes and phenotypes, suggesting that even genotypes of the immune genes did not provide a solid basis for establishing of B-cell or T-cell origin of neoplastic cells. This assumed that rearrangements of the immune genes occurred stochastically in cells with myeloid and lymphoid differentiation, although the persuasive mechanism causing gene rearrangements is still unknown.

On the other hand, in ALL cells corresponding to the phenotypic discrete stage of early B-cell differentiation, simultaneous rearrangements of IgH and TcR genes were strikingly found in CD20-positive cases, and rarely in ALLs with more immature phenotypes. The presence of Cμ mRNA in these cases indicates that these cells already committed into B-cell lineage at least at the DNA-RNA level, and also that rearrangements of TcR genes in the dual-genotypic leukemic cells occurred as an abortive genomic event. This suggests the high accessibility of IgH and TcR genes toward a common recombinase in a particular stage of early B-cell differentiation,[27] probably in a CD20-positive stage, relating dynamic DNA recombinations for making functional Variable (V), Diversity (D), or Joining (J) segments. ALL cells are considered as clonal expansion of cells arrested at a certain developmental stage of lymphocyte differentiation. B-cell progenitor cell leukemia, therefore, provides a useful model system for understanding early B-cell development.

MATURE LYMPHOID NEOPLASMS

In the mature type lymphoid neoplasms, results showed that the genomic studies for Ig and TcR genes were very useful tools for concurrently determining the cellular origin and the clonality of tumor cells. Most of B-cell and T-cell neoplasms had the clonally rearranged Ig and TcR genes, respectively, and the dual-genotype was found only in one B-NHL case and one B-CLL case (Table 1-2). A particular pattern of gene rearrangements was not demonstrated in each phenotypical subtype of mature lymphoid neoplasms. Besides, one or 2 rearranged bands were shown on Southern-blotting of all cases examined, suggesting that these neoplasms developed from clonal expansion of a single cell.

In T-cell neoplasms, it is very difficult to determine the clonality of tumor cells, even with a panel of monoclonal antibodies. Tumor cells from every CD3 positive case had the clonal and simultaneous rearrangements of TcRγ and TcRβ genes, indicating that genomic study is a powerful diagnostic tool for T-cell neoplasms. Also, note that the phenotypic study was necessary to identify the T-cell subtypes of tumor cells, since there was no subtype-specificity between TcRγ and TcRβ in comparison with Ig light chain gene rearrangements in B-cell neoplasms.

Large Granular Lymphocyte (LGL) Lymphoproliferative Disorder

LGLs are considered the major cells responsible for natural killar (NK) activity or anti-

TABLE 1-2
Genotypes of Mature Type Lymphoid Neoplasms

		IgH	Igκ	TcRγ	TcRβ
B-cell type:					
NHL:	sIg(+)	8 / 8	5 / 5	1*/ 8	1*/ 8
	sIg(−)	8 / 8	5 / 5	0 / 8	1†/ 8
CLL		11 / 11	5 / 5	0 / 11	1 / 11
MM/WM		0 / 5	5 / 5	0 / 5	0 / 5
T-cell type:					
NHL:	CD4(+)	0 / 10		9 / 10	9 / 10
	CD8(+)	0 / 4		3 / 4	3 / 4
ATL		0 / 9		8 / 9	8 / 9
CLL:	CD4(+)	0 / 7		7 / 7	7 / 7
	CD8(+)	0 / 1		1 / 1	1 / 1
LGL:	CD3(+)††	0 / 3		3 / 3	3 / 3
	CD3(−)	0 / 7		0 / 7	0 / 7
Others:§		0 / 1		1 / 1	1 / 1

MM, multiple myeloma; WM, Waldenstrom macroglobulinemia.
*: A case of composite lymphoma
†: A case with simultaneous rearrangements of Ig and TcR genes
††: One case was positive for CD8
§: An immunoblastic sarcoma case co-expressing CD5 and CD13

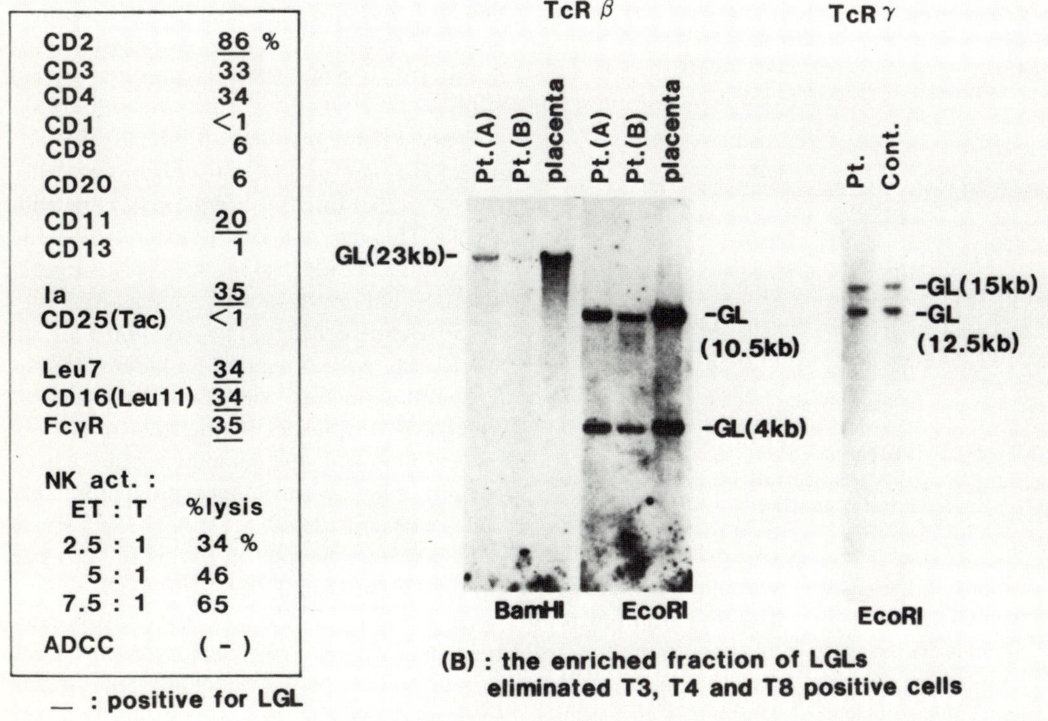

Fig. 1-3. Phenotype and genotype of LGL leukemia. Pathologic cells were positive for CD2, 11, 16, and Leu7, and showed marked NK activity. In addition to the whole fractions of mononuclear cells (A), Southern-blot was performed by using the LGL-enriched fraction (B) eliminated CD3, 4, and 8 positive cells. In each fraction, both TcRγ and TcRβ genes were in germ line.

body-dependent cell mediated cytotoxicity, but their cellular origin in relation to other cell lineages is still undetermined.[28] Seven CD3-negative and 3 CD3-positive cases with Tγ/LGL LPD were examined, and the leukemic cells revealed morphologic, phenotypical, and functional properties corresponding to those of LGL cells. All CD3-negative cases had leukemic cells with the germ line genotypes of both TcRγ and TcRβ (Table 1-2 and Fig. 1-3), and CD3-positive the rearranged genotypes of both TcRγ and TcRβ. This indicates that Tγ/LGL LPD consists of heterogenous populations, and suggests that CD3-negative LGLs do not belong to ordinary T-cell populations undergoing the genetical constriction for immunological specificity in the thymus.

AILD AND HODGKIN'S DISEASE

Angioimmunoblastic Lymphoadenopathy

Phenotypically, undetermined cases of the mature type LPD consisted of 20 AILD and 10 HD cases, and the results were shown in Table 1-3. In mononuclear cells in lymph nodes of AILD and HD, T-cell populations were predominant, whereas B-cells occupied only a part of lymph node cells. One half of the AILD cases showed several clusters of cells with atypia or "clear cells",[14] which allowed the authors to conjecture the presence of neoplastic components in lymph nodes. The other half of AILD cases showed little or slight proliferation of such cells. In the

TABLE 1-3
Clonal Rearrangements of Ig or TcR genes in AILD and HD Cases

	IgH	TcR
AILD: A)	0 / 10	1 / 10
B)	1*/ 10	7 / 10
HD	1†/ 11	4 / 11

A) Cases without cellular atypia
B) Cases with moderate or marked cellular atypia
*: with clonal TcR gene rearrangements
†: A cell line KMH-2 established from HD case

former, CD4 T-cells were more numerous than CD8 ones, and cells with atypia, including clear cells, were frequently found in CD4 populations. In the latter, the ratio of CD4 and CD8 cells varied among T-cell populations. Clonal rearrangements of TcRβ genes were found in 8 of AILD cases, and those of Ig genes were not seen in any AILD cases. Thus, there is a good relationship between clonal bands of TcRβ genes and the existence of cells with atypia in lymph nodes. Even in the cases with the clonally rearranged TcR genes, the intensity of bands was weaker than in the other typical T-cell malignancies (Fig. 1-4).

There has been much discussion about the etiology of AILD. A half of AILD cases tested showed the clonally rearranged band(s) of TcRβ genes on Southern-blotting. Histological pictures of lymph nodes in these cases commonly showed moderate or marked proliferation of cells with atypia such as clusters of clear cells resembling those in IBL-like T-cell lymphoma.[16] Therefore, at least a part of AILD cases represent a continuous disease spectrum to T-NHL. Besides, the number of CD4 cells with atypia increased in comparison with that of CD8 cells, suggesting that CD4 cells were a candidate for cells with the clonally rearranged TcR genes. To concern the precise cellular origin of the clonally proliferating cells, however, gene analysis for each fraction of CD4 or CD8 cells should be carried out.

Other AILD cases showed no clonal bands of TcRβ genes, and also, the histological pictures revealed little proliferation of cells with atypia. This may not always mean that AILD without the cellular atypia is a non-neoplastic disorder, but might result from the sensitivity of Southern-blotting. The existence of an AILD case with 5 single-cell karyotypic abnormalities suggests that clonal expansion of T-cells as neoplastic components might not play a main role for pathogenesis of AILD, because a single-cell karyotypic abnormality can not be considered as definitive karyotypic evidence of a neoplasm. Actually, the size of the tumor population within the lymph nodes, even in cases having the clonally rearranged bands of TcR genes, was too small to interpret all of the histologic and clinical features of AILD.

Clinical manifestations and lymph node pictures of AILD such as hypergammaglobulinemia, eosinophilia, infiltration of heterogenous inflammatory cells in lymph nodes, and proliferation of small vessels are thought to be caused by inflammatory reactions rather than by neoplastic events. The study for Ig producing B-cells in an AILD lesion showed the existence of strong and nonspecific stimulation of polyclonal Ig production in B-cells,[29] suggesting that T-cells, probably CD4 cells in this lesion play a main role in B-cell proliferation. Actually, numerous Ia positive CD4 cells, some CD25 positive, and even IL-2 producing T-cells indicative of activated T-cells were occasionally seen in AILD lesion. Recently, several T-cell factors have been isolated at the DNA level,[30,31] and their multifunctions in blood cells were clarified, such as simultaneous T-cell replacing activity and eosinophil growth activity of IL-5.[31] Therefore, investigations on the immunoregulatory system in relation to T-cell activation may contribute to understand the pathogenesis of AILD.

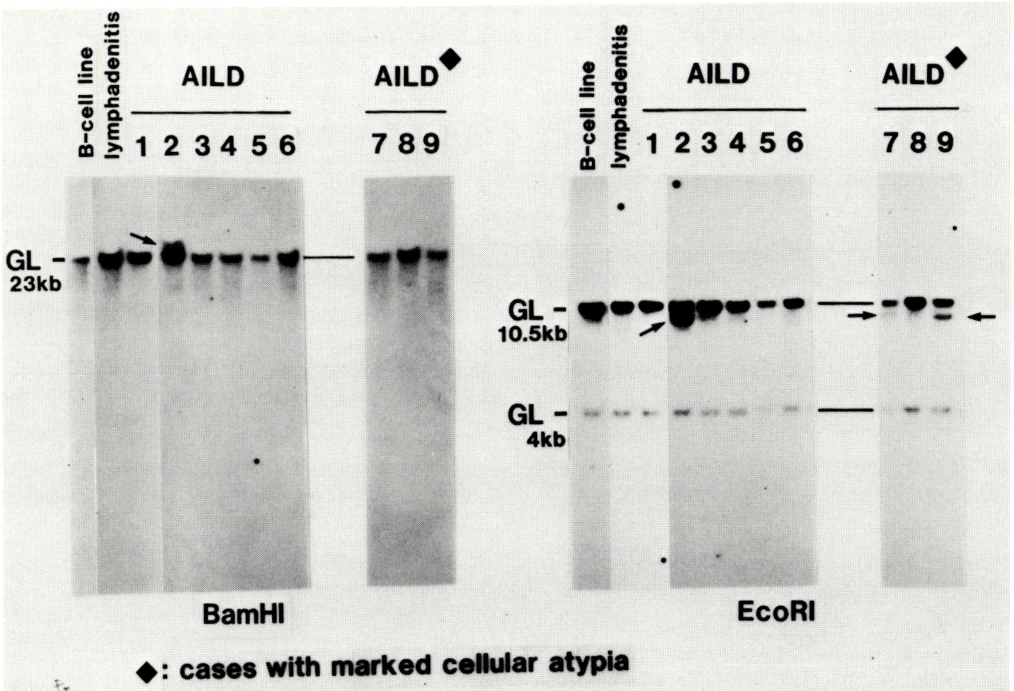

Fig. 1-4. Southern-blot of TcRβ genes of AILD cases. Arrows indicates the rearranged bands. As shown in lanes 7 and 9, the rearranged bands were rather weak, suggesting that clonally proliferative populations occupied only a part of lymph node cells.

Hodgkin's Disease

HD cells commonly reacted with CD15 (LeuM1), CD30(Ki-1), CD25(anti-Tac), and anti-Ia antibody,[18] but were negative for any anti-T-cell and anti-B-cell antibodies. CD4 positive T-cells without atypia were predominant in lymph nodes. Thus, in HD cases, immunophenotyping failed to identify the neoplastic and clonal features of lymph node cells. Four of 10 HD cases examined showed one of two clonally rearranged bands of TcRβ genes without those of Ig genes. On the other hand, a cell line KMH-2 established from HD[32] had sole rearrangements of Ig genes. Similar to most AILD cases showing the TcR-rearranged genotype, the rearranged bands of TcR genes in HD were rather faint.

The cellular origin of HD cells is still obscure despite many histochemical and immunological studies.[17,18,32,33] In the authors' study, the clonally rearranged bands of TcRβ genes were demonstrated in 4 of 10 HD cases examined, although these bands were very faint. HD cells were negative for T-cell antigens by immunohistochemical stainings in these cases, and no cellular atypia of T-cells in lymph nodes were found. Therefore, it is still difficult to decide that HD cells were derived from a T-cell, although a clonal T-cell population actually existed in lymph nodes of these cases. Since HD cell leukemia and HD derived cell line KMH-2 were reported to have the clonally rearranged Ig genes, HD might not only consist of T-cell origin cases, but also B-cell origin ones, as previously pointed out by Stein et al.[18]

ACKNOWLEDGMENTS

The authors thank Drs. T. Honjo (Kyoto University) and T. H. Rabbitts (MRC Laboratory of Molecular Biology, Cambridge, UK) for providing DNA probes; Dr. T. Uchiyama (Kyoto University) for providing monoclonal antibodies; Dr. S. Fukuhara (Kyoto University) for referring of karyotypic analysis; and Drs. M. Hatanaka, S. Doi, and Y. Arita (Kyoto University) for kind and critical advice to the molecular genetic and immunohistochemical studies.

This work was supported in part by Grants-in-Aid for Scientific Research from the Ministry of Education, Science, and Culture, and by Grants-in-Aid for Cancer Research from the Ministry of Health and Welfare of Japan.

REFERENCES

1. Korsmeyer SG, Hieter PA, Raveth JV, et al: Developmental hierarchy of immunoglobulin gene rearrangements in human leukemic pre-B-cells. Proc Natl Acad Sci UAS 78:7096, 1981
2. Royer HD, Acuto O, Fabbi M, et al: Gene encoding the Tiβ subunit of the antigen/MHC receptor undergo rearrangement during intrathymic ontogeny prior to surface T3-Ti expression. Cell 39:261, 1984
3. Waldmann TA, Davis MM, Bongivanni KF, Korsmyer SJ: Rearrangments of genes for the antigen receptor on T cells as marker of lineage and clonality in human lymphoid neoplasms. N Engl J Med 313:776, 1985
4. Pellichi PG, Knowles DM, Favera RD: Lymphoid tumor displaying rearrangements of both immunoglobulin and T cell receptor genes. J Exp Med 162:1015, 1985
5. Brack C, Hirama M, Schuller R, Tonegawa S: A complete immunoglobulin gene created by somatic mutation. Cell 15:1, 1978
6. Honjo T, Kataoka T: Organization of immunoglobulin heavy chain genes and allelic deletion model. Proc Natl Acad Sci USA 75:2140, 1978
7. Yanagi Y, Yoshikai Y, Legett K, et al: A human T cell-specific cDNA clone encodes a protein having extensive homology to immunoglobulin chains. Nature 308:145, 1984
8. Royer HD, Ramarli D, Acute O, et al: Genes encoding the T-cell receptor β and γ subunits are transcribed in an ordered manner during intrathymic ontogeny. Proc Natl Acad Sci USA 82:5510, 1985
9. Taylor CR: An immunological study of follicular lymphoma, reticulum cell sarcoma and Hodgkin's disease. Europ J Cancer 12:61, 1976
10. Greaves MF, Janossy G: Patterns of gene expression and the cellular origin of human leukemias. Biochem Biophys Acta 516:193, 1978
11. Foon KA, Schroff RW, Gale RP: Surface markers on leukemia and lymphoma cells: Recent advances. Blood 60:1, 1982
12. Kita K, Nasu K, Kamesaki H, et al: Phenotypic analysis of acute lymphoblastic leukemia (ALL) cells which are classified as non-T non-B and negative for common ALL antigen. Blood 66:47, 1985
13. Frizzera G, Moran EM, Rappaport H: Angio-immunoblastic lymphadenopathy with dysproteinemia. Lancet 1:1070–1073, 1974
14. Suchi T: Atypical lymph node hyperplasia with fetal outcome. A report on the histopathological, immunological and clinical investigations of the cases. Recent Adv RES Res 14:13, 1974
15. Lukes RJ, Tindle BH: Immunoblastic lymphadenopathy: A hyperimmune entity resembling Hodgkin's disease. N Engl J Med 292:1, 1975
16. Shimoyama M, Minato K, Saito H, et al: Immunoblastic lymphadenopathy (IBL)-like T-cell lymphoma. Jpn J Clin Oncol 9:347, 1979
17. Kadin ME, Stitel DP, Levy R, Warnke R: Exogenous immunoglobulin and the macrophage origin of Reed-Sternberg cells in Hodgkin's disease. N Engl J Med 299:1208, 1978
18. Stein H, Manson DY, Gerdes J, et al: The expression of the Hodgkin's disease associated antigen Ki-1 in reactive and neoplastic lymphoid tissue: Evidence that Reed-Sternberg cells and histiocytic malignancies are derived from activated lymphoid cells. Blood 66:848, 1985
19. Miwa H, Konishi H, Kobayashi N, et al: The T-cell receptor gene rearrangements in T-lineage tumors without OKT-3,4,6,8 markers. J Mol Cell Immunol 3:37, 1987
20. Kobayashi N, Konishi H, Sabe H, et al: Genomic structures of HTLV (human T-cell leukemia virus): Detection of defective genome and its amplification in MT-2 cells. EMBO J 3:1339, 1984
21. Greenberg JM, Quertermous T, Seidman JG, Kersey JH: Human T cell γ-chain gene rearrangements in acute lymphoid and nonlymphoid leukemia: Comparison with the T cell receptor β-chain gene. J Immunol 137:2043, 1986
22. Tsujimoto Y, Finger L, Yunis J, et al: Molecular genetics of follicular lymphoma: Cloning of the chromosome breakpoint of neoplastic B-cells with the t(14;18) chromosome translocation. Science 226:1097, 1984
23. Rovigatti U, Mirro J, Kitchingman G, et al: Heavy chain immunoglobulin gene rearrangement in acute nonlymphocytic leukemia. Blood 63:1023, 1984
24. Kichingman GR, Rovigatti U, Mauer AM, et al: Rearrangement of immunoglobulin heavy chain genes in T-cell acute lymphoblastic leukemia. Blood 65:725, 1985
25. Nadler LM, Korsmeyer SJ, Anderson KC, et al: B cell origin of non-T cell acute lymphoblastic leukemia: A model for discrete stages of neoplastic and normal pre-B cell differentiation. J Clin Invest 74:332, 1984
26. Reinherz EL, Kung PC, Goldstein G, et al: Discrete stages of human intrathymic differentiation: Analysis of normal thymocytes and leukemic lymphoblasts of T-cell lineage. Proc Natl Acad Sci USA 77:1588, 1980
27. Yancopoulos GD, Blackwell TK, Suh H, et al: Introduced T-cell receptor variable region gene segments recombine in pre-B cells: Evidence that B and T cells used a common recombinase. Cell 44:251, 1986
28. Reynolds CW, Foon KA: Tγ-lymphoproliferative

disease and related disorders in humans and experimental animals: A review of the clinical, cellular, and functional characteristics. Blood 64:1146, 1984

29. Ohno T, Kita K, Miwa H, Shirakawa S: Immunophenotypical and molecular genetical examination of angio-immunoblastic lymphadenopathy. Acta Haematol Jpn 50:1657, 1987
30. Noma Y, Sideras P, Naito T, et al: Cloning of cDNA encoding the murine IgG1 induction factor by a novel strategy using SP6 promorter. Nature 319:640, 1986
31. Kinashi T, Harada N, Severinson, et al: Cloning of complementary DNA encoding T-cell replacing factor and identity with B-cell growth factor II. Nature 324:70, 1986
32. Kamesaki H, Fukuhara S, Tatsumi E, et al: Cytochemical, immunologic, chromosomal, and molecular genetic analysis of a novel cell line derived from Hodgkin's disease. Blood 68:285, 1986
33. Knowles II DM, Neri A, Pelicci PG, et al: Immunoglobulin and T-cell receptor β-chain gene rearrangement analysis of Hodgkin's disease: implication for lineage determination and differential diagnosis.

2

Rearrangements of Antigen Receptor Genes in Lymphoid Neoplasia

Jeffrey Sklar

Abstract

Detection of rearranged antigen receptor genes in lymphoid tissue biopsy specimens by means of Southern blot hybridization can be a sensitive method for assessing the clonality, lineage, and malignancy of cells within these tissues. This technique, however, is subject to a number of limitations and problems requiring appropriate caution in the interpretation of results. Detection of intragenic rearrangements—those involved in assembly of potentially functional antigen receptor genes—reflects the presence of clonal proliferations of lymphocytes, but is not specific for malignancy since certain clincally benign lesions display clonal rearrangements. Conversely, rare T-cell lymphomas lack all detectable rearrangements of the T-cell receptor genes tested so far. Configuration of DNA in rearranged genes provides markers for individual lymphocytic clones, but these markers are not completely stable, since somatic mutation of rearranged immunoglobulin genes occurs in some B-cell lymphomas. Intergenic rearrangements—those involving recombination between antigen receptor gene DNA and other sites in the genome outside of these genes—are more specific for malignancy, although they may be more difficult to detect due to the frequent heterogeneity of breakpoints found among intergenic rearrangements of any one type. Conclusive explanations why particular portions of the genome recombine in intergenic rearrangements and for the effect that such rearrangements have on gene expression are at present not possible, but these questions will undoubtedly be investigated intensively in coming years.

Analyses of antigen receptor gene rearrangements over the last few years have provided an important new approach to the diagnosis and characterization of lymphoid neoplasms. These rearrangements involve DNA of subunit genes for both immunoglobulins (including the heavy chain gene and the two light chain genes, kappa and lambda) and T-cell receptors (alpha, beta, gamma, and delta genes). Lymphoid neoplasms have been most extensively studied by analyzing intragenic rearrangements of antigen receptor DNA—that is, the joining by genetic recombination of single variable, diversity, and joining region sequences within antigen receptor genes to construct transcriptionally active templates for antigen receptor subunits synthesis. Less thoroughly studied to date are intergenic rearrangements involving antigen receptor genes. Some of these intergenic rearrangements have been recognized for a number of years as cytogenetic abnormalities and may play a part in the primary transformation of normal lymphocytes to their neoplastic counterparts.

While analyses of antigen receptor genes have, over a rather short period of time, made an impressive impact on the study of lymphoid neoplasia, this review will discuss only a few areas in which the study of antigen receptor genes have contributed to this field. Most of this presentation will focus on some of the less straightforward aspects of gene rearrangement analysis by reviewing several problems and ambiguities that have arisen in this work during investigations carried out by the author's laboratory and in the laboratories of other investigators.

The configurations of rearranged DNA at each rearranged antigen receptor gene offers a unique marker for individual lymphocytes and any clonal progeny of that lymphocyte. These configurations of rearranged genes can be conveniently assessed by way of the Southern blot hybridization procedure, which detects, in its simplest form, one or two non-germline autoradiographic bands, depending whether one or both alleles for a given antigen receptor subunit are rearranged, in the DNA of tissue specimens that contain a monoclonal proliferation of lymphocytes.[1–5] Since there is usually no dominant clone in reactive processes, this technique fails to detect rearranged, non-germline bands in such tissues, permitting distinction between neoplasia and hyperplasia. Together with immune phenotyping, this approach has proved valuable as an adjunct to conventional morphologic analysis for the detection of lymphoma and leukemia in biopsy specimens. The major virtues of the technique include high sensitivity (down to 1% neoplastic cells in the author's experience), the requirement for very small amounts of starting material (about 10^5 cells per analysis) and the opportunity to confirm a result using multiple restriction enzymes or different DNA hybridization probes for different antigen receptor genes. In the case of T-lineage lesions, analysis of T-cell receptor gene rearrangements provides a method for detecting clonality, for which there is no immunophenotypic alternative, such as detection of immunoglobulin light chain restriction for determining clonality of B-lineage lesions.

Antigen Receptor Gene Rearrangements Used to Assess Clonality and Malignancy

Examples of situations in which the author and his colleagues have found analysis of antigen receptor genes particularly useful for assessing clonality include angioimmunoblastic lymphadenopathy (AILD) and dermatopathic lymphadenopathy in mycosis fungoides (MF). Several years ago the author's laboratory examined antigen receptor gene rearrangements in cases of AILD, and found that the majority contained clonal T-cell receptor gene rearrangements, indicating that lesions in most cases probably represent T-cell lymphomas, as had earlier been suggested based on morphologic analysis.[6] Also found, however, were occasional cases lacking detectable T-cell receptor gene rearrangements, including one case that showed distinct clonal rearrangements in a subsequent biopsy. Therefore, AILD seems to represent a rare inflammatory disorder that may evolve to T-cell lymphoma. Recently, one patient who had earlier been found to evolve to lymphoma died and gene rearrangements analysis of autopsy tissues disclosed both T- and B-cell lymphomas at different sites.* Apparently, while development of T-lineage tumors is far more common,

*Sklar J, et al: unpublished observations

patients with AILD are also at risk for development of B-lineage tumors.

Dermatopathic lymphadenopathy in the setting of MF can present difficult diagnostic problems for the surgical pathologist restricted to morphologic evaluation of enlarged lymph nodes removed from such patients. Weiss et al. have found that analysis of T-cell receptor genes is significantly more sensitive than morphology for detecting MF in lymph nodes.[4] This is true even for some cases in which relatively intense rearranged bands compared to much less intense unrearranged germline bands suggest that the majority of cells within the lymph node are neoplastic, despite a morphologic diagnosis of benign dermatopathic change.

An approach which has proved useful in assessing dermatopathic lymph nodes, or in other comparable situation where multiple biopsy specimens are available, has been to compare the pattern of rearranged bands obtained from tissue showing unequivocal morphologic involvement by tumor to the bands obtained from a tissue under investigation. This permits assurance that the bands represent a malignant process and concurrently permits greater sensitivity, since particular attention can be given to specific regions of the autoradiogram for the possible presence of diagnostic bands.

This type of comparative analysis, in which results are compared from morphologically malignant tissue to those from tissue for which a diagnosis is in question, is particularly valuable because detection of clonal antigen receptor gene rearrangements is not specific for malignancy. Detection of rearranged bands is specific for clonality, and malignant processes are clonal, so that detection of rearranged bands is consistent with malignancy. However, it now seems clear that certain clinically benign disorders may involve clonal lymphoproliferative lesions. The author and his colleagues have studied a number of such diseases arising or manifest in the skin. Among these is lymphomatoid papulosis (LP), a condition characterized by recurrent development of crops of papules that ulcerate and heal over a several week course, leaving behind small scars. Patients often have clinical histories of this disease spanning several decades. A minority of such patients may eventually develop lymphomas of the skin. Histologically, lesions from these patients show an infiltrate of the dermis and epidermis consisting of benign-appearing lymphocytes admixed with large, highly atypical lymphoid cells, all of which immunophenotype as T-lineage. Despite the benign clinical course that most patients experience, Weiss et al. have found that the majority of lesions from patients with LP contain clonal T-cell receptor gene rearrangements, indicating the presence of clonal T-cell populations within involved tissue.[7] Similarly, lesions from *pityriasis lichenoides et varioliformis acuta* (Mucha-Habermann disease), a disorder with features similar to LP but lacking the same degree of histologic atypia,[8] and pagetoid reticulosis (Woringer-Kolopp disease), another cutaneous disorder associated with lymphocytic infiltration of the skin, show clonal T-cell receptor gene rearrangements.[9] Thus, there is a group of diseases, formerly considered inflammatory in nature, which, by gene rearrangement analysis, contain clonal lymphocytic proliferations. This fact demonstrates that detection of non-germline bands for antigen receptor DNA within Southern blot autoradiograms cannot be taken as definitive evidence of malignancy, but rather must be evaluated in the context of clinical and histopathologic information.

While detection of clonal antigen receptor gene rearrangements in non-malignant tissue represents a kind of false-positive result, the author recently encountered cases of lymphoma in which analyses of antigen receptor genes yielded apparently false-negative results. These lymphomas, which are clearly malignant as determined by morphologic criteria and clinical behavior, fail to show clonal antigen receptor gene rearrangements in careful analyses with multiple DNA hybridization probes and restriction enzymes. Some of these tumors neoplasms are probably true histiocytic.[10,11] However, in addition, Weiss et al have studied a small group of mature T-cell neoplasms that apparently lack clonal rearrangements for any of the antigen receptor genes tested (all immunoglobulin genes and the β and γ T-cell receptor genes).[12] Cells in most of these tumors expressed relatively few T-cell antigens, but all expressed the most specific antigen known for T-lineage differentiation, CD2, the sheep erythrocyte rosette receptor. Many of these tumors appear to arise in the upper respiratory passages, but this fact may simply reflect the high incidence of T-cell lymphomas at this site in general. In any event, these results indicate that absence of detectable clonal antigen receptor gene rearrangements cannot be regarded as sufficient evidence to exclude malignancy in a tissue biopsy specimen.

Multiclonal Lymphoid Neoplasms

All of the applications described above for antigen receptor gene rearrangements to lymphoid neoplasia have been based upon the appearance of non-germline bands in Southern blot autoradiograms. The precise position of these bands is also often useful in investigating lymphoid neoplasia, since it provides a specific marker for an individual clone. For instance, the authenticity of a cell line derived from a lymphoid tumor specimen may be confirmed by showing that the tissue and the cell line share the same antigen receptor gene rearrangements.[13] Another area of investigation in which this feature of antigen receptor gene rearrangements has been utilized concerns apparent multiclonal neoplasms. These neoplasms show patterns of gene rearrangements that suggest the existence of more than one clone in a single patient. The author and co-workers have studied this phenomenon in several different settings. Several years ago, they found that different lesions from immunosuppressed transplant patients with Epstein-Barr virus-associate lymphoproliferative disorders showed different patterns of immunoglobulin light and heavy chain gene rearrangements when the lesion came from different sites in individual patients. Each lesion appeared monoclonal (no more than two clonal rearranged bands for either the heavy or light chain gene), but in most instances, there were no common bands between any two lesions from the same case.[14–17]

Together with Dr. Ronald Levy at Stanford, Sklar et al. also investigated possible multiclonality in non-immunosuppressed patients with various low-grade lymphomas.[18] A small set of such patients were discovered in whom two populations of neoplastic B-cells could be separated using anti-idiotype antibody in a fluorescence-activated cell sorter. Different patterns of immunoglobulin heavy and light chain gene rearrangements were detected in the separated populations, again suggesting two different lines of neoplastic B-cells within single patients. Similar results were also found when multiple biopsy specimens were analyzed from patients who showed several different histologic subtypes of lymphoma either concurrently or at separate points in their disease.[19]

Subsequent studies have shown that multiclonality assessed by antigen receptor gene rearrangements can be a rather complicated matter. The principal problem with this work is that the positions of rearranged bands in a Southern blot autoradiogram do not appear to be an absolutely stable clonal marker because, at least in follicular B-cell lymphomas, rearranged immunoglobulin genes are subjected to continuous somatic point mutations, very similar to the point mutations that arise in immunoglobulin genes of B-cells participating in normal immune responses.[20,21] Occasionally these mutations affect restriction sites, which in turn may change the position of a rearranged band in a Southern blot autoradiogram. This has been directly shown in some cases of follicular lymphoma by molecularly cloning and sequencing rearranged immunoglobulin genes to demonstrate that different bands contain the same V-D-J gene segments joined at the same sites.[22] In other cases, use of chromosome 18 DNA hybridization probes to detect the position of recombination in t(14;18) chromosomal translocations has shown that both apparent clones of a putative biclonal follicular lymphoma contain the same translocation breakpoint, indicating that both clones probably derive from the same transformed progenitor cell.[22] In these cases the two presumptive clones may represent sublines of the one tumor clone distinguished only by somatic mutations superimposed on the same immunoglobulin gene rearrangements.

Despite the foregoing results, there do appear to be situations in which multiclonal patterns of antigen receptor gene rearrangement actually reflect differences in the manner by which these tumors develop, compared to the way that the majority of tumors develop. For example, the multiclonality of lymphoproliferative lesions in immunosuppressed transplant patients has been confirmed using DNA hybridization probes for the termini of the Epstein-Barr virus (EBV) genome. Upon infection of cells by this virus, the linear genome circularizes through homologous recombination between DNA of tandemly repeated 500 basepair sequences contained within the terminal portions of the EBV genome. The number of tandem repeats included in the circular genome is a marker for the original circularization event and it is transmitted to all clonal progeny produced from the original infected cell. This marker can be analyzed by the Southern blot procedure using a hybridization probe for the 500 basepair tandem repeats and restriction enzymes that flank the fused terminal region containing the repeated elements.[23] When such analyses were carried out on multiple lymphoproliferative lesions from individual transplant patients, the positions of the fused terminal bands within Southern blot autoradiograms differed from lesion to lesion, thereby indicating that each lesion arose from a separately infected B-cell.[24] This finding is consistent with multiclonality.

Mention was made earlier of a patient with AILD who subsequently developed both B- and T-cell tumors. Hu et al. have described an additional patient with eosinophilic fasciitis who also developed both B- and T-cell tumors, in this case two possible B cell tumors with different patterns of immunoglobulin gene rearrangement (although the possibility of somatic mutation complicates this interpretation) and two T cell tumors with different patterns of beta and gamma T-cell receptor gene rearrangements.[25] These cases are clearly multiclonal in the sense that they are multilineage; however, no evidence precludes their origin from a transformed stem cell lacking any antigen receptor gene rearrangements.

Multiclonality also seems possible in one of our original low-grade lymphomas described as a biclonal lymphoma.[18] In this tumor, a small lymphocytic lymphoma, the two presumptive clones expressed different immunoglobulin light chain classes and produced different rearranged immunoglobulin heavy chain bands in Southern blot autoradiograms. The author and colleagues have cloned DNA corresponding to the rearranged heavy chain bands from this case and find that indeed they arise from different V-D-J rearrangements.* Furthermore, by comparing the same rearrangements from several different cells in the tumor, it was found that somatic mutation does not appear to occur in this lymphoma. A similar situation seems to pertain in common acute lymphoblastic leukemias (cALL). Bird et al. found that about 30% show three or more rearranged heavy chain bands in Southern blot autoradiograms.[26] Cloning and sequence analysis of immunoglobulin heavy chain bands in two such cases (one showing three rearranged heavy chain bands and the other showing seven rearranged heavy chain bands) indicates that the bands represent different V-D-J rearrangements and that somatic mutation of immunoglobulin genes is absent or at least very low in such tumors. As in the earlier examples of multilineage lymphomas and the apparently biclonal small lymphocytic lymphoma, these results may be due to origin of these leukemias from transformed stem cells lacking gene rearrangements. Since analysis of G6PD variant enzyme forms in

*Sanjanwala, M, et al: unpublished observation

cALL from female G6PD heterozygotes shows monoclonality in virtually all such tumors, this possibility seems particularly likely.[26a] This interpretation is also supported by the recent finding that some cases of cALL show different patterns of immunoglobulin heavy chain rearrangement in the original diagnostic bone marrow and bone marrow biopsied at relapse.*

Antigen Receptor Gene Rearrangements Used to Assess Lineage

Several different tumors have been described above in which analysis of antigen receptor gene rearrangements has been instrumental in assigning B- or T-lineage to lymphomas or subpopulations within lymphomas. This type of application is another major area in which antigen receptor gene rearrangements have significantly contributed to the study of lymphoid neoplasia. Some of the more important examples of this type of work have involved the description of clonal immunoglobulin gene rearrangements in hairy cell leukemia,[27,28] verifying the B-cell character of this neoplasm despite certain monocytic features exhibited by hairy leukemic cells; the frequent presence of clonal T-cell receptor gene rearrangements and apparent T-cell origin in many cases of morphologically histiocytic tumors;[10,11] and the detection of clonal immunoglobulin gene rearrangements in tissues from a subset of Hodgkin's disease cases.[29] The latter study requires particular caution in interpretation since the cellular composition of involved tissues in Hodgkin's disease is so heterogeneous. However, in the author's experience, detection of clonal immunoglobulin gene rearrangements in Hodgkin's disease is far more frequent in cases containing large numbers of Reed-Sternberg cells, suggesting that the rearranged immunoglobulin genes are contained within these cells, the origin of which has been historically uncertain. Studies by other workers on tissues containing large numbers of Reed-Sternberg cells or on subfractions of Hodgkin's tissues enriched in vitro for Reed-Sternberg cells have supported this general conclusion.[30,31]

While analysis of antigen receptor gene rearrangements may be useful in assigning lineage, this approach (to lineage assignment) must keep in mind that rearrangements of any one type of antigen receptor gene are not specific for B- or T-lineage differentiation. Antigen receptor gene rearrangements have been found in occasional hematopoietic tumors that show predominantly myelocytic differentiation,[32–34] and coexisting rearrangements of immunoglobulin and T-cell receptor genes have been demonstrated in both phenotypic B-lineage neoplasms and T-lineage neoplasms.[35] Despite these problems, the detection of coherent patterns of rearrangement for multiple immunoglobulin genes or T-cell receptor genes in the absence of any rearrangements for genes of the opposite lineage provides strong evidence for B- or T-cell differentiation. For instance, together with Dr. James Jones of the National Jewish Hospital in Denver, Colorado, the author recently studied a small set of lymphomas that contained Epstein-Barr virus (EBV) DNA and arose in patients with chronic active EBV infections. These tumors showed clonal rearrangements of T-cell receptor genes in the absence of immunoglobulin gene rearrangements, indicating that these tumors are T-cell lymphomas latently infected and perhaps primarily transformed by EBV.[36]

Summarizing the foregoing information on intragenic antigen receptor gene rearrangements, it is now clear that several potential problems must be considered when applying intragenic rearrangements to the diagnosis and characterization of lymphoid neoplasia. First, detection of clonal rearrangements is not specific for malignancy, but only for clonal proliferation, and such proliferations can be found in certain clinically benign disorders. Second, rare lymphomas, primarily up to this point certain ones showing T-lineage differentiation, appear to lack all detectable rearrangements of antigen receptor genes tested so far,

*Gocke C, et al: unpublished observation

indicating that absence of detectable genes is not tantamount to absence of neoplasia. Third, rearrangements of any one antigen receptor gene is not specific for a single lymphocytic lineage. Finally, rearranged bands for antigen receptor genes in Southern blot autoradiograms may not be completely stable clonal markers, at least in follicular B-cell lymphomas, because of somatic mutation of rearranged immunoglobulin genes. Nevertheless, despite all of these complicating issues, judicious application of antigen receptor gene rearrangements, particularly taking into account available clinical and histological data, has offered and will continue to offer an important new method for investigating lymphoid neoplasia.

Intergenic Rearrangements of Antigen Receptor Genes

Like intragenic antigen receptor gene rearrangements, intergenic rearrangements also provide a valuable means for study of lymphoid neoplasia, but are associated with a number of limitations and apparent ambiguities, at least from the current perspective.

Recent cytogenetic and molecular investigations have revealed that chromosomal rearrangements (i.e., translocations primarily, but also inversions) frequently involved sites of antigen receptor gene DNA in lymphoid neoplasms.[37] DNA containing chromosomal breakpoints from about a dozen such chromosomal rearrangements have been molecularly cloned and analyzed, confirming the cytogenetic suggestion that DNA in antigen receptor genes is joined to DNA from elsewhere in the genome in these chromosomal rearrangements. DNA hybridization probes constructed from DNA closely linked to the non-antigen receptor breakpoint in these rearrangements can be used in Southern blot analyses to quickly assess the presence and structure of intergenic rearrangements in these tumors.

Rearranged bands in Southern blot autoradiograms for intergenic rearrangements offers a clonal marker similar to the rearranged bands for intragenic rearrangements detected with antigen receptor DNA probes. Unlike the latter bands, however, these markers appear to be specific for malignancy because they have not been detected in any non-malignancy process thus far. Furthermore, because recurrent chromosomal rearrangements are characteristically associated with different types of lymphoid neoplasms, such bands are also markers for different histologic subtypes of lymphoma and leukemia.

Despite advantageous properties of intergenic rearrangements for diagnosing lymphoid neoplasia, the breakpoints in non-antigen receptor DNA involved in chromosomal rearrangements may be quite heterogeneous, making detection of rearranged bands difficult with limited sets of DNA hybridization probes and restriction enzymes. To a certain extent, this problem is mitigated by the clustering of breakpoints in certain regions of DNA, (i.e., as in the example of the t(14;18) chromosomal translocation present in over 90% of follicular B-cell lymphomas.[38–40]) In the future, gel electrophoresis techniques, such as pulsed field gels,[41] designed to separate very large fragments of DNA may permit scanning of long stretches of DNA with single combinations of DNA hybridization probes and restriction enzymes, reducing the difficulty posed by breakpoint heterogeneity for detecting intergenic antigen receptor gene rearrangements.

At the present time, some of the most confusing issues surrounding intergenic antigen receptor gene rearrangements relate to the basic biology of these acquired DNA changes in human tumors. One such issue concerns the mechanisms underlying the generation of these rearrangements. Some investigators have hypothesized that these rearrangements occur randomly and that cells acquiring them are at a relative growth advantage, probably because of transcriptional changes occurring in critical genes near the breakpoint. Another hypothesis suggests that the lymphocyte recombinase system implicated in catalyzing normal intragenic rearrangements may rarely join non-antigen receptor DNA to antigen receptor DNA,[37,42] and that on occasions where critical genes are juxtaposed to antigen receptor DNA, these changes induce or contribute to uncontrolled proliferation of the cell. The latter hypothesis is based on the assertion that certain signal sequences, notably the consensus heptamer CACNGTG, which flank sites of normal intragenic recombination, are often found in germline DNA near sites of intragenic rearrangement. However, the existence of such sequences near chromosomal breakpoints has been highly variable. In the author's experience, such sequences are most often lacking in DNA near the chromosome 18 breakpoint of the t(14;18) translocation of follicular lymphoma, a result that seems consistent with the heterogeneity of breaks within these translocations. On the other hand, researchers in the author's laboratory seem to have found opposite results in two t(7;9) chromosomal translocations, each of which may be present in as many as 10–15% of T-lymphoblastic neoplasms.[43,44] Both of these translocations have breakpoints within the beta T-cell receptor DNA at chromosome position 7q34, while one has a breakpoint at chromosome 9q32 and the other at chromosome 9q34.3. Analysis of DNA at both the 9q32 and 9q34.3 sites show consensus heptamers—in fact, tandem consensus heptamers at the 9q32 site. Examination of 9q32 DNA from t(7;9) translocations of three separate tumors suggests that the breaks occur very close together, if not at identical sites, supporting a possible role for lymphocyte recombinase in creating these translocations.

A second major issue that has been the subject of considerable speculation and investigation in intergenic antigen receptor gene rearrangements concerns activation of genes in non-antigen receptor DNA near the rearrangement breakpoint. The existence of transcription units near these breakpoints does in fact appear universal. Often transcription in the rearranged chromosome spans the site of recombination, as appears frequently to be the case in the t(14;18) chromosomal translocation of follicular B-cell lymphoma[45] and in the t(7;9)(q34;q32) translocation of T-lymphoblastic neoplasms. More directly relevant to the biological effect of these translocations is whether or not the protein products of these genes are modified qualitatively or quantitatively as a result of chromosomal rearrangement. Since the coding sequence of the protein associated with the t(14;18), chromosomal translocation (the so-called bcl-2 gene product) is not altered as a result of translocation, possibly changes in regulation of gene expression through altered stability of the modified transcript may be critical in this translocation.[44] However, generalizations based on these or any other results seem premature at this point. This point is underscored by recent results from analysis of transcription near the chromosome 9q32 breakpoint* An abundant 1.6 kb transcript is detected in cells carrying this translocation. Nucleotide sequence analysis of a cDNA for this transcript has failed to show an open reading frame consistent with a protein of any significant size. Therefore, the role of gene transcription near this breakpoint is obscure. Clearly, this and other molecular aspects of intergenic antigen receptor gene rearrangements bear further investigation, both because of the relevance of these rearrangements to the basic biology of lymphoid neoplasia, and because of their potential importance in the diagnosis of lymphoid biopsy specimens.

ACKNOWLEDGMENTS

The author wishes to thank his coworkers whose data have been described in this presentation: Michael Cleary, Lawrence Weiss, Naomi Galili, Eddie Hu, Benjamin Tycko, Madhusadan Sanjanwala, Christopher Gocke, Thomas Reynolds, Jeffrey Bird, and Leif Ellisen; and his colleagues: Roger Warnke, Stephen Smith, Michael Link, Ronald Levy, Ronald Dorfman, and James Jones.

Research described was supported by grants from the National Institutes of Health and the National Foundation for Cancer Research.

*Tycko, B., et al: unpublished observations

REFERENCES

1. Cleary ML, Chao J, Warnke R, Sklar J: Immunoglobulin gene rearrangement as a diagnostic criterion of B cell lymphoma. Proc Natl Acad Sci USA, 81:593–597, 1984
2. Arnold A, Cossman J, Bakhshi A, et al: Immunoglobulin gene rearrangement as unique clonal markers in human lymphoid neoplasms. N Engl J Med 309:1593–1598, 1983
3. Flug F, Pelicci PG, Bonetti R, et al: T-cell receptor gene rearrangements as markers of lineage and clonality in T-cell neoplasms. Proc Natl Acad Sci USA, 82:3460–3464, 1985
4. Weiss LM, Hu E, Wood GS, et al: Clonal rearrangements of T-cell receptor genes in mycosis fungoides and dermatopathic lymphadenopathy. N Engl J Med 313:537–544, 1985
5. Waldmann TA, Davis MM, Bongiovanni KF, Korsmeyer SJ: Rearrangements of genes for the antigen receptor on T cells as markers of lineage and clonality in human lymphoid neoplasms. N Engl J Med 313:776–783, 1985
6. Weiss LM, Strickler J, Dorfman R, et al: Clonal T cell populations in angioimmunoblastic lymphadenopathy and angioimmunoblastic lymphadenopathy-like lymphoma. Am J Pathol 122:392–398, 1986
7. Weiss LM, Wood G, Trela M, et al: Clonal T cell populations in lymphomatoid papulosis: Evidence for a lymphoproliferative origin for a clinically benign disease. N Engl J Med 315:475–479, 1986
8. Weiss LM, Wood GS, Reynolds TC, et al: Clonal T cell populations in *pityriasis lichenoides et varioliformis acuta* (Mucha-Habermann Disease). Am J Path 126:417–422, 1987
9. Wood GS, Weiss LM, Hu CH, et al: T-cell antigen deficiencies and clonal T-cell receptor gene rearrangements in pagetoid reticulosis (Woringer-Kolopp Disease). N Engl J Med 318:164–167, 1988
10. Weiss LM, Trela M, Turner R, et al: Frequent immunoglobulin and T cell receptor gene rearrangements in 'histiocytic' neoplasms. Am J Path 121:369–373, 1985
11. Weiss LM, Picker LJ, Warnke R, Sklar J: Large cell hematolymphoid neoplasms of uncertain lineage. Hum Path 19:967–973, 1988
12. Weiss LM, Picker LJ, Grogan TM, et al: Absence of clonal beta and gamma T-cell receptor gene rearrangements in a subset of peripheral T-cell lymphomas. Am J Path 130:436–442, 1988
13. Smith SD, Morgan R, Galili N, et al: Establishment and characterization of a common acute lymphoblastic leukemia cell line with a deletion of chromosome 3 band q26. Cancer Res 47:1652–1656, 1987
14. Cleary ML, Warnke R, Sklar J: Monoclonality of lymphoproliferative lesions in cardiac transplant recipients: Clonal analysis based on immunoglobulin-gene rearrangements. N Engl J Med 310:477–482, 1984
15. Cleary ML, Sklar J: Lymphoproliferative disorders in cardiac transplant recipients are multiclonal lymphomas. Lancet 2:489–493, 1984
16. Shearer WT, Ritz J, Finegold MJ, et al: Epstein-Barr virus-associated B cell proliferations of diverse clonal origins after bone marrow transplantation in a 12-year-old patient with severe combined immunodeficiency. N Engl J Med 312:1151–1159, 1985
17. Cleary ML, Dorfman RF, Sklar J: Failure in immunological control of Epstein-Barr virus infection: Post transplant lymphomas, in Epstein MA, Achong BG (eds), The Epstein-Barr Virus: Recent Advances, London, Heinemann, 1986, 163–181
18. Sklar J, Cleary ML, Thielemanns K, et al: Biclonal B cell lymphoma. N Engl J Med 311:20–27, 1984
19. Siegelman M, Cleary ML, Warnke R, Sklar J: Frequent biclonality and immunoglobulin gene alterations among B cell lymphomas that show multiple histologic forms. J Exp Med 161:850–863, 1985
20. Cleary M, Meeker T, Levy S, et al: Clustering of extensive somatic mutations in the variable region of an immunoglobulin heavy chain gene from a human B cell lymphoma. Cell 44:97–106, 1986
21. Levy R, Levy S, Cleary ML, et al: Somatic mutation in human B cell tumors. Immunol Rev 96:44–58, 1987
22. Cleary ML, Galili N, Trela M, et al: Single cell origin of bi-genotypic and bi-phenotypic B-cell proliferations in human follicular lymphomas. J Exp Med 167:582–597, 1988
23. Raab-Traub N, Flynn K: The structure of the termini of the Epstein-Barr virus as a marker of clonal cellular proliferation. Cell 47:883–889, 1986
24. Cleary ML, Nalesnik MA, Shearer WT, Sklar J: Clonal analysis of transplant-associated lymphoproliferations based on the structure of the termini of the Epstein-Barr virus. Blood 72:349–352, 1988
25. Hu E, Weiss LM, Warnke R, Sklar J: Non-Hodgkin's lymphoma containing both B and T cell clones. Blood 70:287–292, 1987
26. Bird J, Galili N, Link M, et al: Continuing rearrangement but absence of somatic hypermutation in immunoglobulin genes of human B cell precursor leukemias. 168:229–245, 1988

26a. Dow LW, Martin P, Moohr J, et al: Evidence for clonal development of childhood acute lymphoblastic leukemia. Blood 66:902–907, 1985

27. Korsmeyer SJ, Greene WC, Cossman J, et al: Rearrangement and expression of immunoglobulin genes and expression of Tac antigen in hairy cell leukemia. Proc Natl Acad Sci 80:4522–4526, 1983
28. Cleary ML, Wood GS, Warnke J, et al: Immunoglobulin gene rearrangement in hairy cell leukemia. Blood 64:99–104, 1984
29. Weiss LM, Hu E, Warnke RA, Sklar J: Immunoglobulin gene rearrangements in Hodgkin's disease. Hum Path 17:1009–1014, 1986
30. Brinker MGL, Poppema S, Buys CHCM, et al: Clonal immunoglobulin gene rearrangements in tissues involved by Hodgkin's disease. Blood 70:186–191, 1987
31. Sundeen J, Lipford E, Uppenkamp M, et al: Rearranged antigen receptor genes in Hodgkin's disease. Blood 70:96–103, 1987
32. Ha K, Minden M, Hozumi N, Gelfand EW: Immunoglobulin gene rearrangement in acute myelogenous leukemia. Cancer Res 44:4658–4660, 1984
33. Cheng G, Minder M, Toyonaga B, et al: T cell receptor and immunoglobulin gene rearrangements in acute meyloblastic leukemia. J Exp Med 163:414–424, 1986

34. Rovigatti U, Mirro J, Kitchingman G, et al: Heavy chain immunoglobulin gene rearrangement in acute non-lymphocytic leukemia. Blood 63:1023–1027, 1984
35. Pelicci PG, Knowles DM, II, Dalla-Favera R: Lymphoid tumors displaying rearrangements of both immunoglobulin and T cell receptor genes. J Exp Med 162:1015–1024, 1985
36. Jones JF, Shurin S, Abramowsky C, et al: Development of T-cell lymphomas containing Epstein-Barr viral DNA in patients with chronic Epstein-Barr virus infection. N Engl J Med
37. Croce CM: Role of chromosome translocations in human neoplasia. Cell 49:155–156, 1987
38. Cleary ML, Sklar J: Nucleotide sequence of a t(14:18) chromosomal breakpoint in follicular lymphoma and demonstration of a breakpoint cluster region near a transcriptionally active locus on chromosome 18. Proc Natl Acad Sci 82:7439–7443, 1985
39. Cleary ML, Galili N, Sklar J: Detection of a second t(14;18) breakpoint cluster region in human follicular lymphomas. J Exp Med 164:315–320, 1986
40. Weiss LM, Warnke R, Sklar J, Cleary ML: Molecular analysis of the t(14;18) chromosomal translocation in malignant lymphoma. N Engl J Med 317:1185–1189, 1987
41. Schwartz DC, Cantor CR: Separation of yeast-chromosome-sized DNAs by pulsed field gradient gel electrophoresis. Cell 37:67–75, 1984
42. Finger LR, Harvey RC, Moore RCA, et al: A common mechanism of chromosomal translocation in T- and B-cell neoplasia. Science 234:982–985, 1986
43. Reynolds TC, Smith SD, Sklar J: Analysis of DNA surrounding a breakpoint of chromosomal translocations involving the beta T cell receptor gene in human lymphoblastic neoplasms. Cell 50:107–117, 1987
44. Tycko B, Reynolds TC, Smith SD, Sklar J: Consistent breakage between consensus recombinase heptamers of chromosome 9 DNA in a recurrent chromosomal translocation of human T-cell leukemia. J Exp Med 169:369–377, 1989
45. Cleary ML, Smith SD, Sklar J: Cloning and structural analysis of cDNAs for the *bcl*-2 and a hybrid *bcl*-2/immunoglobulin transcript resulting from t(14;18) chromosomal translocation. Cell 47:19–28, 1986

3

A Novel Antigen Expressed in the HTLV-1-Infected Cells Detected with a Monoclonal Antibody

Y. Namba
F. Tsubai
Zu You-Li
M. Kohno
S. Hanada
M. Hanaoka

Abstract

A monoclonal antibody, FTF-148, was prepared by immunizing BALB/c mice with the cultured cells derived from an adult T-cell leukemia (ATL) patient (KUT-2 cell). This monoclonal antibody reacted with all of the human T-cell leukemia virus 1 (HTLV-I)-infected cell lines tested but did not react with other T-cell lines, B-cell lines or other non-T/non-B-cell lines. This antibody was not directed to viral antigens because it reacted equally well with almost all KUT-2 and MT-1 cells, only 1%–3% of which were ATL-associated antigen-positive. This antibody precipitated 50k and 74k proteins and the antigen was different from the IL 2-receptor. This antigen was also different from the product of the Xs gene of HTLV-1. This antigen was also expressed in IL 2-dependent cells infected with HTLV-1, suggesting that its expression was not responsible for cell transformation, but probably responsible for cell immortalization.

From IL-2-dependent HTLV-1 infected cells, one IL-2 independent convertant was obtained. The proteins of the convertant and the original cell line were compared with the result that two out of four proteins, which were usually phosphorylated by IL 2-stimulation, were autonomously phosphorylated, and one protein not found in IL 2-dependent cells was expressed in IL 2-independent convertant.

Adult T-cell leukemia (ATL), a particular type of T-cell malignancy, was first reported by Takatsuki et al[1]. It is endemic in the southwestern part of Japan. Clinical features of ATL include high white cell counts, frequent skin lesions, hepatosplenomegaly, lymphadenopathy, and a rapidly fatal terminal course. The human type C-retrovirus was first isolated from a cultured T-cell derived from a patient with a cutaneous T-cell lymphoma (mycosis fungoides), and subsequently, isolated from cell lines derived from ATL patients.[2–4] Seroepidemiologic studies indicated that almost all of the ATL patients possess antibodies reactive with cell lines established from ATL patients. These antigens, termed ATL-associated antigen (ATLA), were found to include gag proteins and env proteins.[5–6] Studies revealed, however, that this virus does not have cell-derived oncogenes and the integration site of the virus genome varies from one patient to another.[7,8] Therefore, the mechanism of leukemogenesis by HTLV-1 still remains to be clarified. One of the unique features of HTLV-1 is the genome's pX region, which is located between the 3′ end of the env gene and the 5′ end of U3-R of the LTR. Several groups reported evidence for expression of the pX IV region of HTLV-1 in human cells and its products (tat) enhance the transcription of its own LTR.[9,10] This protein might also activate cellular gene expression, and this activation might be associated with T-cell transformation. In order to identify the cellular gene product, which is necessary to maintain the proliferation of ATL cells, the authors made two experiments. First, they tried to obtain monoclonal antibodies that react specifically with ATL-derived cells irrespective of the production of HTLV-1 virus. Second, they compared proteins of IL 2-dependent ATL-derived cells and the IL 2-independent convertant. The comparison was especially made of the phosphorylation reaction of proteins induced by IL 2.

PREPARATION AND CHARACTERIZATION OF THE MONOCLONAL ANTIBODY

The monoclonal antibodies were prepared by hybridizing murine myelomal cells (NS-1) and spleen cells of BALB/c mice immunized with cultured cells derived from ATL patient (KUT-2 cells). From approximately 1,200 hybridoma clones, two clones (FTF-148 and FTG-193) were selected by their specific reactivity with ATL-derived cell lines. Although these clones were obtained independently, the staining pattern of the immunofluorescence was almost the same, and the antigen reactive with FTF-148 antibody was characterized. The reactivity of this monoclonal antibody with various kinds of human cell lines was examined by an immunofluorescence method (Table 3-1). The FTF-148 antibody reacted with all of the HTLV-1-infected cell lines, but did not react with other T-cell lines derived from non-ATL patients. The antibody also did not react with EBV-transformed B-cell lines and other non-T/non-B-cell lines. The only exception was a Raji cell line in which approximately 1% of the cell population was positively stained by a membrane immunofluorescence method. The possibility that this antigen, mainly expressed on the cell membrane, is identical with the IL 2-receptor molecules expressed in abundance in HTLV-1-infected cells was ruled out because normal peripheral blood leukocytes stimulated with phytohemagglutinin or concanavalin-A reacted with a monoclonal antibody against the IL 2 receptor but did not react with FTF-148 monoclonal antibody. The expression of the antigen detected with this antibody correlated well with the integration of HTLV-1 proviral DNA in the cells, but it did not correlate with the expression of the ATLA that was detected with anti-ATLA-positive human serum (Table 3-2). As shown in this table, FTF-148 antibody reacted with more than 90% of KUT-2 and MT-1 cells, of which only 1%–3% of the cells expressed the ATLA. This antibody also reacted with

TABLE 3-1
Reactivity of FTF-148 Antibody with Human Hematopoietic Cell Lines*

Cell line	% Fluorescence-stained cells with FTF-148
ATL derived T-cell lines	
MT-1	>90
MT-2	>90
HUT-102	>90
KUT-1	>90
KUT-2	>90
UW-4	>90
ATL derived B-cell lines	
KUT-3	80
ATL-B-1	75†
ATL-B-2	80†
non-ATL T-cell lines	
HSB-2	0
CCRF-CEM	0
Molt-4	0
Jurkat	0†
non-ATL B-cell lines	
Raji	1–2
EBV-1	0
B-ALL-1	0†
B-CLL-1	0†
non-ATL non T/non B cell line	
K-562	0
U-937	0†

* Percent positive cells were determined by an indirect immunofluorescence method using aceton-fixed smeared cells. FITC-conjugated IgG of rabbit against human IgG or mouse IgG were used as second antibodies.
† Determined by surface immunofluorescence method.

more than 90% of KUT-1 cells in which ATLA-positive cells were not detected. As anti-ATLA positive antiserum mainly detects env and gag proteins, FTF-148 antibody may not be directed to the viral antigen of HTLV-1.

For the biochemical analysis, KUT-2 cells were labeled with ^{3}H-leucine for 16 hr, lysed and immunoprecipitated with this antibody and subjected to SDS-polyacrylamide gel electrophoresis. The fluorographic patterns of SDS-PAGE revealed that two proteins were specifically precipitated by this antibody (Fig. 3-1). These proteins had apparent molecular weights of 74,000 and 50,000. The treatment of KUT-2 cells with tunicamycin did not reduce the apparent molecular weights of these proteins, suggesting that these proteins did not have long N-linked carbohydrate chains. From the ^{125}I surface-labeled material, these two proteins were also specifically precipitated, thus suggesting that at least a part of these proteins was exposed to the exterior of the plasma membrane. The relationship between these two proteins is still unclear.

The other proteins encoded by the genome of HTLV-1 virus are the *pol* and Xs genes. The *pol* gene protein of the retrovirus that is known as reverse transcriptase is in general synthesized as a *gag-pol* read-through product and is often detected as a 180K–200K polyprotein.[11,12] The nucleotide sequence of HTLV-1 suggested that the *pol* gene of this virus could code for a 99,000-dalton protein. Neither *gag-pol* product nor *pol* gene product has been identified yet in HTLV-1-infected cells, though the enzyme activity was demonstrated on HTLV-1 virion particles. One of the unique features of HTLV-1 is its gene termed Xs, which resides downstream of the *env* gene and is flanked by 3'LTR. Recently,

TABLE 3-2
Reactivities of FTF-148 Antibody and anti-ATLA Positive Human Serum with ATL Derived T-cell Lines*

Cell line	% Immunofluorescence-stained with: anti-ATLA	FTF-148
MT-1	1–3	>90
MT-2	90	>90
HUT-102	ND†	>90
KUT-1	0	>90
KUT-2	1–3	>90
UW-4	1–2	>90

* Percent positive cells were determined by an indirect immunofluorescence method using acetone-fixed smeared cells. FITC-conjugated IgG of rabbit against human or mouse IgG were used as second antibodies.
† Not determined

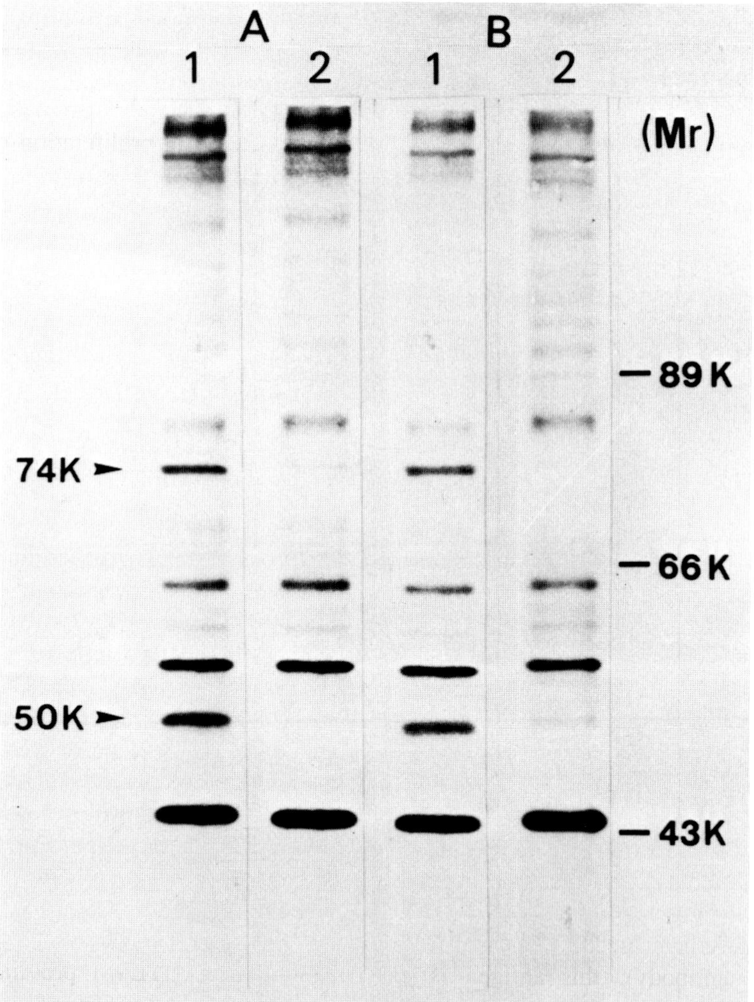

Fig. 3-1A & B. Immunoprecipitation and SDS-PAGE analysis of ^{3}H-leucine-labeled KUT-2 cells. The cells were labeled with ^{3}H-leucine for 16 hours and subjected to immunoprecipitation with FTF-148 antibody (A-1) or with normal mouse IgG (A-2); (B) KUT-2 cells were incubated with tunicamycin (0.8 μg/ml) for one hour followed by ^{3}H-leucine labeling for 15 hours. The cells were subjected to immunoprecipitation with FTF-148 antibody (B-1) or normal mouse IgG (B-2).

using rabbit antibodies to the synthetic oligopeptide specific to the predicted amino acid sequences of the product of the Xs region, 40K proteins were detected in HTLV-1-infected cells.[13] The authors prepared a monoclonal antibody (MI-73) against the synthetic oligopeptide of the COOH terminal region of pX IV (tat) that specifically reacted with this 40K protein. By an immunofluorescence method, this 49K protein was found to be distributed in the cytoplasm (polysome) and nucleus of the major population of HUT-102, KUT-1, and KUT-2 cells in which the expression of ATLA was in a minor population (HUT-102, KUT-2) or not expressed at all (KUT-1). Therefore, the antigen detected with FTF-148 was considered to be different from that protein. The pX III protein (27K protein) was recently found in the ATL-derived cells and this protein was found to change the splicing mode of HTLV-1 messenger RNA in favor of the production of the viral structure proteins. Taken together, the antigen detected with FTF-148 antibody is not the protein encoded by the viral genome.

REACTIVITY OF FTF-148 ANTIBODY WITH PBL AND LYMPH NODE CELLS OF ATL PATIENTS

The reactivity of this antibody to fresh PBL obtained from ATL patients was examined by a viable cell surface immunofluorescence method. In some cases a significant percentage of PBL reacted with this antibody (Table 3-3). In most cases, however, the ATL cells in the peripheral blood did not express this antigen in vivo, thereby making it necessary to elucidate the expression of this antigen in relation to the proliferation of ATL cells. The authors then examined the lymph nodes of ATL patients by an immunohistochemical method with the result that in three patients out of four more than 10% of the lymph node cells expressed this antigen, thus indicating that in the tissue in which ATL cells are actively proliferating (as checked with Ki-67 monoclonal antibody), this antigen is expressed in a high percentage of ATL cells. In the lymph nodes of ATL patients, the structure proteins of HTLV-1 were not expressed, as evidenced by nonreactivity of the cells with the monoclonal antibodies to these proteins. These results suggest that this antigen may be related to the proliferation of ATL cells and is a product of certain cellular genes activated by some transacting factor (e.g., *tat*) produced by HTLV-1 infecton.

BIOCHEMICAL ASPECTS OF TRANSFORMATION OF ATL CELLS

The antigen detected by FTF-148 antibody is also expressed in the cell lines derived from ATL patients, which still depend on the presence of IL-2 for its proliferation. There is still a controversy as to whether ATL cells depend on IL-2 or not. The PBL from the ATL patients proliferate very well in the presence of IL-2, and from almost all cases IL 2-dependent permanent cell lines are established. This phenomenon is in high contrast to cultures of PBL from normal persons because the proliferation of the latter cells gradually decreased and it is hard to establish a permanent cell line. This phenomenon suggests that ATL cells are immortalized by the integration of HTLV-1 proviral DNA. The antigen detected by FTF-148 antibody may be related to cell immortalization.

TABLE 3-3

Reactivity of FTF-148 Antibody with Fresh PBL of ATL Patients*

		% positive cells in PBL			
Source of PBL	No. of cases	0–1	1–5	5–10	>10
ATL patients	18	7	3	4	4†
Healthy adults of non-endemic area	11	11	0	0	0
Blood donors in endemic area	27	24	1	2‡	0

* PBL were separated from peripheral blood with Ficoll-Paque and percent positive cells was determined by an indirect immunofluorescence method.

† More than 40% of PBL were positively stained in two out of four cases.

‡ Anti-ATLA positive adults. Another seropositive adult in this group did not have any positively stained cells in PBL.

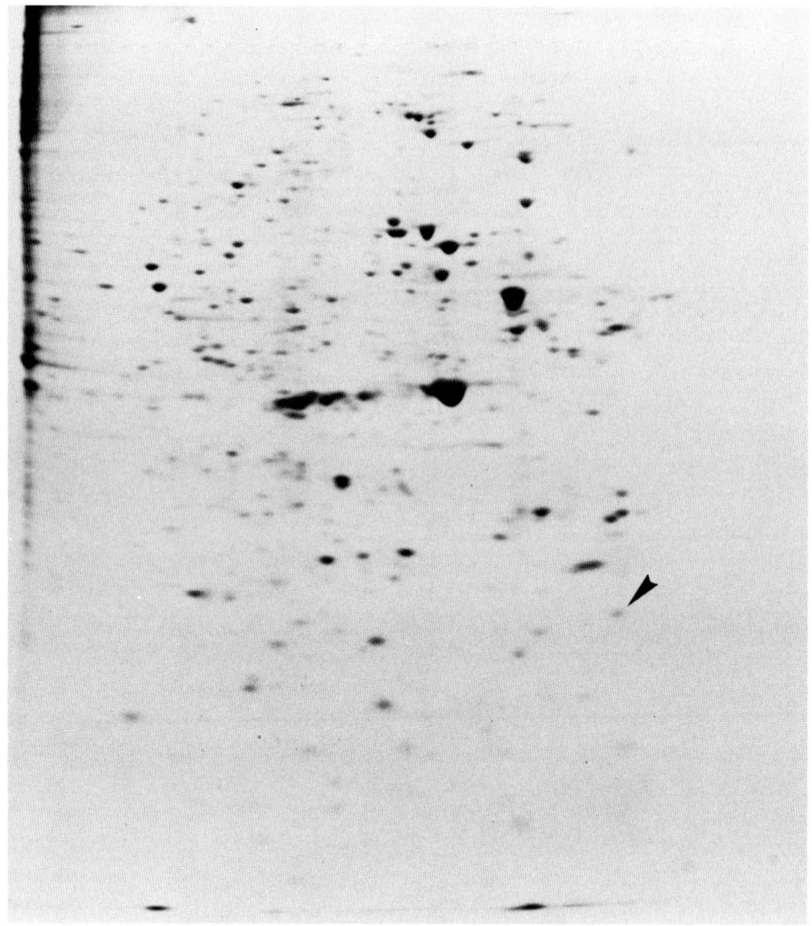

Fig. 3-2. Proteins of UW-4X cells were metabolically labeled with ^{3}H-leucine, lysed, and analyzed by two-dimensional gel electrophoresis. The gel was fixed, stained, and treated with enhancer. The gel was dried and exposed to X-ray film for seven days at −70°C. Arrowheads indicate the protein with Mr value of 30,000 (30K).

From the IL 2-dependent cells derived from ATL lymphocytes, the conversion to IL 2-independent cells rarely occurs. This conversion may correspond to the change from a smoldering or chronic type to an acute type of ATL. The authors analyzed the biochemical changes corresponding to this conversion. First, an ATL-derived IL 2-dependent cell line (UW-4B) and its IL 2-independent convertant (UW-4X) were labeled with ^{3}H-leucine and analyzed by two dimensional gel electrophoresis. The distribution of protein spots of these two cell lines were extremely similar and only one spot newly appeared in the IL 2-independent cell line (Fig. 3-2). This protein that has an apparent molecular weight of 30,000 may be responsible for the conversion from an IL 2-dependent state to an IL 2-independent state and its function should be clarified. It has been reported that IL 2 induces phosphorylation of some cellular proteins.[14,15] The phosphorylation pattern of UW-4B and UW-4x cells was compared with or without IL 2 addition. When IL 2 was added to IL 2-dependent cell (UW-4B), four proteins were newly phosphorylated (Fig. 3-3). The phosphorylation reaction was very rapid and the reaction was saturated within 15 minutes. The analysis of protein phosphorylation of IL 2-independent cells (UW-

Fig. 3-3. Phosphoproteins of UW-4B cells. IL 2-arrested cells were labeled with ^{32}P for 30 min, treated with 20 units/ml of human recombinant IL 2 (rIL 2) for 15 minutes, lysed and analyzed by two-dimensional gel electrophoresis. The gel was fixed, stained, dried and exposed to X-ray film for four days at −70°C. Arrowheads indicate the positions of the proteins with Mr value of 70K, 65K, and two proteins of Mr value of 20–25K.

4X) revealed that two proteins (70K and 65K) out of the four proteins were autonomously phosphorylated without addition of IL 2 (Fig. 3-4). The possibility that UW-4X became IL-2 independent, but the acquisition of the ability to produce IL 2 was ruled out, because IL 2 activity was not detected in the culture supernatant of UW-4X and two other proteins (20–25K proteins) were additionally phosphorylated by IL 2 addition. It is highly probable that the autonomous phosphorylation of 70K and 65K proteins are related to the IL 2-independent proliferation of UW-4X cells. The mechanism of this autonomous phosphorylation reaction must be made clear. The 30K proteins that were newly synthesized in IL 2-independent cells may be related to or responsible for this reaction.

REFERENCES

1. Uchiyama T, Yodoi J, Sagawa K, et al: Adult T cell leukemia; clinical and hematologic feature of 16 cases. Blood, 50:481, 1977
2. Poiesz BJ, Ruscetti FW, Gazder AF, et al: Detection and isolation of type-C retrovirus particles from fresh and cultured lymphocytes of a patient with cutaneous T-cell lymphoma. Proc Natl Acad Sci, 77:7415, 1980
3. Hinuma Y, Nagata K, Hanaoka M, et al: Adult T-cell leukemia; antigen in an ATL cell line and

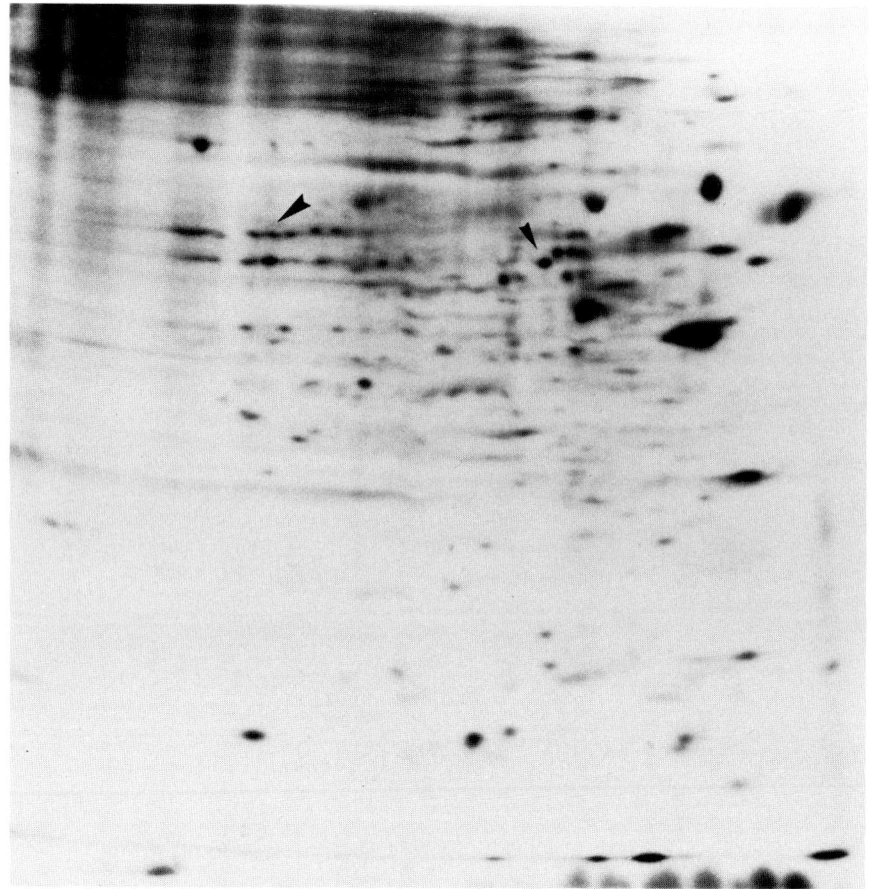

Fig. 3-4. Phosphoproteins of UW-4X cells. The cells were labeled with ^{32}P for 30 min, lysed, and analyzed as in Fig. 3-3. Arrowheads indicate the positions of proteins with Mr value of 70K and 65K.

detection of antibodies to the antigen of human sera. Pro Natl Acad Sci, 78:6476, 1981

4. Yoshida M, Miyoshi I, Hinuma Y: Isolation and characterization of retrovirus from cell lines of human adult T-cell leukemia and its implication of the disease. Proc Natl Acad Sci, 79:2031, 1982
5. Yamamoto N, Hinuma Y: Antigens in an adult T-cell leukemia virus-producer cell line; reactivity with human serum antibodies. Int J Cancer, 30:289, 1982
6. Kobayashi N, Yamamoto N, Koyanagi Y, et al: Translation of HTLV (human T-cell leukemia virus) RNA in a nuclease-treated rabbit reticulocyte system. EMBO J, 3:321, 1984
7. Seiki M, Hattori S, Hirayama Y, Yoshida M: Human adult T-cell leukemia virus: Complete nucleotide sequence of the provirus genome integrated in leukemia cell DNA. Pro Natl Acad Sci, 80:3618, 1983
8. Seiki M, Eddy R, Shows TB, Yoshida M: Nonspecific integration of the HTLV provirus genome into adult T-cell leukemia cells. Nature 309:640, 1984
9. Kiyokawa T, Seiki M, Imagawa K, et al: Identification of a protein ($p40^x$) encoded by a unique sequence pX of human T-cell leukemia virus type I. Gann 75:747, 1984
10. Sodroski JG, Rosen CA, Haseltine WA: Trans-acting transcriptional activation of the long terminal repeat of human T lymphotropic viruses in infected cells. Science 225:381, 1984
11. Opperman H, Bishop JM, Varmus HE, Levintow L: A joint product of the genes gag and pol of avian sarcoma virus. A possible precursor of reverse transcriptase. Cell 12:993, 1977
12. Hayman NJ: Synthesis and processing of avian sarcoma virus glycoprotein. Virology 85:475, 1978
13. Miwa M, Shimotohno H, Fujino M, Sugimura T: Detection of pX proteins in human T-cell leukemia virus (HTLV)-infected cells by using antibody against peptide deduced from sequences of X-IV DNA of HTLV-1 and Xc DNA of HTLV-II proviruses. Gann 75:752, 1984
14. Kohno M, Kuwata S, Namba Y, Hanaoka M: Interleukin 2 induces rapid phosphorylation of cellular proteins in murine T-lymphocytes. FEBS Letters 198:33, 1986
15. Ishii T, Sugamura K, Nakamura M, Hinuma Y: Interleukin (IL-2) rapidly induces phosphorylation of a cellular protein, pp67, in an IL-2 dependent murine cell line. Biochem Biophys Res Commun, 135:487, 1986

4

Roles of T3-T Cell Receptor Complexes for Leukemogenesis of Adult T-Cell Leukemia

Toshio Hattori
Masao Matsuoka
Seiko Yamamoto
Hitoshi Sakano
Yuji Wano
Kiyoshi Takatsuki

Abstract

The role of the T3-T cell receptor (TCR) complex in leukemogenesis of adult T-cell leukemia (ATL) cells was studied. The density of T3-TCR comlexes on ATL cells was low, but protein synthesis and gene expression of T3-TCR complexes in ATL cells were higher than in T4 chronic lymphocytic leukemia. Configurations of TCR β chain genes were heterogenous and Vβ genes of ATL belonged to different Vβ families. These findings support the idea that T3-TCR complexes on ATL cells are stimulated and this stimulation may be one of the primary causes of activation of ATL cells. This stimulation was found not to be mediated by specific Vβ genes. In addition interleukin 1 production by ATL cells was observed, and its biological significance was discussed.

Adult T-cell leukemia (ATL) is known to be etiologically associated with human T-cell leukemia virus type 1 (HTLV-1).[1–4] Morphologic studies of leukemia cells showed that ATL cells are larger than normal lymphocytes, have typical lobulated nuclei, and slightly basophilic cytoplasm. Surface marker studies of ATL cells revealed that ATL cells are positive for CD2, CD3 and CD4 antigens and lack CD1 and CD8 antigens, suggesting that they are derived from mature helper T cells. In addition, ATL cells expressed CD25 antigen,[5] the interleukin 2-receptor.[6] In contrast to ATL, CD4-antigen-bearing chronic lymphocytic leukemia (T4-CLL) cells usually do not express these activated T-cell markers. Therefore, the expression of CD25 antigen is a feature of leukemia cells that may be caused by HTLV-1 infection. Thus, analyses of the mechanisms of abnormal expression of the CD25 antigen would help in interpreting of leukemogenesis of ATL. The primary physiological signals for activation of T-cells are mediated by the T-cell receptor (TCR) and its associated molecules, a complex of T3 proteins.[7,8] Therefore, the surface expression of T3-TCR complexes were examined, as were configurations of TCR β chain genes,[9,10] in order to clarify whether T3-TCR complexes are involved in the leukemogenesis of ATL.

Furthermore, clinical features of ATL were studied from the point of view that secreted lymphokines from ATL cells might modify pathophysiology of ATL patients. Because one of the main causes of death of patients with ATL is hypercalcemia, and microscopic observations of postmortem individuals showed bone resorptions and osteoclast activation. Recently, it was noted that ATL derived factor (ADF) induced proliferations of acute myelogenous leukemia cells.[11] A similar factor, interleukin 1 (IL-1), has been reported to have multiple biological activities. For example, IL-1 is well known to induce CD25 antigen on cells, and has an osteoclast activating activity. In addition, IL-1 causes neutrophilia in mice when administered intravenously.[12] These findings prompted further investigation to determine whether patients with ATL show neutrophilia and ATL cells produce IL-1 or not.

MATERIALS AND METHODS

Neutrophilia and Hypercalcemia in ATL

The numbers of neutrophils and platelets, and the serum Ca levels at the time of initial diagnosis have been investigated in 35 patients with leukemic type ATL. Twenty-two patients with acute lymphocytic leukemia (ALL) were studied as controls. The student's t-test was employed for statistical analyses.

Interleukin 1 Production by ATL Cells

Macrophages and monocytes were depleted from fresh peripheral blood mononuclear cells (PBMC) of patients with ATL and normal volunteers, and residual cell suspensions were cultured for 18 hours. IL-1 activities of collected culture supernatants were measured by a thymocyte proliferation assay using thymocytes from C3H/HeN mice. In order to clarify whether produced IL-1 belong to IL-1α or IL-1β, effects of anti-IL-1α or anti-IL-1β on IL-1 activities in culture supernatants were examined.

Cell Surface Marker Analyses

Cell surface markers were analysed with a laser flow cytometer (Ortho Diagnostic Systems, Westwood, MA). The monoclonal antibodies (mAb) used in this study were WT31 or OKT3 mAbs, which identify a frame work epitope of TCR and TCR associated molecules, respectively. Second antibodies were fluorescein isothiocyanate (FITC) conjugated $F(ab)'_2$ fragments of goat anti-mouse immunoglobulin (IgG). Leukemic cells from 12 patients with ATL and peripheral blood lymphocytes from 8 normal individuals were examined. The data were expressed as percentages of immunofluorescence (IF)-positive cells, and also as mean fluorescence intensity (MFI), the density of cell surface antigens.

Southern Analysis of DNA

DNA was prepared from the leukemia cells of each patient by proteinase-K digestion followed by phenolchloroform extraction. DNA was then digested with restriction enzymes, electrophoresed in a 0.8% agarose gel, and blotted to a nitrocellulose filter. The membrane filter was then hybridized to a nick-translated DNA probe. The Tβ probe was a 3 kilobase (kb) EcoRI/Hind III fragment con-

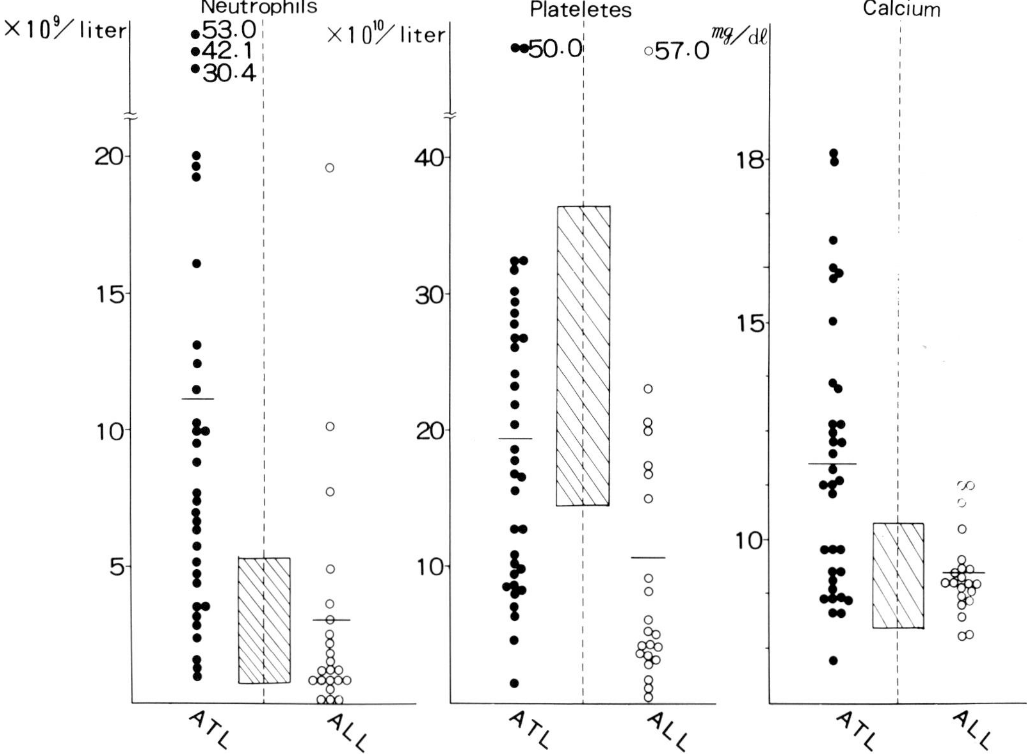

Fig. 4-1. The numbers of neutrophils and platelets and the serum Ca levels of patients with leukemic-type ATL (closed circle) and ALL (open circle). Thirty-five patients with leukemic-type ATL (23 males and 12 females; mean age ± SD is 59 ± 13) and 22 patients with ALL (13 males and 9 females; mean age ± SD is 42 ± 23) were studied. Values of mean ± 2SD for each parameter in 30 healthy persons (15 males and 15 females; mean age ± SD is 47 ± 11) are indicated by hatched regions.

taining the Jβ gene fragments. The T-cell receptor β-chain gene has two sites of joining gene clusters each with their own constant genes, Cβ1 and Cβ2. The Cβ1 probe detects two hybridizing bands of 10.2 and 4.2 kilobase (kb) in EcoRI digests of germline DNA. The 10.2 kb band contains Cβ1, while the 4.2 kb band cross-hybridizes with the Cβ2 gene. No evidence of polymorphism was found in the EcoRI digests of the population tested. The Jβ2 gene probe detects a 4.0 kb band in EcoRI digests of germline DNA.

Vβ Sequences of Functionally Rearranged ATL

The specific decrease of T3-TCR expression on ATL cells suggests that T3-TCR complex on these cells is stimulated in vivo. Such stimulation may cause uncontrolled proliferation of HTLV-1 infected T-cells, resulting in leukemia. The authors therefore studied the DNA sequences of functionally rearranged Vβ genes in leukemic cells from two ATL patients and one with T-cell acute lymphocytic leukemia (T-ALL), the latter serving as a control. To make DNA libraries, 10 μg of each patient's DNA were digested with a restriction enzyme, EcoRI, ligated with 5 μg of Charon 4A arm DNA, and then packaged in vitro by the method of Hohn. DNA clones were isolated and analyzed by standard methods.

RESULTS

Neutrophilia in ATL

Clinical studies revealed that absolute neutrophilia as well as hypercalcemia were frequently observed in ATL (Fig. 4-1).[13] The numbers of neutrophils and the serum Ca levels of leukemic-type ATL were significantly ($P < 0.01$) higher than those of ALL. The numbers of platelets were significantly ($P < 0.05$) different between leukemic-type ATL and ALL. This difference, however, could be explained by frequent bone marrow involvement in ALL, because the numbers of platelets were significantly ($P < 0.01$) lower than normal in ALL.

IL-1 Production by ATL Cells

A control supernatant obtained from normal PBMC did not promote significant ^{3}H-thymidine incorporation by murine thymocytes, while both purified recombinant IL-1α and IL-1β significantly enhanced thymocyte proliferation in a dose dependent manner. Most of the culture supernatants from ATL patients and that from a case with T4-CLL contained IL-1 activity (Table 4-1).[14] The results showed that most IL-1 activity was suppressed by the addition of anti-IL-1β and not by anti-IL-1α. Interleukin-1 gene expression in ATL was also confirmed by northern blotting methods. A distinct gene expression of IL-1β was found in RNA from tumor T cells, but only a small amount of transcript of IL-1β was detected in RNA from HTLV-1 infected cell lines.[14] Wano et al.'s data clearly indicate the secretion of IL-1 by ATL cells. An association between serum Ca levels with IL-1 production by ATL cells was not observed.[14] The other undefined lymphokines secreted from ATL cells could be responsible for this clinical feature.

Cell Surface Marker Analyses of ATL

MFI of T3 and WT31 antigens on ATL cells were 46.1 ± 11.4 and 29.9 ± 7.8, respectively. Those of normal T-cells were 105.4 ± 8.3 and 87.9 ± 5.8, respectively.

TABLE 4-1
Thymocyte DNA Synthesis in Tumor Cell Culture Supernatants

Experiment	Final dilution or concentration	^{3}H-TdR incorporation (mean ± 1 SD cpm)	% Suppression* anti-IL-1α	anti-IL-1β	NRS†
1. Control	1:4	650 ± 100			
2. rIL-1α	10u/ml	8,400 ± 850	47.6	−12.5	−3.0
	100u/ml	26,650 ± 880			
3. rIL-1β	1u/ml	3,710 ± 120			
	10u/ml	14,910 ± 2,610	−1.5	38.9	9.2
	100u/ml	27,760 ± 5,470			
4. T4-CLL	1: 4	31,100 ± 2,210	7.9	47.8	−5.4
	1:12	23,800 ± 1,510			
	1:36	9,620 ± 570			
5. ATL case 1	1: 4	32,250 ± 6,710	23.0	53.0	2.6
	1:12	19,250 ± 1,450			
6. ATL case 2	1: 4	8,370 ± 2,880			
	1:12	1,050 ± 190			
7. ATL case 3	1: 4	3,250 ± 1,790	57.8	66.3	7.2
8. ATL case 6	1: 4	4,620 ± 820			
	1:12	2,840 ± 990			
	1:36	1,220 ± 230			
9. ATL case 7	1: 4	20,200 ± 1,440	28.1	78.2	10.7

* % Suppression: (1-CPM plus serum/CPM no serum) × 100
† Anti-IL-1 heteroantibodies and NRS were used at a final dilution of 1:1,000.

These results confirmed that the density of T3-TCR complex on ATL cells was low compared with normal T-cells. The low density of T3-TCR complexes could not be explained by leukemic changes, because T4-CLL cells had a normal density of T3-TCR complexes on their surface.[9] Analyses with OKT3 mAb showed that incubation of ATL cells with OKT3 mAb caused a further decrease of T3 antigen density, associated with an increase of CD25 antigen, when examined with FITC-conjugated anti-CD25 mAb, suggesting that T3-TCR complexes were not frozen by leukemic changes but were subject to regulation.[9]

Southern Blotting Assay

Southern blotting analyses of ATL cells with the probes described in "materials and methods" revealed that all samples displayed DNA rearrangements in one or both alleles of the Tβ gene. A variety of rearranged bands were detected both in ATL and non-ATL samples. In addition, there were no preferential rearrangements of Cβ1 or Cβ2 genes in either ATL or non-ATL T4-CLL cells. Representative data of southern blot analyses are presented in Figure 4-2. As controls, data obtained with non-ATL samples were also

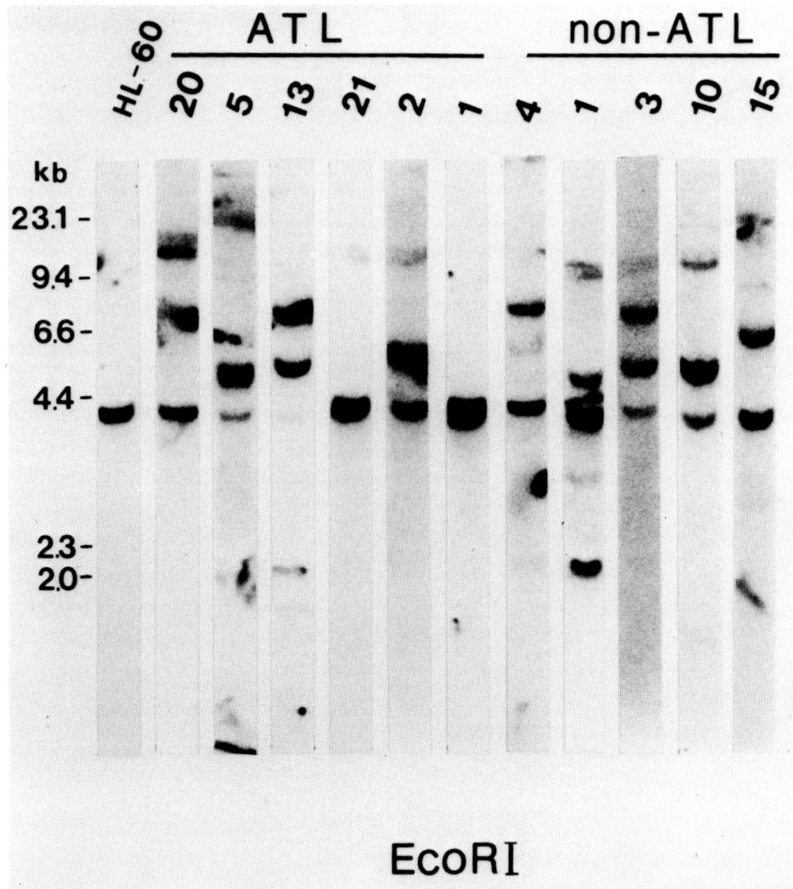

Fig. 4-2. Tβ gene rearrangement in ATL and non-ATL samples. The probe used was Jβ2. As a control, genomic DNA of HL-60 cells, a human promyelocytic leukemia cell line, was used.

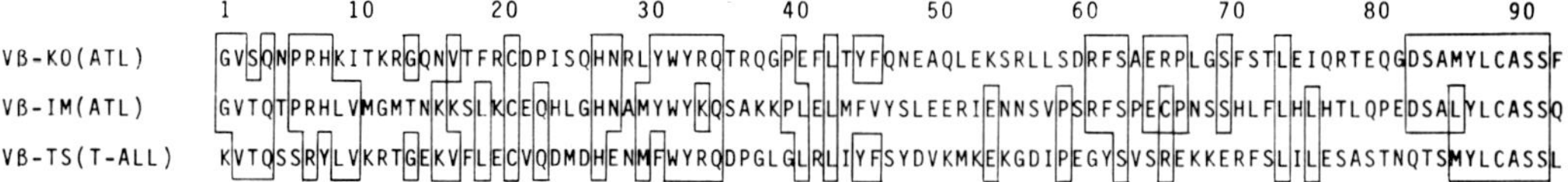

Fig. 4-3. Deduced amino acid sequences of functional Vβ genes in 2 ATL and one non-ATL case. Each amino acid is represented as a single letter. Boxes indicate homologous regions.

included. In some cases, one rearranged Cβ1 gene and two rearranged Cβ2 genes were detected. These were probably the result of sister-chromatid exchanges that duplicated part of the gene loci, followed by subsequent rearrangement of the gene. Alternatively, additional chromosomal abnormalities such as trisomy 7, may have contributed to the observed excessive Tβ gene bands, though abnormalities of chromosome 7 could not be detected in these cases.[10]

Vβ Sequences of Functionally Rearranged Genes in ATL

Vβ genes joining the Jβ1 gene were isolated from the genomic DNA libraries of DNA from two ATL samples (Patient IM; Patient KO) and were then sequenced. The Vβ gene of DNA from cells of a patient with T-ALL (Patient TS) was also sequenced. According to Concannon et al.,[16] Vβ-IM, Vβ-TS and Vβ-KO belong to Vβ7, Vβ3 and Vβ6 gene families,[10] respectively. Deduced amino acid sequences of the Vβ gene products are shown in Figure 4-3. The homology between Vβ-IM and Vβ-KO was 33.3%, that of Vβ-IM and Vβ-TS at 30.1%, and that of Vβ-KO and Vβ-TS at 25.8%. Thus, it was concluded that there were no specific structures common to the Vβ genes in ATL cells.

DISCUSSION

It has become clear that ATL cells belong to the group of activated T-cell neoplasms, although the mechanisms which activate ATL cells is not clear. We studied whether T3-TCR complexes on ATL cells play a role in the activation of tumor T-cells, because these complexes are primary signals for T-cell proliferation. The surface expression of T3-TCR complexes on all ATL cells was low, when examined by flow cytometry. In contrast, RNA levels of these antigens were not low or even higher than those of T4-CLL. It was also found that protein levels of T3 antigen are not suppressed in ATL (unpublished observations). Previously, we noted that T3 complexes on ATL cells were not arrested at low levels, but still subject to regulation.[9] Taken together, it is quite likely that T3-TCR complexes were stimulated by unknown mechanisms. If the agents that stimulate T3-TCR complexes on ATL cells are the same, it is likely that rearranged patterns of Tβ genes might be common, alternatively ATL might use similar Vβ genes. Southern blotting analyses of Tβ genes of ATL showed that there were no consistent profiles of rearrangements of Tβ genes in ATL.[10] In addition, sequences of Vβ genes showed that ATL cells used different families of Vβ genes. These findings do not support the concept that T3-TCR complexes on ATL cells are stimulated. However, elevations of RNA and protein levels of T3-TCR complexes suggest that T3-TCR complexes on ATL cells are stimulated, although the stimulation is not mediated by a specific Vβ gene.

REFERENCES

1. Takatsuki K, Uchiyama T, Sagawa K, Yodoi J: Adult T-cell leukemia in Japan, in Seno S, Takaku F, Irino S (eds): Topics in Hematology Excepta Medica, Amsterdam, 1977, 73–77
2. Uchiyama T, Yodoi J, Sagawa K, et al: Adult T-cell Leukemia: Clinical and hematologic features of 16 cases. Blood 50:481–492, 1977
3. Poiesz BJ, Ruscetti FW, Fazdar AF, et al: Detection

and isolation of type C retrovirus particles from fresh and cultured lymphocytes of a patient with cutaneous T-cell lymphoma. Proc Natl Acad Sci 78:1887–1881, 1981
4. Hinuma Y, Nagata K, Hanaoka M, et al: Antigen in an adult T-cell leukemia cell line and detection of antibodies to the antigen in human sera. Proc Natl Acad Sci 78:6476–6481, 1981
5. Hattori T, Uchiyama T, Toibana T, et al: Surface phenotype of Japanese adult T-cell leukemia cells characterized by monoclonal antibodies. Blood 58:645–647, 1981
6. Leonard WJ, Depper JM, Uchiyama T, et al: A monoclonal antibody that appears to recognize the receptor for T cell growth factor: Partial characterization of the receptor. Nature 300:267–269, 1982
7. Reinherz EL, Meuer S, Fitzgerald KA, et al: Antigen reaction by human T lymphocytes is linked to surface expression of the T3 surface molecular complexes. Cell 30:735–741, 1982
8. Meuer SC, Fitzgerald KA, Hussey RE, et al: Clonotypic structures involved in antigen specific human T cell function. Relationship to the T3 molecular complex. J Exp Med 157:705–712, 1983
9. Matsuoka M, Hattori T, Chosa T, et al: T3 surface molecules on adult T cell leukemia cells are modulated *in vivo*. Blood 67:1070–1076, 1986
10. Matsuoka M, Hagiya M, Hattori T, et al: Gene rearrangements of T cell receptor β and γ chains in HTLV-I infected primary neaplastic T cells. Leukemia 2:84–90, 1988
11. Yamamoto S, Hattori T, Matsuoka M, et al: Induction of TAC antigen and proliferation of myeloid leukemic cells by ATL-derived factor: comparison with other agents that promote differentiation of human myeloid or monocytic leukemic cells. Blood 67:1714–1720, 1986
12. Oppenheim JJ, Kovacs EJ, Matsushima K, Durum SK: There is more than one interleukin 1. Immunol Today 7:45–56, 1986
13. Yamamoto S, Hattori T, Asou N, et al: Absolute neutrophilia in adult T cell leukemia. Jpn J Cancer Res (Gann) 77:858–861, 1986
14. Wano Y, Hattori T, Matsuoka M, et al: Interleukin 1 gene expression in adult T cell leukemia. J Clin Invest 80:911–916, 1987
15. Maniatis T, Fitch E, Sambroox J: Molecular cloning: A laboratory manual (Cold Spring Harbor Laboratory, Cold Spring Harbor, NY)
16. Concannon P, Pickering LA, Kung P, Hood L: Diversity of human T-cell receptor β-chain variable region genes. Proc Natl Acad Sci 83:6598–6602, 1986

5

Chromosome Translocations in Human B-Cell Malignancies

Yoshihide Tsujimoto
Carlo M. Croce

Abstract

It is generally accepted that tumors arise through the accumulation of several genetic changes that affect the control of cell growth. To date, the most well characterized changes are the chromosome abnormalities, in particular translocations and inversions, often associated with hematopoietic tumors.

The frequent involvement of the immunoglobulin loci in the chromosome translocations found in B-cell tumors has allowed both structural and functional studies of these translocations. Based on such studies of the t(11;14) translocation in chronic lymphocytic leukemia, the t(14;18) translocation in follicular lymphoma, and the t(8;14) translocation in Burkitt's lymphoma, especially the endemic type, Tsujimoto and Croce proposed that these translocations arise during immunoglobulin gene rearrangement by mistakes in the VDJ joining recombination machinery.

Analysis of the t(14;18) translocation has also led us to identify a new putative oncogene, bcl-2, which might play a crucial role in the development of follicular lymphoma. Such studies demonstrate the power of an approach based on analysis of chromosome translocation in identifying new oncogenes involved in hematopoietic malignancies.

Chromosome translocations have been studied extensively in two tumor systems: Burkitt's lymphomas with the t(2;8), t(8;14), and t(8;22) translocations involving the c-myc proto-oncogene;[1] and chronic myelogenous leukemia with the t(9;22) translocation, which directly involves the c-abl oncogene.[2] Analysis of these two different tumors led to the concept that activation of cellular proto-oncogenes by specific chromosome translocations results in the neoplastic transformation of cells.

In human B-cell tumors, chromosome translocations involving the immunoglobulin heavy chain (IgH) locus on chromosome 14q32 are very common.[3] The authors have

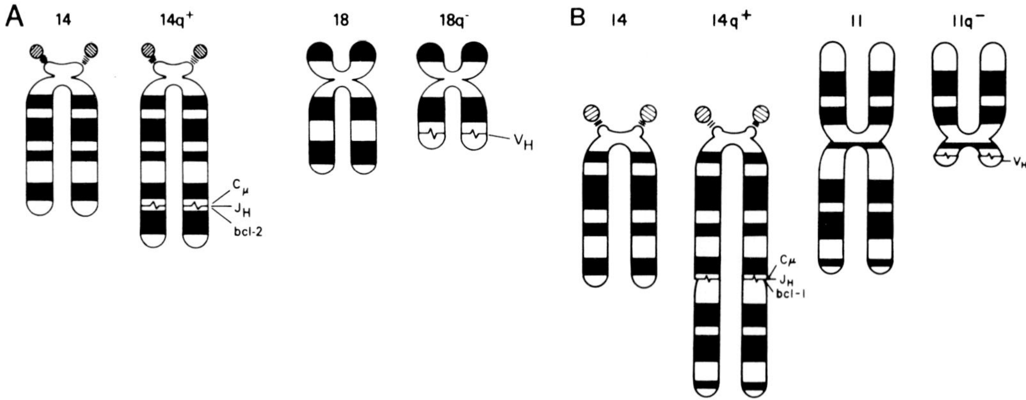

Fig. 5-1. Diagrams of the t(14;18) and t(11;14) translocations. Genes for the constant regions of the IgH gene remain on the involved chromosome 14, whereas V_H genes translocate to the involved chromosome 14 or 11. The bcl-1 (putative) and bcl-2 gene are juxtaposed to the J_H region.

focused on the t(11;14) (q13;q32) translocation, associated with some cases of chronic lymphocytic leukemia (CLL) and diffuse B-cell lymphoma,[4] on the t(14;18) (q32;q21) translocation, the hallmark of follicular lymphoma (FL), and one of the most common hematopoietic malignancies in the U.S.A.,[4] and on the t(8;14) (q24;q32) translocation, characteristic of Burkitt's lymphoma and of some acute lymphocytic leukemias (ALL).[5] The t(11;14) and t(14;18) translocations are diagrammed in Figure 5-1. Because no cellular homolog of a viral oncogene maps to chromosome 11q13 and chromosome 18q21, Tsujimoto and Croce proposed new oncogenes, designated bcl-1 and bcl-2, respectively.

In this paper, the authors describe their progress in the last few years concerning the chromosome translocations that occur in B-cells and the characterization of the bcl-2 proto-oncogene.

Most of Chromosome Translocation Associated with B-cell Tumors Occur During VDJ Recombination of the Immunoglobulin Genes.

Tsujimoto and Croce exploited the involvement of the IgH locus in the translocations in B-cells[6] to clone and characterize the joining regions of two chromosomes.[7,8] Figures 5-2 and 5-3 summarize the results of these studies on the t(11;14)[9] in CLLs and the t(14;18)[10–12] in FLs, respectively. The breakpoints on chromosome 11 of two cases of CLL were found to be only 7 bp apart from each other (Fig. 5-2).[9] In the case of the t(14;18) translocation, two hot spots for the breakpoints on chromosome 18 have been described (Fig. 5-3A),[13] one (60% of cases) within the 3′ noncoding region of the 2nd exon of the bcl-2 gene, and the other (10%), about 15 kbp downstream. The DNA sequence of the major breakpoint region within the bcl-2 2nd exon is shown in Figure 5-3B. Thus, in both the t(11;14) and t(14;18) translocations, the breakpoints are tightly clustered within a very small stretch of DNA, indicating the potential usefulness of the DNA probes derived from the breakpoint regions on chromosomes 11 and 18 as diagnostic tools for B-cell malignancies with these translocations. Chromosomes 11 and 18 are joined to the 5′ end of J_H segments.[9–12] Since the 5′ end of J_H segments is also the site of normal D segment rearrangement during immunoglobulin gene assembly,[14] the structures of the breakpoints of the t(11;14) and t(14;18) translocations immediately suggested that these translocations occur during VDJ recombination, possibly by a mistake of VDJ recombina-

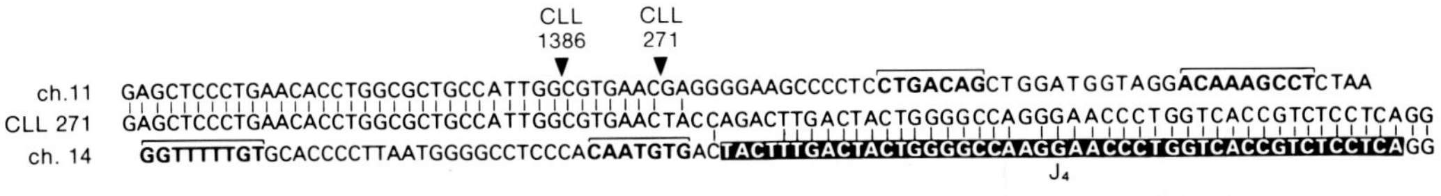

CLL 1386 CLL 271

ch.11 GAGCTCCCTGAACACCTGGCGCTGCCATTGGCGTGAACGAGGGGAAGCCCCTCCTGACAGCTGGATGGTAGGACAAAGCCTCTAA

CLL 271 GAGCTCCCTGAACACCTGGCGCTGCCATTGGCGTGAACTACCAGACTTGACTACTGGGGCCAGGGAACCCTGGTCACCGTCTCCTCAGG

ch. 14 GGTTTTTGTGCACCCCTTAATGGGGCCTCCCACAATGTGACTACTTTGACTACTGGGGCCAAGGAACCCTGGTCACCGTCTCCTCAGG

J_4

Fig.5-2. DNA sequences of the joining site between chromosomes 11 and 14 in CLL 271 and of the corresponding normal chromosome 11. Identical nucleotide sequences are shown by vertical lines. The filled triangle indicates the breakpoint of another CLL case 1386. The boxed region indicates the J_H coding segment of the IgH gene on chromosome 14. The 7mer-9mer sequences for recognition by VDJ joining recombinase are shown by brackets.

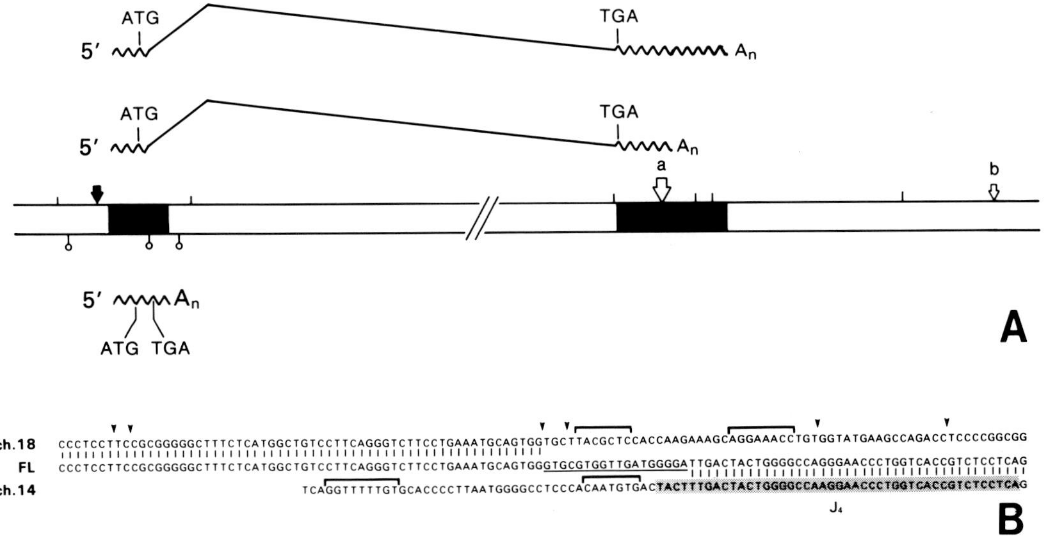

Fig. 5-3. (A) Structure of the human bcl-2 gene. The filled boxes represent two exons of the bcl-2 gene. The distance between two exons is more than 50 kb. Wavy lines indicate three different mRNAs (3.5 kb, 5 kb and 8 kb). Open arrows indicate breakpoint hot spots of the t(14;18) translocation and filled arrow indicates the region, which was rearranged in one case of follicular lymphoma.[32] Restriction sites are shown by tick marks with open circles (BamHI) and tick marks without circles (HindIII). (B) DNA sequences of the breakpoints of the t(14;18) translocation. The top line represents normal chromosome 18 sequences. Triangles indicate the breakpoints on chromosome 18 from $14q^+$ chromosome in 6 cases of follicular lymphoma. The middle and bottom line are a respresentative t(14;18) breakpoint sequences and J4 segment sequences, respectively. N-region-like sequences are underlined.

tion machinery.[9–10] This hypothesis was strengthened by the findings[9,10] of stretches of DNA at the breakpoint regions on chromosomes 11 and 18, with sequences similar to the 7mer-9mer sequences[14] required for VDJ recombination, and also the existence of extra nucleotides at the breakpoints derived from neither chromosome, but resembling the N-region sequences added during VDJ recombination, possibly by deoxyterminal transferase.[15] Similar observations have been made with the t(8;14) translocations associated with endemic Burkitt's lymphoma and with some cases of ALL.[16] Since some of the t(18;14) translocations in sporadic Burkeitt's lymphoma have been shown to break at switch regions, the translocation in these cases seems to occur during isotype switching of the IgH gene. This clearly illustrates the molecular difference between sporadic and endemic Burkitt's lymphomas, in addition to phenotypic and immunological differences described previously.

The Reciprocal Partners of the t(11;14) and t(14;18) Translocations (18q- and 11q-) Involve the D_H Region.

Tsujimoto and Croce have also characterized the structure of the reciprocal partners of translocations, that is, the joinings of the 11q-chromosome resulting from the t(11;14) translocation and the 18q-chromosome of the t(14;18) translocation. DNA sequencing studies of these joining regions, combined with analysis of chromosome $14q^+$ joining sequences revealed that two chromosome translocations, t(11;14) and t(14;18), occur in a nearly balanced manner on chromosomes 11 and 18 but not on chromosome 14. Extensive deletions were observed between the D region and the J_H region of the IgH locus (Fig. 5-4).[17,18] The breakpoint of one case of t(11;14) translocation and of two cases of the

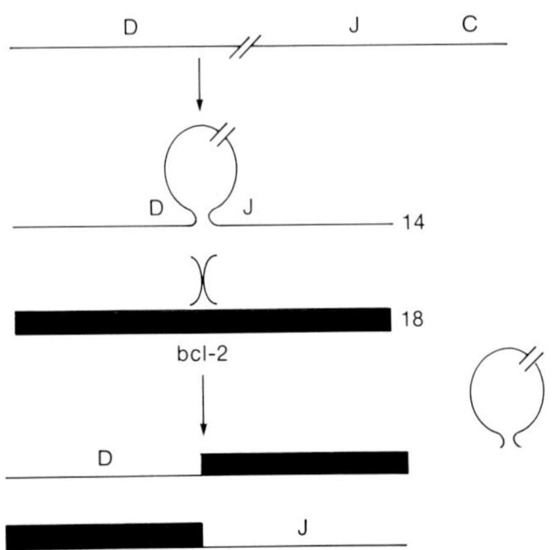

Fig. 5-4. Scheme of the t(14;18) translocation in which D, J, and C represent diversity segment, joining segment and constant region, respectively. The translocation occurs on chromosome 18 in an almost balanced manner, while on chromosome 14, a DNA segment between the D and J regions is deleted.

t(14;18) translocations map within the previously described D_H region, [19] but do not directly involve previously identified D segments (D1 and D4).[19] However, DNA sequences encompassing the breakpoints are characteristically flanked by 7mer-9mer sequences and appear to be arranged in the same way as D_H segments, suggesting the presence of additional functional D segments in the human IgH gene and preferential usage of some of them for the chromosome translocations. More detailed data are forthcoming.[17]

bcl-2 Gene in Follicular Lymphoma

By analogy to the c-myc gene in Burkitt's lymphoma and the c-abl gene in CML, the t(14;18) translocation is proposed to activate an oncogene that plays a crucial role in follicular lymphomagenesis. The transcriptionally active region, which Tsujimoto and Croce named bcl-2 (B cell lymphoma/leukemia) and that resides at the breakpoint region of the t(14;18) translocation, appears to be the most likely candidate for the oncogene involved in the t(14;18) translocation, because most t(14;18) translocations disturb this gene and also elevate transcription levels from this region.[10,13]

The bcl-2 gene consists of two exons[20,21] and is transcribed into three mRNA species.[20] The smallest mRNA (about 3 kb) is derived from the 1st exon, and the larger mRNAs (5 and 8 kb) are produced by splicing two-thirds of the 1st exon to the 2nd exon of the bcl-2 gene and by differential selection of polyadenylation sites.[20] Since the splicing donor signal is within the open reading frame, two bcl-2 proteins α and β, are expected. These are identical except at the carboxyl terminal portion.[20]

The bcl-2α protein derived from the spliced mRNAs, has been detected in human B-cells by immunoprecipitation using rabbit polyclonal antibodies raised against a bcl-2/β gal fusion protein expressed in *E. coli* (Fig. 5-5).[22] Subcellular fractionation of total cellular proteins into nuclear, cytosolic, and mem-

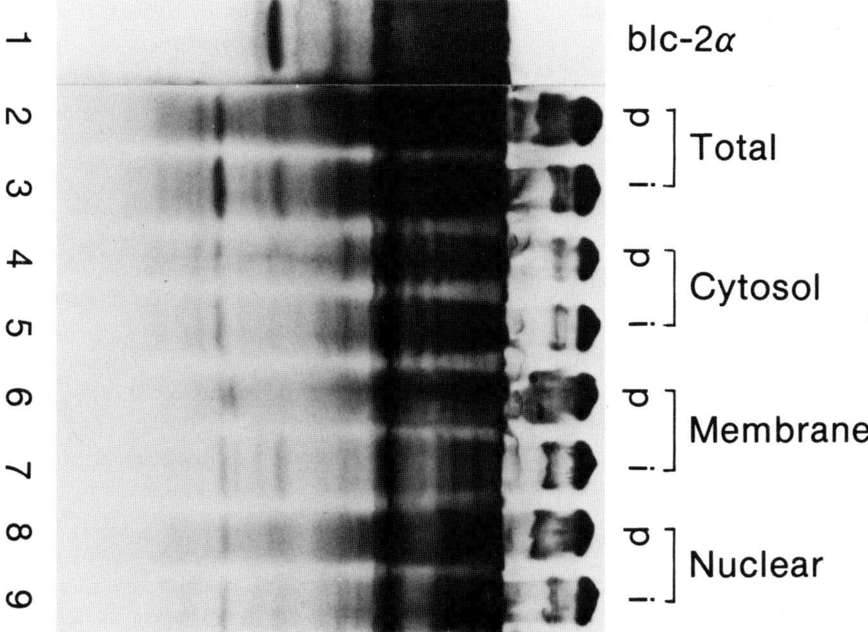

Fig. 5-5. Immunoprecipitation of the bcl-2α protein from subcellular fractions of human B-cells analyzed on 12.5% polyacrylamide/SDS gel. Each fraction (cytosolic, membrane and nuclear), equivalent to 10^7 cells, was immunoprecipitated with pre-immune serum (lanes 2, 4, 6, and 8) and antiserum (lanes 3, 5, 7, and 9). Lane 1, in vitro translated bcl-2α protein.

brane fractions, followed by immunoprecipitation revealed the bcl-2α protein in the membrane fraction.[22] Since the amino acid sequence of the bcl-2α protein deduced from the DNA sequences does not indicate either a signal peptide or a transmembrane domain,[20,21] the bcl-2α protein seems to be located at the inner side of the cytoplasmic membrane where it might function in signal transduction.

The mouse homolog of the human bcl-2 gene has been cloned and characterized.[23] The organization of the mouse bcl-2 gene (mbcl-2) is the same as that of the human gene.[23] A mouse bcl-2 DNA probe was used to demonstrate the tissue-specific expression of this gene; mbcl-2 is highly expressed in lymphoid tissues such as spleen and thymus but is either absent or expressed at very low levels in the other tissues such as heart and kidney, and excepting brain.[23]

Analyses of the human bcl-2 gene have revealed high level expression in mitogen-activated B- and T-cells; bcl-2 in mRNA appears in these cells after 6–8 hr of mitogenic stimulation.[24] No bcl-2 gene expression is detectable in resting B- and T-cells.[24] These results suggest the possible involvement of the bcl-2 gene product in cell growth. To test this possibility, an antisense oligonucleotide complementary to the region encompassing the initiation codon (AUG) of bcl-2 mRNA was introduced into a human pre-B cell line (697) and the growth of these cells was monitored. Both cell growth and DNA synthesis were inhibited.* Thus, the bcl-2 protein appears to play a role in cell growth, and the disturbance in bcl-2 gene expression is follicular lymphoma could be an important step in follicular lymphomagenesis.

---

* J. Reed et al: unpublished

It should be noted that the normal bcl-2 gene is expressed at very low levels (less than 1⁄10) as compared with expression of the rearranged bcl-2 gene.* Since bcl-2 gene expression is high at the pre-B cell stage, it must be lowered during B-cell differentiation toward FL cells. However, in the rearranged bcl-2 gene, the juxtaposed immunoglobulin locus acts to maintain expression at high levels.

Tsujimoto and Croce recently analyzed an interesting clinical case in which the patient was diagnosed as having follicular lymphoma and who later developed acute pre-B cell leukemia.[25] Unfortunately, no DNA sample could be obtained from the follicular lymphoma specimen; however, DNA extracted from acute leukemia cells showed bcl-2 gene rearrangement at the major breakpoint clustering region with the 5′ end of J_H segment and also rearrangement of the c-myc gene at the 5′ flanking region with the switch region of the IgH locus.** This observation strengthens the authors' previous model of tumor progression in which activation of the bcl-2 gene by the t(14;18) translocation led to a low-grade malignancy such as FL, and subsequent activation of the c-myc gene by the t(8;14) translocation results in a more aggressive malignancy.[5] Since FL cells are more differentiated than pre-B cells, it should be noted that FL patients might have pre-B cells carrying the t(14;18) translocation.

Epilogue

Tsujimoto and Croce have taken advantage of IgH involvement in the translocations in B-cell neoplasms to analyze the structure of the t(11;14), t(14;18) and t(8;14) translocations and have also identified a putative oncogene, bcl-2, which is directly involved in the t(14;18) translocation in follicular lymphoma and ALL. This is a powerful approach to identify the oncogenes activated by specific chromosomal abnormalities. A similar approach using T-cell surface antigen receptor (TcR) genes as probes has been taken to analyze the chromosome abnormalities in human T-cell neoplasia and in other T-cell disorders, such as ataxia telangiectasia.[26–28] Most translocations and inversions in both B- and T-cell neoplasms seem to occur during Ig and TcR gene rearrangement. It would be then interesting to learn the mechanisms responsible for the chromosome changes observed in non-B and non-T cell tumors.

It is clear that specific chromosome abnormalities play a crucial role in tumor development in humans. It has been suggested, however, from experiments using transgenic mice[29,30] that activation of a single oncogene by the chromosome translocation is not sufficient. This is compatible with a multi-step model of tumor development. What additional factors might be required for full expression of the neoplastic phenotype? Even in follicular lymphoma cells, there is evidence of some recurring chromosome changes in addition to the t(14;18) translocation,[31,32] which might activate another oncogene. The present and future efforts to gather more information on pre-neoplastic cells will also help to answer these questions.

* Y. Tsujimoto, unpublished data
** C. Gauwerky et al., unpublished

REFERENCES

1. Haluska F, Tsujimoto Y, Croce CM: Oncogene activation by chromosome translocation in human malignancy. Ann Rev Genetics 21:321–345, 1987
2. Groffen J, Stephenson JR, Heisterkamp N, et al: The human c-abl oncogene in the Philadelphia translocation. J Cell Physiol (suppl) 3:179–191, 1984
3. Levine EG, Arthur DC, Frizzera G, et al: There are differences in cytogenetic abnormalities among histologic subtypes of the non-Hodgkin's lymphomas. Blood 66:1414–1422, 1985
4. Yunis JJ: The chromosomal basis of human neoplasia. Science 221:227–236, 1983
5. Pegoraro L, Palumbo A, Erikson J, et al: A 14;18 and an 8;14 chromosome translocation in a cell line derived from an acute B-cell leukemia. Proc Natl Acad Sci 81:7166–7170, 1984
6. Erikson J, Finana J, Tsujimoto Y, et al: The chromosome 14 breakpoint in neoplastic B cells with the t(11;14) translocation involves the immunoglobulin heavy chain locus. Proc Natl Acad Sci 31:4144–4148, 1984

7. Tsujimoto Y, Yunis J, Onorato-Showe L, et al: Molecular cloning of the chromosomal breakpoint of B-cell lymphomas and leukemias with the t(11;14) chromosome translocation. Science 224: 1403–1406, 1984
8. Tsujimoto Y, Finger LR, Yunis J, et al: Cloning of the chromosome breakpoint of neoplastic B cells with the t(14;18) chromosome translocation. Science 226:1097–1099, 1984
9. Tsujimoto Y, Jaffe E, Cossman J, et al: Clustering of the breakpoints on chromosome 11 in human B-cell neoplasms with the t(11;14) chromosome translocation. Nature 315:340–343, 1985
10. Tsujimoto Y, Gorham J, Cossman J, et al: The t(14;18) chromosome translocations involved in B-cell neoplasms result from mistakes in VDJ joining. Science 229:1390–1393, 1985
11. Bakhshi A, Jersen JP, Goldman P, et al: Cloning the chromosomal breakpoint of t(14;18) human lymphomas: clustering around JH on chromosome 14 and near a transcriptional unit on 18. Cell 41:899–906, 1985
12. Cleary ML, Sklar J: Nucleotide sequence of a t(14;18) chromosomal breakpoint in follicular lymphoma and demonstration of a breakpoint-cluster region near a transcriptionally active locus on chromosome 18. Proc Natl Acad Sci 82:7439–7443, 1985
13. Tsujimoto Y, Cossman J, Jaffe E, Croce CM: Involvement of the bcl-2 gene in human follicular lymphoma. Science 228:1440–1443, 1985
14. Tonegawa S: Somatic generation of antibody diversity. Nature, 302:575–581, 1983
15. Desiderio SV, Yancopoulos GD, Pasking M, et al: Insertion of N regions into heavy-chain genes is correlated with expression of terminal deoxytransferase in B cells. Nature 311:752–755, 1984
16. Haluska FG, Finver S, Tsujimoto Y, et al: The t(8;14) chromosomal translocation occurring in B-cell malignancies results from mistakes in V-D-J joining. Nature 324:158–161, 1986
17. Tsujimoto Y, Louie E, Bashir MM, Croce CM: The reciprocal partners of both the t(14;18) and the t(11;14) translocations involved in B-cell neoplasms are rearranged by the same mechanism. Oncogene 2:347–351, 1988
18. Bakhshi A, Wright JJ, Graninger W, et al: Mechanism of the t(14;18) chromosomal translocation: structural analysis of both derivative 14 and 18 reciprocal partners. Proc Natl Acad Sci 84:2396–2400, 1987
19. Siebenlist U, Ravetch JV, Korsmeyer S, et al: Human immunoglobulin D segments encoded in tandem multigenic families. Nature 294:631–635, 1981
20. Tsujimoto Y, Croce CM: Analysis of the structure, transcripts, and protein products of bcl-2, the gene involved in human follicular lymphoma. Proc Natl Acad Sci 83:5214–5218
21. Cleary ML, Smith SD, Sklar J: Cloning and structural analysis of cDNA for bcl-2 and a hybrid bcl-2/immunoglobulin transcript resulting from the t(14;18) translocation. Cell 47:19–28, 1986
22. Tsujimoto Y, Ikegaki N, Croce CM: Characterization of the protein product of bcl-2, the gene involved in human follicular lymphoma. Oncogene 2:3–7, 1987
23. Negrini M, Silini E, Kozak C, et al: Molecular analysis of mbcl-2: Structure and expression of the murine gene homologous to the human gene involved in follicular lymphoma. Cell 49:455–463, 1987
24. Reed JC, Tsujimoto Y, Alpers JD, et al: Regulation of bcl-2 proto-oncogene expression during normal human lymphocyte proliferation. Science 236: 1295–1299, 1987
25. Gauwerky CE, Hoxie J, Nowell PC, et al: Pre-B-cell leukemia with a t(8;14) and a t(14;18) translocation is preceded by follicular lymphoma. Oncogene 2:431–435, 1987
26. Denny CT, Yoshikai Y, Mak T, et al: A chromosome 14 inversion in a T-cell lymphoma is caused by site-specific recombination between immunoglobulin and T-cell receptor loci. Nature 320:549–551, 1986
27. Mengle-Gaw L, Willard HF, Smith CIE, et al: Human T-cell tumors containing chromosome 14 inversion or translocation with breakpoints proximal to immunoglobulin joining regions at 14q32. EMBO J 6:2273–2280, 1987
28. Reynolds TC, Smith SD, Sklar J: Analysis of DNA surrounding the breakpoints of chromosomal translocations involving the β T cell receptor gene in human lymphoblastic neoplasms. Cell 50:107–117, 1987
29. Stewart TA, Pattengale PK, Leder P: Spontaneous mammary adenocarcinomas in transgenic mice that carry and express MTV/myc fusion genes. Cell 38:627–637, 1984
30. Adams JM, Harris AW, Pinkert CA, et al: The c-myc oncogene driven by immunoglobulin enhancers induces lymphoid malignancy in transgenic mice. Nature 318:533–538, 1985
31. Yunis JJ, Frizzera G, Oken MM, et al: Multiple recurrent genomic defects in follicular lymphoma. A possible model for cancer. N Engl J Med 316:79–84, 1987
32. Tsujimoto Y, Bashir MM, Givol I, et al: DNA rearrangements in human follicular lymphoma can involve the 5′ and 3′ region of the bcl-2 gene. Proc Natl Acad Sci 84:1329–1331, 1937

6

Molecular, Cytogenetic, and Clinical Studies in Japanese 14q+ Marker-Positive Lymphoma

Shirou Fukuhara
Hitoshi Ohno

Structural rearrangements of the long arm of chromosome 14 (14q) in B-lymphoid malignancy are associated primarily with a 14q32 band involved in translocations, which have been identified as a 14q+ marker chromosome. Fukuhara and Rowley proposed earlier that the presence of a 14q translocation might be important for distinguishing among morphologically different, but functionally comparable subgroups of lymphoid malignancies,[1–5] and that 14q+ marker-positive cancer should be phylogenetically and clinically divided into subclasses according to the 14q32 translocations.[6–8] A scheme of the 14q+ marker-positive cancer, given in Fig. 6-1,[8] is comparable with the systemic tree illustrating the principle of the evolutional (differentiated) genesis of Vertebrate:[7] a translocation having a consistent breakpoint at band 14q32 can be one indication of a common progenitor, and the variability in the translocation and the subsequent chromosome changes can reflect the evolutional process of the progenitor cell.[2] The proposal appears to be supported

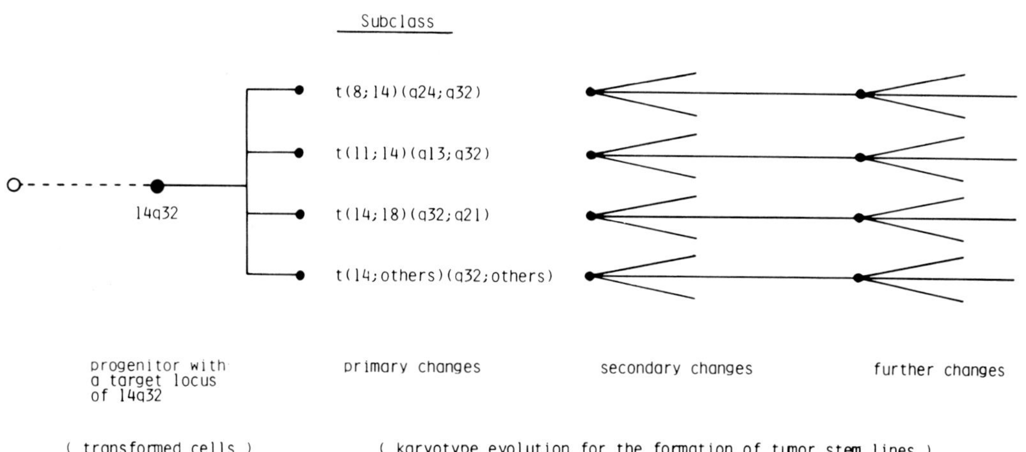

Fig. 6-1. Diagrammatic representation of the karyotype evolution in $14q^+$ marker-positive cancer.[8]

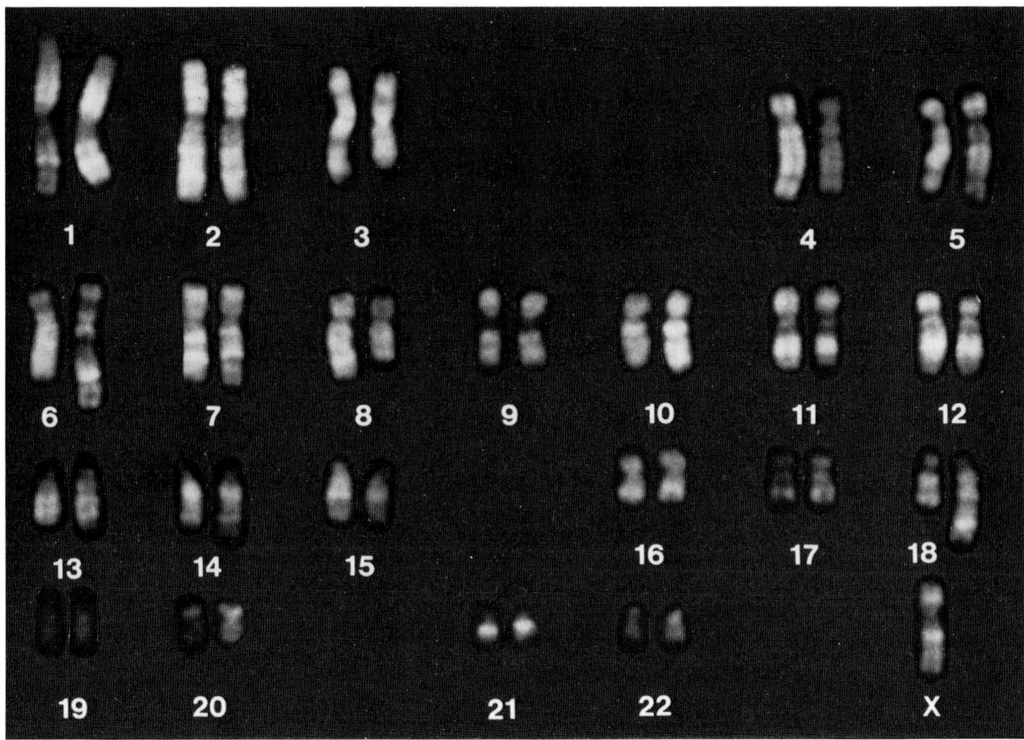

Fig. 6-2. Karyotype of a cell from a Burkitt cell line (KS-Bu3): 45,X,−X,−3,−6,−18, t(1;7)(q25;q22),+der(3)t(3;?),+der(6) t(1;6) (q21;q15),t(8;14) (q24.1;q32.3).+der(18)t(18;?)(q23;?). The cell line was established from a patient with t(8;14)-positive cancer [46,XX,−6,t(1;7), +der(6),t(8;14)].

by the recent findings in molecular genetics that the genesis of 14q+ marker-positive cancer is closely associated with molecular recombination of an immunoglobulin heavy chain gene located on chromosome 14 band q32 and a cellular oncogene mapped on the "donor" chromosome,[9] which had evolutionally been conserved.

In order to explore further the significance of 14q+ marker-positive cancer, molecular, cytogenetic and clinical findings of the two subclasses in Japan are presented here, namely t(8;14)-positive cancer (Fig. 6-2) and t(14;18)-positive cancer (Fig. 6-3).

Molecular Genetics of Two Subclasses in Japanese 14q+ Marker-Positive Cancer

The authors examined the involvement of a human c-myc gene and a putative oncogene, termed bcl-2, in the two subclasses of Japanese 14q+ marker-positive cancer. A panel includes newly established 9 cell lines having a 14q+ marker, derived from malignant lymphoma: 5 Burkitt's lymphoma-leukemia (BLL); 3 follicular small cleaved-cell lymphoma (FSCL); and 1 diffuse large-cell lymphoma (DLL) developed from FSCL. A 14q+ marker chromosome in 3 of 5 BLL-derived cell lines was the result of a t(8;14) (q24.1;q32.3) chromosome translocation, however, the origin of a 14q+ marker in 2 others was undetermined because of the absence of an 8q- chromosome. Genomic DNAs from these cell lines were subjected to Southern blot hybridization with radiolabeled probes corresponding to c-myc gene (first and second exon) and J segment of IgH genes (JH). Rearrangement of c-myc gene was observed in 4 adult cell lines including one cell line with a 14q+ marker of unknown origin,

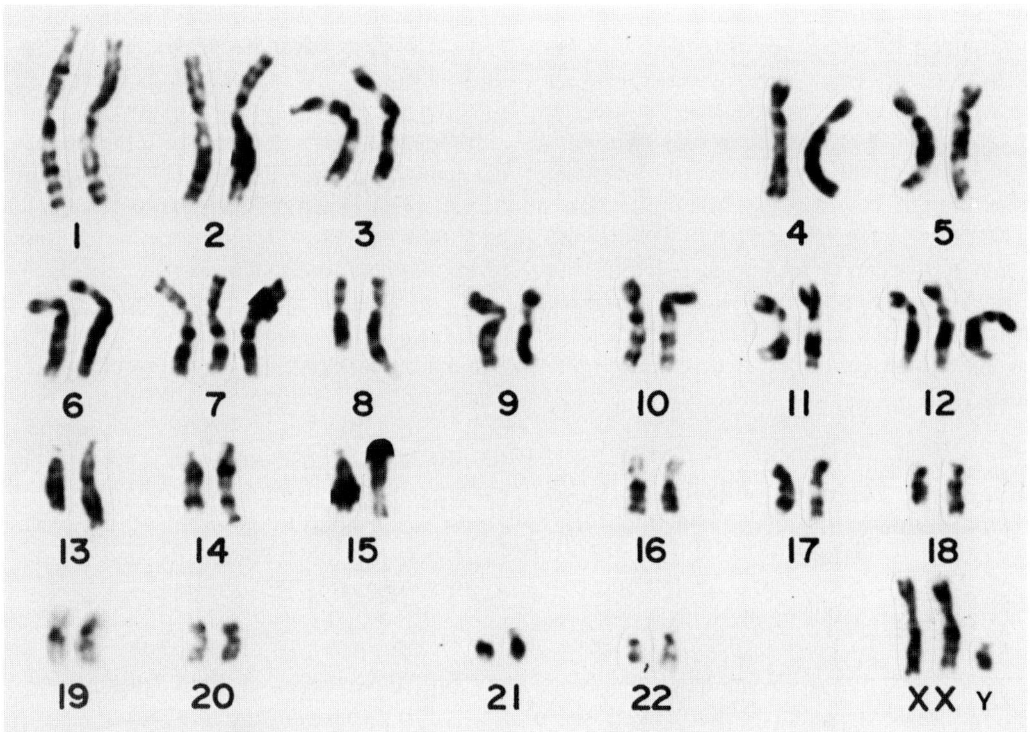

Fig. 6-3. Karyotype of a cell from a patient with t(14;18)-positive cancer: 49,XY,+X,+7,+12,dir ins(13;8)(q14;q22q24),t(8;22)(q24;q13.1),t(14;18)(q32.3;q21.3).

and the structural alterations occurred within a 5′ region of the gene. The rearranged fragments migrated with one of two rearranged JH containing fragments. In a infantile cell line with a 14q+ marker of unknown origin, any rearranged c-myc containing fragment was not detected and a copy of the germline was increased. These findings suggest that the unknown material of a 14q+ marker in the two cell lines originates from a no. 8 chromosome band q24, and the chromosome breakage in most of Japanese BLL with a t(8;14) occurs at the site of sporadic BLL,[10] although the endemic site[10] of the breakpoint could also be found (Table 6-1.).

Two genes of c-yes-1 and bcl-2 have been independently mapped at the same position of a no. 18 chromosome band q21.3, which is a breakpoint in a t(14;18) (q32.3;q21.3) chromosome translocation.[11,12] Genomic DNA's and mRNA from 2 follicular lymphoma cell lines carrying a t(14;18) were analyzed by using probes specific for yes and bcl-2 gene. There was no detectable c-yes rearrangements or transcription, whereas the two cell lines had a rearranged bcl-2 contain-

TABLE 6-1
Frequency of Structural Rearrangements of c-myc in Burkitt's Lymphoma[10]

Burkitt's Lymphoma (BL)	c-myc locus rearrangements*
endemic BL	
fresh samples	0/12
cell lines	2/6
sporadic BL	
fresh samples	7/7
cell lines	7/7
Japanese BL (present study)	
cell lines	4/5

* Values express the frequency of rearrangement detected by both EcoRI and Hind III restriction enzyme digestions.

ing a fragment that migrated with one of two rearranged JH-containing fragments, as well as other two t(14;18) bearing cell lines. The active transcription was observed at a higher level than in lymphoma cell lines without a t(14;18) used as control.[13] These findings indicate that the c-yes-1 is not involved in a t(14;18), and suggest that a t(14;18) chromosome translocation in Japanese lymphomas causes molecular recombination of the bcl-2 gene and the J region of IgH genes, such as the translocation in American lymphomas.[14–16]

Karyotype Evolution of Two Subclasses in Japanese 14q+ Marker-Positive Cancer[17,18]

The authors investigated whether the two subclasses of Japanese 14q+ marker-positive cancer have a different route of the karyotype evolution. Of 16 patients with t(8;14)-positive cancer, 15 had additional chromosome changes and 11 had structural rearrangements of the long arm of chromosome 1 (1q). These rearrangements were composed of a tandem duplication of 1q and a translocation involving 1q each in 6. Except for one, they were exclusively associated with a trisomy for a region 1q25 to 1q32 and the trisomic 1q was a single prominent change. On the other hand, of 13 patients with t(14;18)-positive cancer, 11 had additional chromosome changes that were extensive. Prominent chromosomes involved in the additional changes were chromosomes 8, 12, and 18, which were found each in 6 of the 9 hyperdiploid patients. The no. 8 chromosomes were structurally rearranged, and the rearrangements occurred at band 8q22 in 2, however, breakpoints in the others appeared to be variable. A complete trisomy 12 (+12) was noted in 5, including 2 who had chromosome 12 involved in translocations. A partial tetrasomy 12 was found in one who had a tandem duplication of 12q, and the tandem duplication was also observed in one of two hypotetraploid patients. Two patients had an extra chromosome 18 and 4 others had one or 2 extra 18q-chromosomes. The extra 18q- had the same banding pattern as that an 18q- derived from a t(14;18), and it was interpreted as being the 18q- in duplication since a 14q+ chromosome derived from the t(14;18) was not duplicated even in 3 patients having the 2 extra 18q-. Two hypotetraploid patients also had the extra 18q- chromosome in addition to the t(14;18) in duplication.

These findings indicate that the two subclasses of t(8;14)- positive and t(14;18)-positive cancer in Japan have a different "major route" of the karyotype evolution (Fig. 6-4). Especially, it is of interest that a duplication of an 18q- derived from a t(14;18) is evolutionally comparable with the second Ph[1] chromosome often found in the blastic phase of chronic myelocytic leukemia marked with a t(9;22)(q34;q11).

Clinical Features of Two Subclasses in Japanese 14q+ Marker Positive Cancer

The clinical features of 29 Japanese patients used in the above study were examined (Fig. 6-5). Sixteen patients with t(8;14)-positive cancer consisted of 12 patients with BLL and 4 with DLL. The median survival was only 7 months from diagnosis. One patient with stage IE disease has a complete remission course over 60 months. The clinical course of 15 others in the advanced stages was highly progressive, with 14 dying within 15 months, and the features were characterized by extranodal expansion including leukemia or leukemic conversion, meningeal involvement, and sarcomatous pleuritis or peritonitis. Thirteen patients with t(14;18)-positive lymphoma included 7 patients with FSCL, five with DLL, and one with diffuse mixed cell lymphoma. Their clinical features were variable and the median survival was 48 months. Three patients with simple karyotypes and 2 with complex karyotypes are still alive with a follow-up ranging from 25 to 106 months. Six of eight others with complex karyotypes had a short clinical course, surviving for 3 to 26

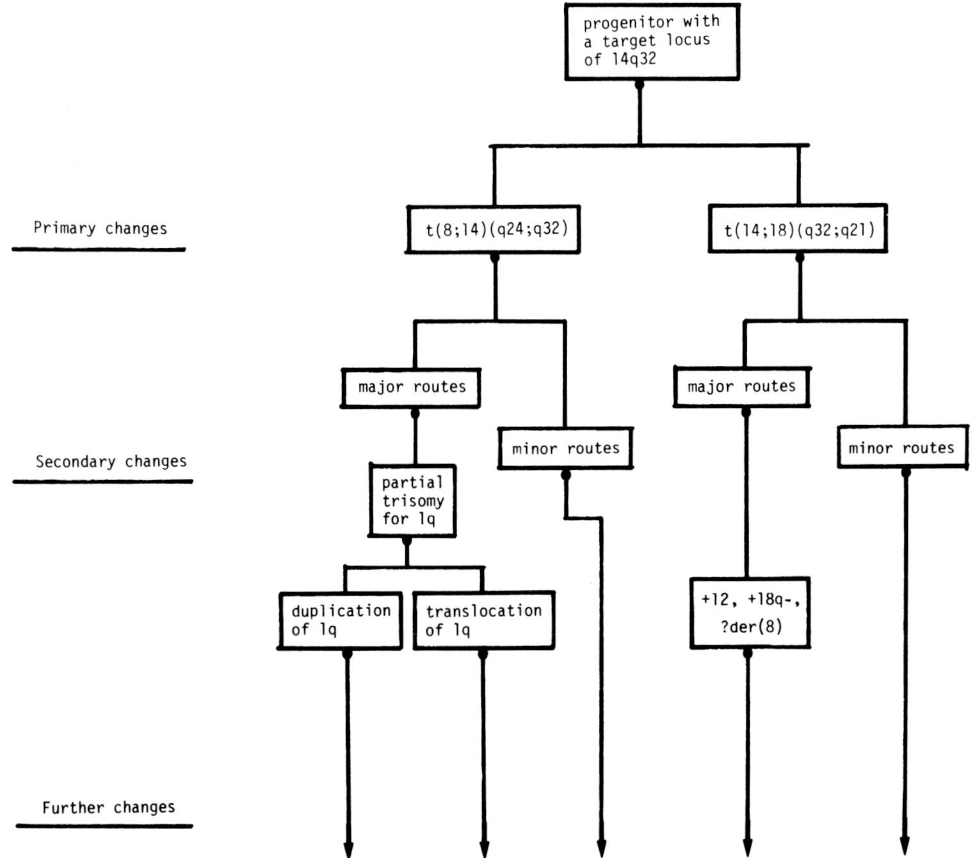

Fig. 6-4. Diagrammatic representation illustrating a different "major route" of the karyotype evolution in two subclasses of Japanese 14q+ marker-positive cancer, which are t(8;14)-positive and t(14;18)-positive cancer.

months, and 2 who died within 2 months after the chromosome study had a clinical course for 48 and 90 months, respectively. Therefore, a clinical course between two groups of patients with t(8;14)-positive and t(14;18)-positive cancer is quite different.

PERSPECTIVES

Geographic differences in incidence of malignant lymphomas have been noted.[19] Fukuhara et al have demonstrated that in t(8;14)-positive cancer the "major routes" of the karyotype evolution are composed of a partial trisomy for 1q and the major routes are absent in African Burkitt's lymphoma (BL) that carries a t(8;14) (q24;q32).[17] The follicular lymphoma group of low-grade malignancies, which is prevalent in the United States, is uncommon in Japan.[19] In a study of 71 American patients with follicular lymphoma, Yunis et al. observed that 85% of the patients had a t(14;18) (q32;q21).[20] However, among a large number of American patients with t(14;18)-positive lymphoma included in this series, an extra 18q- chromosome, which constitutes a "major route" of the karyotype evolution in Japanese t(14;18)-positive lymphoma is extremely rare. The question is therefore whether a different route of the karyotype evolution between endemic and

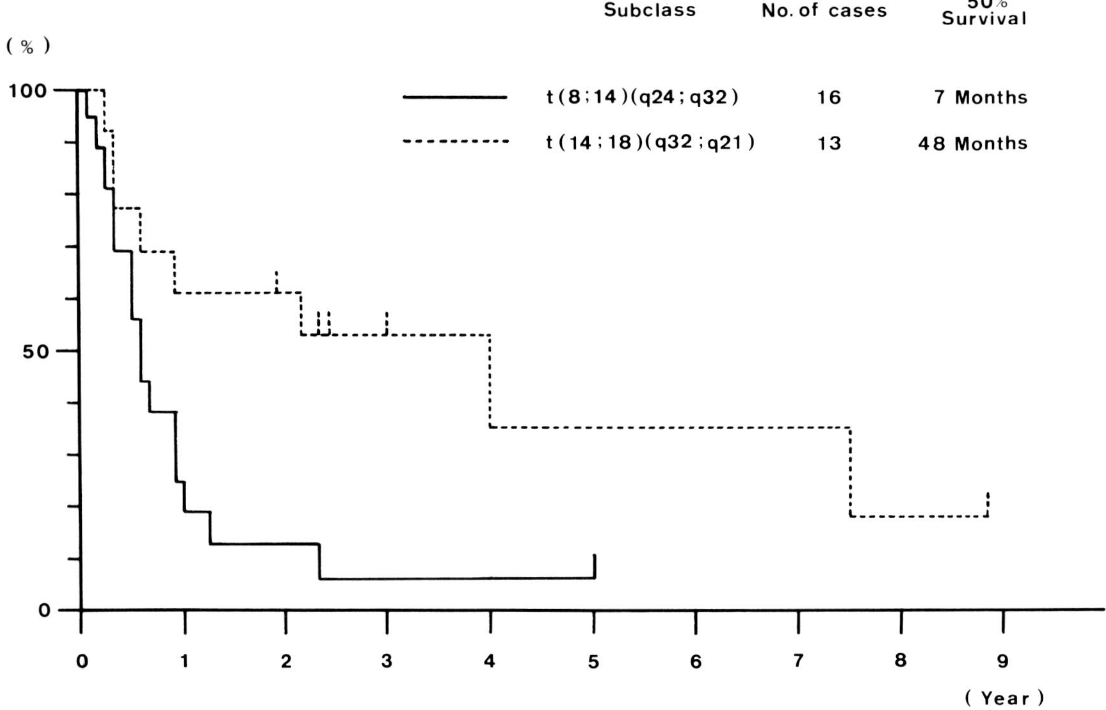

Fig. 6-5. Survival curve for Japanese t(8;14)-positive and t(14;18)-positive cancer.

sporadic t(14;18)-positive cancer could be associated with the peculiar clinicopathologic features. The resolution of this question will provide a significant clue in our further understanding of lymphomagenesis.

ACKNOWLEDGMENTS

We are grateful to doctors who referred patients for this study.

This work was supported by Grants-in-Aid for Cancer Research from the Ministry of Education, Science and Culture, and the Ministry of Health and Welfare of Japan.

REFERENCES

1. Fukuhara S, Rowley JD: Chromosome 14 translocation in non-Burkitt lymphomas. Int J Cancer 22:14–21, 1978
2. Fukuhara S: Significance of 14q translocations in non-Hodgkin lymphomas. Vichows Arch B Cell Path 29:99–106, 1978
3. Fukuhara S, Rowley JD, Variakojis D, Sweet DL: Banding studies on chromosomes in diffuse ''histiocytic'' lymphomas: Correlation of 14q+ marker chromosome with cytology. Blood 52:989–1002, 1978
4. Fukuhara S, Rowley JD, Variakojis D, Golomb HM: Chromosome abnormalities in poorly differentiated lymphocytic lymphoma. Cancer Res. 39:3119–3128, 1979
5. Rowley JD, Fukuhara S: Chromosome studies in non-Hodgkin's lymphomas. Semin Oncol 7:255–266, 1980
6. Fukuhara S, Uchino H: Subclasses of a 14q+ marker-positive lymphoid cancer. N Engl J Med 308:1603–1604, 1983
7. Fukuhara S, Nasu K, Kita K, et al: Cytogenetic approaches to the clarification of pathogenesis in lymphoid malignancies: Clinico-pathologic characterization of 14q+ marker -positive non-T-cell malignancies. Jpn J Clin Oncol 13:461–476, 1983
8. Fukuhara S, Ueshima Y, Kita K, Uchino H: 14q+ marker-positive lymphoid cancer and its subclasses. Acta Haematol Jpn 47:51–62, 1984
9. Croce CM, Nowell PC: Molecular basis human B cell neoplasia, Blood 65:1–7, 1985
10. Pelicci PG, Knowles DM, Magrath I, Dalla-Favera R: Chromosomal breakpoints and structural alterations of the c-myc locus differ in endemic and sporadic forms of Burkitt lymphoma. Proc Natl Acad Sci (Wash) 83:2984–2988, 1986
11. Tsujimoto Y, Finger LR, Yunis J, et al: Cloning

of the chromosome breakpoint of neoplastic B cells with the t(14;18) chromosome translocation. Science 226:1097–1099, 1984
12. Yoshida MC, Sasaki M, Mise K, et al: Regional mapping of the human proto-oncogen c-yes-1 to chromosome 18 at band q21.3. Gann 76:559–562, 1985
13. Ohno H, Fukuhara S, Takahashi R, et al: c-yes and bcl-2 genes located on 18q21.3 in a follicular lymphoma cell line carrying a t(14;18) chromosomal translocation. Int J Cancer 39:785–788, 1987
14. Tsujimoto Y, Cossman J, Jaffe E, Croce CM: Involvement of the bcl-2 gene in human follicular lymphoma. Science 228:1440–1443, 1985
15. Cleary ML, Sklar J: Nucleotide sequence of a t(14;18) chromosomal breakpoint in follicular lymphoma and demonstration of a breakpoint-cluster region near a transcriptionally active locus on chromosome 18. Proc Natl Acad Sci (Wash) 82:7439–7433, 1985
16. Bakhshi A, Jensen JP, Goldman P, et al: Cloning the chromosomal breakpoint of t(14;18) human lymphomas; clustering around JH on chromosome 14 and near a transcriptional unit on 18. Cell 41:899–906, 1985
17. Fukuhara S, Kita K, Nasu K, et al: Karyotype evolution in B-cell lymphoid malignancy with an 8;14 translocation. Int J Cancer 32:555–562, 1983
18. Fukuhara S, Ohno H, Amakawa R, et al: Significance of extra 18q- chromosome in Japanese t(14;18)-positive lymphoma. Blood 71:1748–1751, 1988
19. Kadin ME, Berard CW, Namba K, Wakasa H: Lymphoproliferative diseases in Japan and Western countries Hum Path 14:745-772, 1983
20. Yunis JJ, Frizzera G, Oken MM, et al: Multiple recurrent genomic defects in follicular lymphoma: A possible model for cancer. N Engl J Med 316: 79–84, 1987

7

Chromosome Aberrations in Lymphoid Malignancies and Transforming Gene in Adult T-Cell Leukemia

Nanao Kamada
Kimio Tanaka
Keiko Sakatani
Akira Hasegawa

Abstract

Of 93 untreated patients with lymphoid malignancies that had been phenotypically identified using either monoclonal antibodies or histochemical techniques, 71 (76.3%) were found to have chromosome aberrations in their bone marrow, lymph nodes or peripheral blood. The percentage of patients in which aberrations were detected was 58.6%, 75%, 88.5%, and 86.4% for acute lymphocytic leukemia (ALL:29 patients): T-cell Non-Hodgkin's Lymphoma (NHL-T: 16). B-cell NHL-B (26); and adult T cell leukemia (ATL:22), respectively. Thus the frequencies of aberrations in each of the respective stem lines increased in the order ALL<NHL-T<ATL<NHL-B. Chromosome breaks at 14q32, 6q21, 6q15, 3q21, and 9q34 were frequently observed in these malignant lymphoid malignancies.

To investigate the genetic basis of T-cell leukemogenesis, DNAs were extracted for peripheral blood cells of ATL patients and were used in in vivo selection assays for transforming genes. Tumors developed in nude mice inoculated with transfected NIH3T3 mouse cells containing DNA extracted from the peripheral blood cells of all 5 patients studied. All tumors were shown to contain Alu sequences and the transforming N-ras gene. The biological significance of the chromosome aberrations observed in malignant lymphoid cells and of the transforming gene in ATL patients is discussed.

It has been well documented that most human leukemias are associated with characteristic chromosomal abnormalities,[1] often involving either a reciprocal chromosome translocation, leading to oncogene deregulation, or a deletion of a chromosome band, resulting in the loss of a critical DNA sequence. In the case of malignant lymphomas, a number of findings have been reported over the last few years, including a significant link between karyotype and lymphoma histology. Examples of this link include the translocation between chromosomes 14 and 18 in lymphomas with of a follicular small cleaved histology; trisomy of chromosome 8 in follicular mixed lymphoma; breaks at 6q21 in immunoblastic lymphoma; and translocation 8;14 in small noncleaved lymphoma.[2–6] These associated abnormalities have been found to occur in 30%–70% of malignant lymphoma with any given histology.

There are also geographical and racial differences in the distribution of histologic subtypes and immunophenotypes of lymphomas. In the USA, T-cell lymphomas occur in only 5% of the total number of lymphoma patients, but in Japan it is about 40%. Reports of cytogenetic examinations of T-cell lymphomas are small in number in the literature and provide insufficient data for a statistical analysis of their clinical, cytogenetic, and histologic characteristics. Thus, the accumulation of cytogenetic data for T-cell lymphomas is necessary to understand the pathogenesis of lymphoid malignancy.

Since 1985, Japanese cytogeneticists have collected clinical and cytogenetic data for 114 cases of Adult T-cell leukemia (ATL) and 52 T-cell lymphomas form the main cytogenetic laboratories in Japan and have reviewed the karyotypes in detail. Final conclusions, however, have not yet been reached. In the present study, we investigated the cytogenetic characteristics of lymphoid malignancies in Hiroshima, with special reference to the differences in the cytogenetic findings obtained for T- and B-cell non-Hodgkin's lymphomas (NHL) and ATL.

Although activated transforming genes have been detected in solid tumors and hematologic disorders (mostly of acute myelocytic leukemia and myelodysplastic syndrome), no reports on the transforming genes of ATL have appeared in the literature. For this reason, the preliminary results concerning the ATL cell transforming gene are also reported here.

Chromosome Aberrations in Non-Hodgkin Lymphoma in Hiroshima

Ninety-three patients examined between 1981 and 1986 at Hiroshima University Hospital were studied cytogenetically. They included 29 with acute lymphocytic leukemia (ALL), 22 with ATL, and 42 with malignant lymphomas (ML). The tumors of all patients in this study were examined for phenotype using histochemical and/or monoclonal antibody techniques at the time of diagnosis. Of the 29 ALL patients, 5 had the T-cell type, 14 the B-cell type, and 10 the stem-cell type. Of the 42 ML patients, 16 had the T-cell type, amounting to 38% of the malignant lymphoma patients (Table 7-1). The percentage of patients bearing chromosome abnormalities varied from one disease to another (Table 7-2), being significantly lower among the ALL patients than among those with ATL or malignant lymphoma. It was approximately equal, however, for ATL, T-cell ML(T-ML), and B-cell ML(B-ML). Analysis of the stem cell modal chromosome number detected a high incidence of hyperdiploidy and tetraploidy in patients with malignant lymphoma. The percentage of patients with a hyperdiploid stem line was 3.5 (one out of 29) for ALL, and 15.6 (7 out of 42) for ML. Tetraploid stem lines were found only in ML patients (5 out of 42). Analysis of whole chromosome gain and loss in NHL and ATL revealed a high incidence of +3: while in B-ML, +7 and +18 were detected: and −18, −8, and −9 in ML nonspecific subtypes (Fig. 7-1). Mean numbers of chromosomes gained per

TABLE 7-1
Karyotype of Cases of Lymphoid Malignancies

Case	Sex/Age	Karyotype
		ALL (T cell type)
1	M/14	46,XY/46,XY,del(22)(q11)
2	M/32	46,XY
3	M/29	46,XY
4	M/16	46,XY/47,XY,+19
5	F/41	46,XX,−3,−3,−13,−14,−17,+der(3)t(3;?)(q12;?),+der(3)t(3;?)(q12;?) del(3)(p23),+der(17)t(3;17)(q21;q21),+2mar
		ALL (B cell type)
6	M/37	46,XY,t(9;15)(p22;p11)
7	M/14	46,XY
8	F/30	46,XX
9	M/8	48,XY,+21,del(11)(q13),+mar
10	M/55	46,XY/46,XY,t(8;14)(q24;q32)
11	M/69	47,XY,+3,del(4)(q11),i(8q),del(11)(p12)/46,XY
12	F/43	46,XX
13	M/33	46,XY
14	F/37	49,XX,+1,+2,t(9;22)(q34;q11),r(20)(?),+22q−/46,XX
15	M/34	58,XY,+1,+7,+8,+8,+10,+11,+11,+12,+12,+13q+,+18,+22
16	M/67	46,XY
17	F/68	48,XX,−6,−11,+18,+20,+21,+22,14q+
18	M/43	46,XY
19	M/77	49,XY,+21,+22,t(9;22)(q34;q11),+22q−/46,XY
		ALL (nonT, nonB type)
20	M/15	46,XY,t(4;11)(q21;q23)/46,XY,t(4;11)(q21;q23),t(1;18)(p32;q21)
21	M/16	46,XY,t(11;19)(q23;p13)
22	M/6	46,XY
23	M/14	46,XY
24	F/42	46,XX
25	M/18	46,XY,t(4;18)(q21;p11),t(8;12)(q13;p13),t(7;13)(q32;q14),del(10)(p13)
26	M/52	46,XY
27	M/34	46,XY/46,XY,t(9;22)(q34;q11)
28	M/41	46,XY,−11,+17/46,XY
29	M/34	46,XY,t(9;22)(q34;q11)/49,XY+7,+8,+22q−
		ATL
30	F/41	47,XX,+12
31*	F/64	47,X,−X,−1,−3,−11,−14,−15,−16,−18,−22,+der(3)t(3;?)(q21;?),+der (3)t(3;?)(p25;?),+der(11)t(1;11)(p12;q14),+der(14)t(14;?)(p11;?) ,+der(15)t(1;15)(q21;p11),+der(?)t(1;?)(q25;?),+4mar
32	M/53	45,XY,−8,−14,−14,−18,−20,+4mar
33	M/69	46,XY,+3,−8,−9,−10,−15,−17,−18,del(14)(q11q13),+der(17)t(17;?)(p13;?),+4mar/ 47,XY,+3,−8,−9,−15,−17,−18,del(14)(q11q13),+der(17)t(17;?)(p13;?),+4mar
34*	M/49	47,XY,+17,t(1;12;4)(q41;q13;q31),del(5)(q15q22),del(7)(p14),del(13)(q32)
35	M/66	46,XY,−14,−18,del(6)(q22),t(7;9)(p12;q34),+der(14)t(14;?)(q32;?),del (16)(q22),+der(18)t(18;?)(p11;?)
36	M/68	46,XY/46,XY,t(1;5)(q11;q22)/46,XY,t(3;9)(q21;p22)/47,XY,+18
37*	F/67	46,XX/48,XX,−7,+11,−17,−18,−19,+der(7)t(7;?)(q32;?),+der(19)t(19;?)(q12;?),+3mar

TABLE 7-1 (continued)

Case	Sex/Age	Karyotype
38	M/63	46,XY,dup(4)(p11→p14)/48,XY,+9,del(12)(q15q22),+der(20)t(20;?)(p13;?)/47,XY,+min
39	F/57	46,XX,t(16;20)(q13;p11)/46,XX
40	M/54	46,XY/48,XY,+3,+14,+21,−5,−8,−19,del(6)(q15),t(7;14)(p13;p11),+2mar
41	M/?	46,XY,t(3;7)(q21;q22)
42*	F/52	46,XX
43	M/57	46,XY,/47,XY,+7/48,XY,+3,+7
44	M/48	48,XY,−12,+22,del(6)(q11q21),+der(12)t(7;12)(p15;q24), +mar/ 49,XY,−12,+22,del(6)(q11q21),+der(12)t(7;12)(p15;q24),+2mar
45	F/72	46,X,−X,−2,−3,−3,+7,−9,+der(2)t(2;?)(q33;?),+der(3)t(3;?)(p25;?), del(6)(q21q25),del(10)(pl3),+mar 1,+mar 2/ 47,X,−X,−2,−3,−3,−5,+7,−9,+der(2)t(2;?)(q33;?),+der(3)t(3;?) (p25;?),del(6)(q21q25),del(10)(pl3),+mar 1,+mar 2,+mar 3,+mar 4
46	M/56	47,Y,−X,−10,−13,+15,+der(X)t(X;?)(p22;?),+der(10)t(10;?)(q26;?), +der(13)t(13;?)(q22;?)
47	M/53	46,XY
48	M/18	46,XY
49	F/76	49,XX,+X,+5,+21
50	M/69	47,XY,+Y,−2,+der(2)t(2;14)(q33;q13)
51	M/61	46,XY,t(1;10)(p13;q24),dup(8)(q24.1→ q24.3),t(9;14)(q32;q32),t(11;17)(q21;q11)/ 47,XY,del(9)(q22),+mar/46,XY
		Malignant Lymphoma (T cell type)
52	F/78	85,XX
53	F/66	46,XX,dup(3)(q25→q27)
54	M/65	46,XY,−3,−8,t(1;6)(p36;p21),+der(3)t(3;?)(q29;?),+der(8)t(8;?)(q24;?),del(8)(p21)
55	M/74	46,XX
56	F/78	42,X,−X,−1,−2,−4,−4,−11,−13,−14,−14,−15,−18,−18,del(3)(q22),+der (4)t(4;?)(p16;?),del(8)(p22),+der(13)t(13;?)(q34;?),+der(14)t(14;?)(q32;?),4mar
57	F/49	47,XX,+1,−2,−8,−13,−17,−18,+der(13)t(13;?)(q32;?),+der(17)t(17;?) (p11;?).+der(18)t(18;X)(p11;p11),+der(X)t(X;2)(p11;p11),+2mar
58	M/63	49,XY,+5,+7,+13,del(6)(q13),del(13)(q22)/46,XY
59	F/73	45,XX,−8,−16,+der(16)t(8;16)(q13;q13)/46,XX,del(3)(p13)
60	F/74	46,XX
61	M/38	48,XY,−2,−4,−9,−10,−15,−22,t(2;4)(p11;q11),+der(2)t(2;?)(p11;?), t(3;12)(q21;q13),+5mar
62	M/12	46,XY
63	M/69	46,XY
64	M/19	46,XY/47,XY,+22/50,XY,+9,+10,+21,+r(?)
65	M/67	52,XY,+4,+7,−18,−22,+der(12)t(12;?)(q12;?),+5mar
66	F/4	79,XX,del(6)(q21),+der(13)t(13;?)(q32;?)
67	M/31	46,XY,−20,del(2)(q23),t(6;9)(q15;q32),+mar
		Malignant Lymphoma (B cell type)
68	M/72	48,XY,−1,+4,+22,+der(1)t(1;6)(q32;q21),del(6)(q13),del(9)(p13p23), del(12)(q22q24),del(16)(q22),inv(19)(pl3ql3)/ 46,XY,−1,−9,+22,+der(1)t(1;6)(q32;q21),del(6)(q13),del(9)(p13p23), del(12)(q22q24),inv(19)(p13q13)
69	M/84	49,XY,−4,−5,−14,−16,−17,−18,−20,−21,+11mar
70	F/60	87,XX,+10mar
71	F/48	88,XX
72	M/69	46,XY,−5,−6,−10,−10,i(9q),del(12)(p12),del(22)(q11),+4mar
73	M/70	53,X,+X,−Y,−6,+13,−16,−18,+21,+del(3)(p21),+der(9)t(9;?)(p22;?), +mar1,+mar2,+mar3,+mar4,+2mar5/46,XY
74	F/74	46,XX

TABLE 7-1 (continued)

Case	Sex/Age	Karyotype
75	M/76	50,XY,+3,+7,+10,+22,−4,−5,−8,−8,−15,del(5)(p12),+der(5)t(5;?)(p11;?),+der(21)t(21;?)(q22;?),+3mar
76	F/49	46,XX,−3,−21,inv(2)(q21q31),+der(3)t(3;?)(q21;?),del(6)(q21),t(8;10)(q22;q22),+mar/ 45,XX,−3,−14,−21,inv(2)(q21q31),+der(3)t(3;?)(q21;?),del(6)(q21),t(8;10)(q22;q22),+mar
77	F/46	50,XX,+3,+3,+13,+14,+18,−11,−12,+2mar/46,XX
78	M/60	46,XY,t(9;13)(q13;p11)
79	F/83	51,X,−X,+3,+5,+18,t(3;11)(p13;q23),+3mar
80	M/67	47,XY,+4,+18,−9,−9,−13,t(1;2;6)(q25;q35;q21),der(13)t(9;13)(q13;q22),+mar
81	M/60	50,XY,+5,+9,−2,−6,−15,del(1)(q12),+i(1q),del(3)(q27),+der(6)t(1;6)(p22;q15),+der(6)t(6;?)(q25;?),dup(12)(q13→q24),del(16)(q23),+2mar
82	M/51	48,XY,+18,−3,−8,−10,+der(3)t(3;?)(p21;?),+der(8)t(8;?)(p11;?), del(9)(q11q13,+der(10)t(10;?)(q22;?),del(11)(q23),+mar1/ 48,XY,+18,−3,−8,−10,+der(3)t(3;?)(p21;?),+der(8)t(8;?)(p11;?), del(9)(q11q13).del(11)(q23),+mar1,mar2
83	M/53	49,XY,−1,−12,−14,−15,−17,−18,−19,−20,del(1)(p22),+der(1)t(1;6)(p36;p21),del(1)(p11p22),del(6)(q15q23),+der(11)t(11;?)(p11;?),+ der(12)t(12;?)(p11;?),del(12)(p11),+der(14)t(14;?)(q32;?),+5mar
84	M/58	46,XY,−14,+der(14)t(14;?)(q32;?)/47,XY,−14,+der(14)t(14;?)(q32;?),+mar
85	M/71	48,XY,+3,+18,−8,−9,−14,del(6)(p15),+i(8q),+der(14)t(14;?)(q32;?),+mar
86	M/27	92,XY,+X,+Y,+der(1)t(1;?)(q32;?),der(7)t(7;?)(q22;?),+der(14)t(14;?)(q32;?),+3mar
87	M/47	46,XY/46,XY,t(6;12)(q15;p13)/46,XY,+9,−17
88	F/73	45,XX,−9,−13,−14,−21,dirdup(1)(p26→q32),del(6)(q15q21),+der(18)t(18;?)(q11;?),+2mar
89	F/70	49,X,−X,+12,+21,−2,−7,−18,−20,del(3)(q21),del(5)(p13),del(6)(q21), +der(18)t(18;?)(p11;?)
90	F/68	50,XX,+3,+7,+11,−4,−8,+der(4)t(4;?)(q33;?),+2mar
91	M/46	46,XY
92	F/80	46,XY/46,XX,t(3;11)(p13;q21),del(9)(p22)
93	F/13	46,XX

* Cases submitted to ATL Karyotype Review Committee—1985

TABLE 7-2

Percentage of Patients with Chromosome Abnormalities

	Number of Patients Studied	Cases with Chromosome Abnormlities	Percent of Patients with Chromosome Abnormalities		
ALL-T cell	5	3	60	58.6%	
-B cell	14	8	57		
-stem cell	10	6	60		
				*1	
ATL	22	19	86.4		
ML-T cell	16	12	75.0	83.3%	
-B cell	26	23	88.5		*2

* Fisher's exact test

*1 : p = 0.03, *2 : p = 0.02

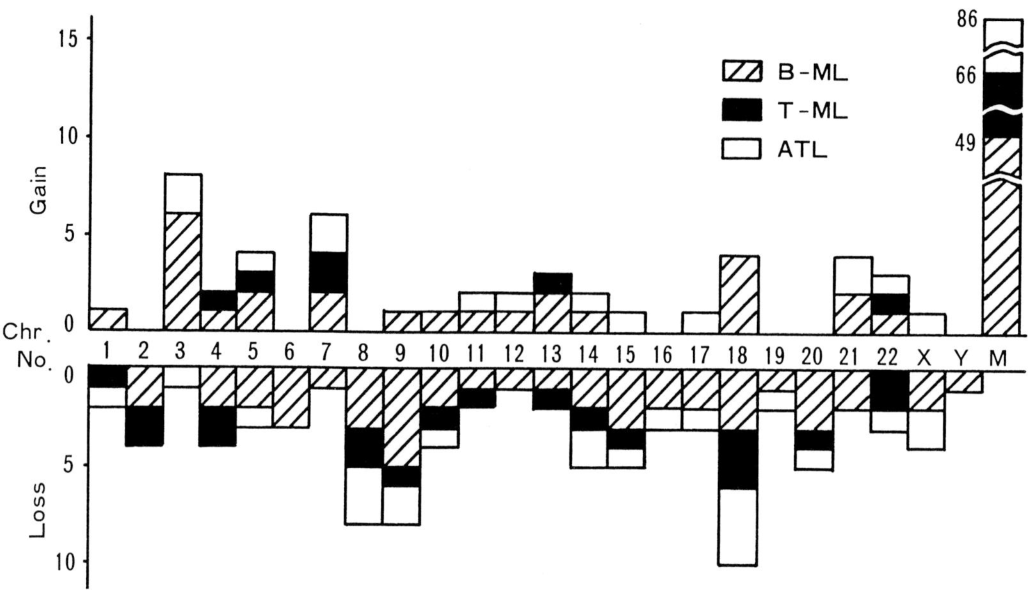

Fig. 7-1. Histogram showing whole chromosome gain and loss in non-Hodgkins lymphoma and ATL cells

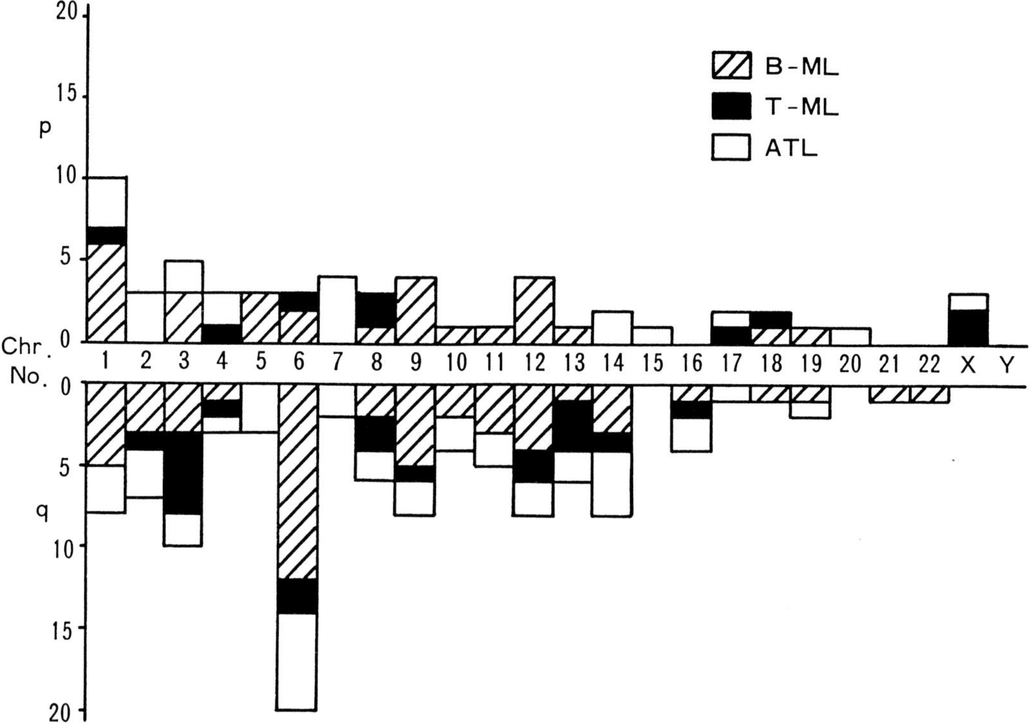

Fig. 7-2. Histogram of structural abnormalities involving each chromosome in non-Hodgkins lymphoma and ATL cells

stem cell line were 3.4 in B-ML, 1.6 in T-ML, and 1.6 in ATL, thus demonstrating a high incidence of gain in B-ML. Chromosome losses in each of the three diseases, however, showed no statistically significant differences. Structural abnormalities in each chromosome, excluding marker chromosomes, are shown in Figure 7-2; the data demonstrate that abnormalities occurred with higher frequencies in chromosome segments 1p, 3q, 6q, 9q, 12q, and 14q. The most commonly rearranged chromosome regions in these lymphoid malignancies were 6q21, 14q32, 11q21–25, and 1p36. Most patients with B-cell NHL had more than 6 chromosome aberrations per stem line, whereas two-thirds of those with T-cell NHL were shown to have less than 5 chromosome aberrations (Fig. 7-3), demonstrating that the percentage of normal metaphases was higher in T-ML than B-ML patients cells, and that B-ML cells had more complicated chromosome aberrations than did ATL or T-ML. It is evident that more cytogenetic information on T cell ML is needed for final conclusions to be reached on the link between T-ML karyotype abnormalities and its histologic types.

Detection of Transforming Genes in DNAs extracted from ATL Cells

To investigate the genetic basis of T-cell leukemogenesis, the transforming activity of DNAs extracted from ATL cells was examined by means of an in vivo selection assay.[7] Patient DNA incorporated into plasmid pSV2Neo DNA was co-transfected into mouse NIH3T3 fibroblasts. Transfected cells were selected with the antibiotic, neomycin, and then injected subcutaneously into nude mice. Tumors appeared 4–8 weeks later. The leukemic cells of 5 ATL patients were examined for the presence of transforming genes. All such patients were male and positive for the human T-cell lymphotropic virus type-1(HTLV-1) genome, and four had acute and one chronic ATL. The percentage of "flower" cells in the peripheral blood ranged from 32% to 87%. Histologic examination of lymph-nodes from 4 patients led to a diagnosis of immunoblastic lymphoma(IBL)-polymorphous for 2, and diffuse mixed(T) and IBL(T) types for each of the other 2. Cytogenetic studies were performed on cells from 3 patients, and 2 were shown to contain com-

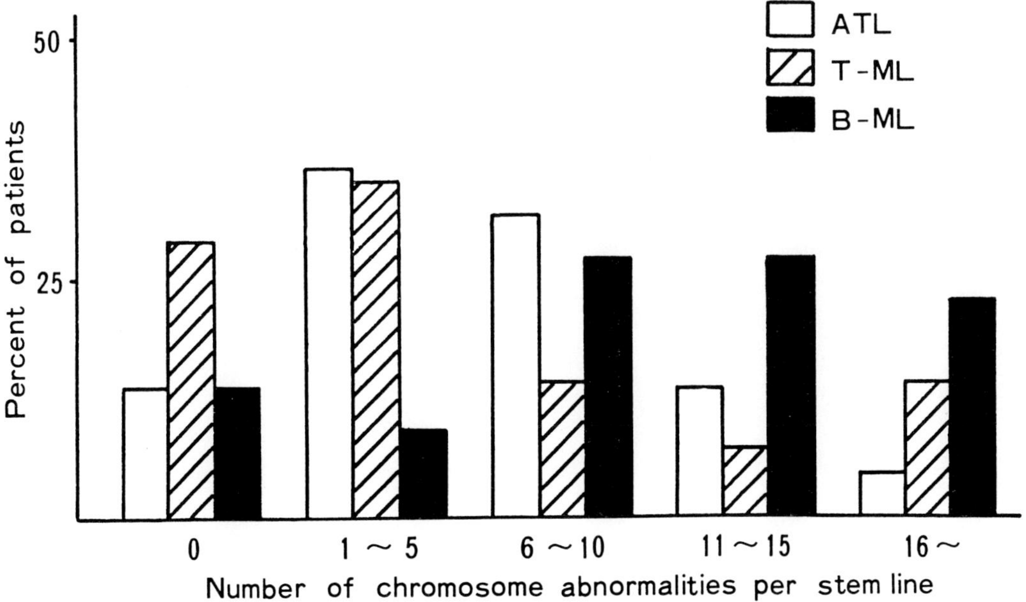

Fig. 7-3. Distribution of patients with chromosome abnormalities

TABLE 7-3
Laboratory Findings for ATL Patients

Case(Age/Sex)	% "Flower Cells" in PB	HTLV-1 Genome	Type of ATL	Type of Histology	Chromosome Abnormalities
1 (60/M)	80	+	Acute	IBL-polymorphous	—
2 (49/M)	87	+	Acute	—	47,XY,+18,−1,−4,−12,+der(1) t(1 ; ?)(q42 ; ?),+der(4)t(4;12) (q31;q13),del(7)(p14),del(13)(q32), +mar
3 (67/M)	71	+	Acute	Diff. mixed(T)	46,XY,t(1;5)(q21;q22)
4 (54/M)	32	+	Acute	IBL-polymorphous	47,XY,+21,−4,−5,−8,−19, +der(3) t(3;?)(p25;?),t(7;14)(p13;p11), del(6)(q15),+der(14)t(14;?)(q32;?), +2mar
5 (46/M)	58	+	Chronic	IBL(T)	—

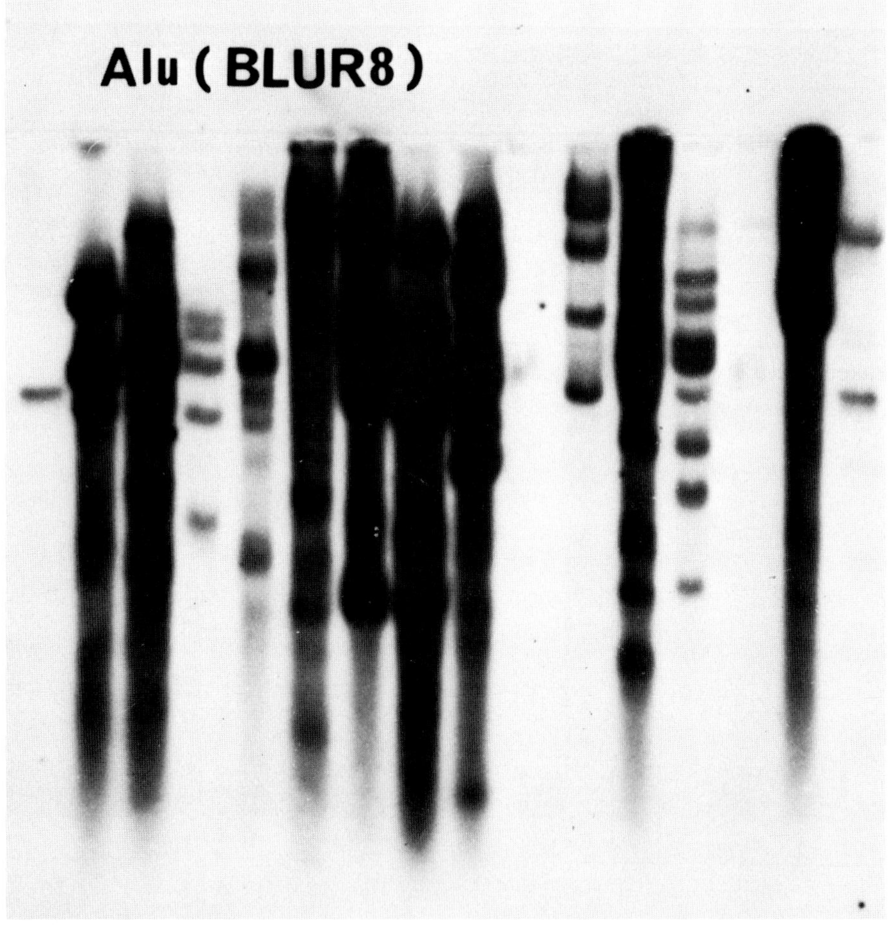

Fig. 7-4. Detection of human DNA sequences in tumors produced following inoculation of transfected cells into nude mice

plicated chromosome abnormalities, as shown in Table 7-3. Tumors, which were histologically fibrosarcoma, were produced following inoculation of NIH3T3 cells transfected with DNA from any of the 5 ATL patients, with 3–4 tumors arising from 4 inoculated sites per animal. DNAs extracted from any of these tumors contained human DNA-specific Alu sequence (Fig. 7-4), and when hybridized with human N-ras genomic DNA, all were found to contain the human N-ras gene.

Transforming Gene in Hematologic Disorders

The development of DNA-mediated gene transfer techniques has provided an approach to the detection of cellular transforming DNA sequences. Using the NIH3T3 cell transfection assay, transforming genes have been detected in diverse human tumors, including carcinomas, sarcomas, and hematopoietic malignancies.[8–13] Studies of the oncogenes of hematopoietic tumors have so far resulted in the detection of transforming DNA sequences in cell lines isolated from T-cell[14,15] and B-cell[15,16] lymphoid malignancies and from acute promyelocytic leukemia,[17] as well as in leukemic cells obtained from acute myelocytic leukemia patients.[18–21] In most cases, the transforming gene detected was N-ras, with mutations occurring at codons 12 or 61.

Detection of the N-ras gene in DNAs from ATL patients is important in understanding the genetic and biologic bases of T-cell lekemogenesis. HTLV-1 provirus contains the pX gene, instead of the oncogene usually found in retroviruses. The pX gene produces three kinds of proteins, named $p40^x$, $p27^x$, and $p21^x$. The p40 protein reacts with the long terminal repeat and activates its transcription, as well as inducing synthesis of the IL-2 receptor. T-cells newly infected with HTLV-1 initially proliferate polyclonally, but then progress to clonal malignancy. Furthermore, activation of the N-ras gene, detected in the authors' present experiments, may be linked to one of the steps in malignant transformation leading to the formation of ATL cells. A more detailed analysis of the site of mutation in the N-ras gene will be reported elsewhere.

ACKNOWLEDGMENTS

This work was supported in part by Grants-in-Aid for Cancer Research from the Ministry of Education, Science, and Culture, from the Japan Medical Association (1986) and from the Japanese Foundation for Multi-Disciplinary Treatment of Cancer (1987).

REFERENCES

1. Rowley JD: Principles of cancer biology: Chromosomal abnormalities, in Cancer-Principles & Practice of Oncology, Devita VR, Hellman S, Rosenbert SA, (eds): 1985 67–78
2. Yunis JJ, Oken MM, Kaplan ME, et al: Distinctive chromosomal abnormalities in histologic subtypes of non-Hodgkin's lymphoma. N Engl J Med, 307:1231–1236, 1982
3. Bloomfield CD, Arthur DC, Frizzera G, et al: Nonrandom chromosome abnormalities in lymphoma. Cancer Res 43:2975–2984, 1983
4. Pandolfi F: T-CLL and allied diseases: New insights into classification and pathogenesis. Diagnostic Immunology 4:75–80, 1986
5. Koduru PRK, Filippa DA, Richardson ME, et al: Cytogenetic and histologic correlations in malignant lymphoma. Blood 69:97–102, 1987
6. Yunis JJ, Frizzera G, Oken MM, et al: Multiple recurrent genomic defects in follicular lymphoma. N Engl J Med, 316:79–84, 1987
7. Southern PJ, Berg P: Transformation of mammalian cells to antibiotic resistance with a bacterial gene under control of the SV40 early region promoter. J Mol Appl Genet, 1:327–341, 1982
8. Perucho M, Goldfarb M, Shimizu K, et al: Human-tumor-derived cell lines contain common and different transforming genes. Cell, 27:467–476, 1981
9. Lane MA, Sainten A, Cooper GM: Stage-specific transforming genes of human and mouse B- and T-lymphocyte neoplasms. Cell 28:873–880, 1982
10. Shih C, Weinberg RA: Isolation of transforming sequence from a human bladder carcinoma cell line. Cell 29:161–169, 1982
11. Pulciani S, Santos E, Lauver AV, et al: Oncogenes in human tumor cell lines: Molecular cloning of a transforming gene from human bladder carcinoma cells. Proc Natl Acad Sci 79:2845–2849, 1982
12. Der CJ, Krontiris TG, Cooper GM: Transforming genes of human bladder and lung carcinoma cell lines are homologous to the *ras* genes of Harvey and Kirsten sarcoma viruses. Proc Natl Acad Sci 79:3637–3640, 1982

13. Shimizu K, Goldfarb M, Perucho M, Wigler M: Isolation and preliminary characterization of the transforming gene of a human neuroblastoma cell line. Proc Natl Acad Sci 80:383–387, 1983
14. Souyri M, Fleissner E: Identification by transfection of transforming sequences in DNA of human T-cell leukemias. Proc Natl Acad Sci 80:6676–6679, 1983
15. Lane MA, Sainten A, Cooper GM: Stage-specific transforming genes of human and mouse B- and T-lymphocyte neoplasms. Cell 28:873–880, 1982
16. Eva A, Tronick SR, Gol RA, et al: Transforming genes of human hematopoietic tumors: Frequent detection of *ras*-related oncogenes whose activation appears to be independent of tumor phenotype. Proc Natl Acad Sci 80:4926–4930, 1983
17. Murray MJ, Shilo BZ, Shih C, et al: Three different human tumor cell lines contain different oncogenes. Cell 25:355–361, 1981
18. Gambke C, Signer E, Moroni C: Activation of N-*ras* gene in bone marrow cells from a patient with acute myeloblastic leukaemia. Nature 307:476–478, 1984
19. Bos JL, Toksoz D, Marshall CJ, et al: Amino-acid substitutions at codon 13 of the N-*ras* oncogene in human acute myeloid leukaemia. Nature 315:726–730, 1985
20. Hirai H, Tanaka S, Azuma M, et al: Transforming genes in human leukemia cells. Blood 66:1371–1378, 1985
21. Bos JL, de Vries MV, van der Eb AJ, et al: Mutation in N-*ras* predominate in acute myeloid leukemia. Blood 69:1237–1241, 1987

8

Chromosome Abnormalities in Malignant Lymphoma in an Area Nonendemic for Adult T-Cell Leukemia-Lymphoma in Japan

Masaharu Sakurai
Nobuo Maseki
Yasuhiko Kaneko

Abstract

Chromosome abnormalities are found in most patients with malignant lymphoma, and some abnormalities have been correlated with certain histologic or immunologic characteristics of lymphoma. Maseki et al.'s recent studies on chromosomes in 92 patients with non-Hodgkin's malignant lymphoma in the northern suburbs of Tokyo indicate a conspicuous difference in the distribution of various karyotypic categories between these patients and similar patients in the United States or Europe. While they had 8q24 translocations in a frequency comparable to those in the western countries, there were fewer lymphomas with t(14;18)(q32;q21) in northern Tokyo area than in western countries. These observations correspond with the already known histologic findings that there are fewer follicular lymphomas and more diffuse lymphomas in Japan than in the U.S. or Europe. Also, there were proportionately more T-lymphomas than in the western countries, although adult T-cell leukemia-lymphoma was not endemic in their area. Thus, Maseki et al. were able to find significant associations between certain chromosome abnormalities and some histologic or immunologic characteristics of lymphoma, such as associations between trisomy 5 and diffuse, mixed lymphoma, and between multiple clones and T-cell lymphomas. The authors hypothesized that factors affecting the lymphomagenesis may be different, or operating in different intensities in different geographic areas.

Chromosome abnormalities are found in most patients with malignant lymphoma (ML). Certain abnormalities have been correlated with histologic[1–5] and immunologic[6] characteristics, and some chromosomal translocations implicated in the genesis of lymphoma.[7]

The majority of chromosome studies in a large series of patients with malignant lymphoma have been carried out in the United States[1–6] where follicular lymphomas are common and T-cell lymphomas are rare in contrast with the situation in Japan. Although chromosomal data on adult T-cell leukemia-lymphoma (ATL), the most common type of ML in southwestern Japan, have been amply reported,[8–12] those on other T- and B-cell lymphomas are scarce in this country.[13] Maseki et al.'s recent studies on karyotypes in non-Hodgkin's ML in patients admitted to a cancer hospital in the northern suburbs of Tokyo[14] indicate a conspicuous difference in the distribution of various karyotypic categories between these patients and ML patients in the United States[1–6] or Europe.[15] Their findings on chromosomes correspond to the findings on histology that are also different between Japan and the U.S., or Europe.[16] In their studies, Maseki et al. have been able to correlate several non-random chromosome abnormalities with certain histologic or immunologic phenotypes of ML. In addition, they suspect that there may be fewer patients with t(14;18) in Japan than in the United States.

Histologic and Immunologic Phenotypes in Malignant Lymphoma in Saitama

Only 11% (10 of 92) of ML patients showed a follicular pattern[17] (Table 8-1). This finding was in sharp contrast to those of other countries. In the U.S., follicular lymphomas constitute almost one half of the total lymphomas,[1–6,16] and the situation in Europe apparently shows a similar tendency.[15–16] Thus, the most common type in their series was diffuse, large cell (DL) lymphoma. Diffuse, mixed, small and large cell (DM) lymphoma and large cell, immunoblastic (IBL) lymphoma were next in frequency. Some patients with diffuse, small cleaved cell (DSC) or IBL lymphoma were also classified as diffuse, medium-sized cell type, or diffuse, pleomorphic type by the Japanese Lymphoma-Study-Group (LSG) classification.[18] These patients were shown to have T-cell lymphoma by immunophenotyping.

Of the patients who had immunologic studies conducted, 48% had B-cell lymphoma,

TABLE 8-1

Cases of Non-Hodgkin's Malignant Lymphoma in Saitama by Histology According to Working Formulation and Immunophenotype[14]

	Working Formulation*										
	B	C	D	E	F	G	H	I	J	Misc	Total
Total number	1	5	3	8	15	32	15	5	6	2	92
Immunophenotype†											
B	1	3	1	3	1	14	5		4	2	34
T				4	9	8	1	3			25

*Malignant lymphoma was diagnosed before therapy for each patient. B, ML, follicular, predominantly small cleaved cell (FSC); C, ML, follicular, mixed small cleaved and large cell (FM); D, ML, follicular, predominantly large cell (FL); E, ML, diffuse, small cleaved cell (DSC); F, ML, diffuse, mixed small and large cell (DM); G, ML, diffuse, large cell (DL); H, ML, large cell, immunoblastic (IBL); I, ML, lymphoblastic (LBL); J, ML, small noncleaved cell (SNC); Misc, miscellaneous. Groups B, C and D constitute follicular lymphomas. No cases had ML, small lymphocytic (SL).

† Determinable cases only.

and 35% had T-cell lymphoma. Thus, although the authors' hospital is located in an area nonendemic for ATL, there have been proportionately more T-cell lymphoma patients in our hospital than seen in the U.S.[1–6] or Europe.[15] Lymphoma cells were CD4-positive and CD8-negative, and were thought to be helper/inducer in all T-cell lymphomas tested.

Only 9% of the patients tested had ATLA antibodies in their serum. This positivity rate is much lower than that in lymphoma patients from the southwestern districts of Japan. All three ATLA-positive patients had T lymphoma; had only one typical ATL.

Chromosome Abnormalities in Malignant Lymphoma in Saitama

Ninety-seven percent of the total 92 patients with non-Hodgkin's ML had clonal chromosome abnormalities at diagnosis or relapse (Table 8-2).

In pseudo- or near-diploid tumors, chromosomes 5, 7, 12, and 18 were most repeatedly found as a supernumerary chromosome (9% each of the total patients). The X chromosome was most frequently lost (11%).

The only translocations that recurred were t(8;14)(q24;q32) and t(14;18)(q32;q21). The paucity of t(14;18) in the Maseki et al. series (only 3%) was conspicuous when compared with its high frequency to those in the series from the western hemisphere.[1–6,15]

The long arm of chromosome 6 was deleted most frequently (22%). Partial deletion of the long arm of chromosome 6 is one of the commonest structural abnormalities in ML, whether B- or T-cell.[1,6,9–12]

Correlation of Karyotype with Histology

Trisomy 5 was significantly associated with DM lymphoma (Table 8-3). In one other patient, a clone with trisomy 5 was found in the tumor after relapse when the histology had transformed from DM to IBL. Trisomy 5 may be correlated with both DM and IBL

TABLE 8-2

A Summary of Chromosomal Findings in 92 Patients with Malignant Lymphoma from Saitama[14]

	No. of cases
No abnormality	3
Numerical abnormalities only	3
Structural abnormalities only	10
Numerical and structural abnormalities	76
Numerical abnormalities (in pseudo- or near-diploid tumors only)	
Trisomy 5	8
Trisomy 7	8
Trisomy 12	8
Trisomy 18	8
Monosomy X	10
Structural abnormalities (146 bands were involved in 40 types of translocations, 4 types of inversions, and 62 types of deletions)	
t(8;14)(q24;q32)	5
t(14;18)(q32;q21)	3
14q32 translocations	24
Deletion 6q	20

TABLE 8-3

Correlation of Numerical Chromosome Abnormality with Histology in 64 Untreated Malignant Lymphomas in Saitama[*,14]

Numerical chromosome abnormality	Working Formulation[†]									
	B-D (7)	E (2)	F (11)	G (20)	H (14)	I (3)	J (5)	Misc (64)	Total (64)	P value
+5	1		3		1				5	0.03
−8				5	1			1	7	0.03
−13				3					3	0.03
+18				2	4				6	0.02
+X			1		3				4	0.03

[*] Pseudo- or near-diploid tumors only. Numbers in parentheses indicate total numbers of cases.
[†] For explanation of each group, see footnote for Table 8-1.

TABLE 8-4

Correlation of Structural Chromosome Abnormality with Histology in 71 Untreated Malignant Lymphomas in Saitama[14]

Structural chromosome abnormality	Working Formulation[*]									
	B-D (8)	E (2)	F (12)	G (24)	H (15)	I (3)	J (5)	Misc (2)	Total (71)	P value
8q24 translocations				3	1		3		7[†]	<0.01
t(14;18)(q32;q21)	2							1[††]	3	0.03
Break at 3q21	1			4					5	0.04
7q rearrangements		1	1	6					8	0.02
13q rearrangements				1	3				4	0.03

Numbers in parentheses indicate total numbers of cases.
[*] For explanation of each group, see footnote for Table 1.
[†] Includes 4 patients with t(8;14)(q24;q32), one with t(2;8)(p11;q24), and 2 with other 8q24 translocations.
[††] Composite lymphoma with follicular and diffuse areas.

lymphomas.[3,19] Significant associations were also observed between trisomy 18 or trisomy X, and IBL lymphoma, with loss of a chromosome 8 or a chromosome 13 and DL lymphoma.

Besides the already established associations between specific abnormalities and certain histologic categories, such as 8q24 and SNC lymphoma, and t(14;18)(q32;q21) and follicular lymphomas,[1,2,4,5] correlations were found between some other structural abnormalities and certain histologic categories (Table 8-4). Thus, a break in 3q21 was significantly associated with DL lymphoma. Also, a break in 7q was associated with DL, and a break in 13q with IBL lymphoma.

Correlation of Karyotype with Immunological Phenotypes

Seventy-one percent (10 of 14) of lymphomas with multiple clones and interpretable immunologic examinations were T-cell, and unrelated multiple clones were seen only in T lymphomas (Table 8-5). Thus, the occurrence of unrelated clones was significantly correlated with the T-cell phenotype. Similar findings have been reported by others.[10] Thus, the occurrence of multiple clones, especially unrelated ones, is an important characteristic of T-cell lymphoma.

Although various numerical abnormalities were present in pseudo- or near-diploid tu-

TABLE 8-5
Correlation of Recurrent Chromosome Abnormalities with the Immunophenotype in Malignant Lymphomas in Saitama[14]

Chromosome abnormality	Immunophenotype B (n = 34)	Immunophenotype T (n = 25)	Total	P value
Multiple clones	4	10	14	0.01
−Y	6	0	6*	0.02
4q rearrangements	0	4	4	0.03
7q rearrangements	2	7	9	0.02
15q rearrangements	0	4	4	0.03
Break at 6p21	0	4	4	0.03

* Of 22 B and 17 T lymphomas among 39 male patients with a modal chromosome number in the diploid range.

mors, only the correlation of loss of a Y chromosome with B-cell phenotype in male patients was statistically significant. Structural abnormalities in some chromosome arms, i.e. 4q rearrangements, 7q rearrangements, and 15q rearrangements, were each associated with the T-cell phenotype. The breakpoints tend to cluster in chromosome bands 4q27-q33, 7q32, and 15q24. The association of 7q rearrangements with malignant T-cell diseases has been emphasized.[20] T-cell lymphoma/leukemia cases with rearrangements of 4q and 15q have also been reported.[1,5,6,9,11,19,21]

All lymphomas with a break in 6p21 were of the T-cell phenotype. Association of breaks in 6p and T-cell lymphoma has been reported by Mecucci et al.[22] and by Maseki et al.,[23] whose most recent data confirmed the correlation, and specified the breakpoint in 6p21. Band 6p21 contains the major histocompatibility complex gene cluster and the putative oncogene *pim*.

The Paucity of t(14;18) in Malignant Lymphoma in Japan

The geographical difference in the frequency of t(14;18) is also an important finding in our study (Table 8-6). Maseki et al. compared the frequencies of two common translocations, t(8;14) (q24;q32) and t(14;18) (q32;q21), between patients whose lymph nodes or tumor tissue were studied before therapy in their series[14] and those in the series reported from the University of Minnesota.[1,2,3,4,6] The frequencies of t(8;14) (q24;q32) were similar in both the Saitama and Minnesota series. Lymphomas having t(14;18)(q32;q21), however, were much less frequently observed in Saitama than in Minnesota. Similar findings were obtained in the Fifth International Workshop on Chromosomes in Leukemia-Lymphoma (5th IWCL).[24] These findings obtained by the chromosome studies are consistent with the pathologic data showing the less frequent occurrence of follicular lymphoma in Japan than in the U.S. or Europe,[15] and suggest that factors affecting the lymphomagenesis may be different, or operating in different intensities in different areas.

TABLE 8-6
Incidences of 8q24 Translocation and t(14;18) in Japan and the United States[14]

	Saitama	Minnesota*	P value
Total number	71	142	
t(8;14)(q24;q32)	4	10	NS
t(14;18)(q32;q21)	3	39	<0.01

* Data in five reports[1,2,3,4,6] were combined.

SUMMARY AND CONCLUSION

Maseki et al. demonstrated the correlation of specific chromosome abnormalities with histologic and immunologic phenotypes of non-Hodgkin's ML in Saitama, an area nonendemic for ATL in Japan, and clarified that one of the common translocations, t(14;18), may not occur in Japan as frequently as in the United States. They also found association of several chromosome abnormalities with certain histologic and immunologic phenotypes of ML. The roles of some chromosome translocations in the lymphomagenesis have been recognized by molecular approaches.[7] However, little is known about how most of the chromosome abnormalities described in this report act in the genetic steps toward the development of lymphoma. Epidemiologic and molecular approaches will clarify the enigmas presented by their observations.

REFERENCES

1. Yunis JJ, Oken MM, Kaplan ME, et al: Distinctive chromosomal abnormalities in histologic subtypes of non-Hodgkin's lymphoma. N Engl J Med 307:1231–1236, 1982
2. Bloomfield CD, Arthur DC, Frizzera G, et al: Nonrandom chromosome abnormalities in lymphoma. Cancer 43:2975–2984, 1983
3. Yunis JJ, Oken MM, Theologides A, et al: Recurrent chromosomal defects are found in most patients with non-Hodgkin's-lymphoma. Cancer Genet Cytogenet 13:17–28, 1984
4. Levine EG, Arthur DC, Frizzera G, et al: There are differences in cytogenetic abnormalities among histologic subtypes of the non-Hodgkin's lymphomas. Blood 66:1414–1422, 1985
5. Koduru PRK, Filippa DA, Richardson ME, et al: Cytogenetic and histologic correlations in malignant lymphoma. Blood 69:97–102, 1987
6. Levine EG, Arthur DC, Gajl-Peczalska KJ, et al: Correlations between immunologic phenotype and karyotype in malignant lymphoma. Cancer Res 46:6481–6488, 1986
7. Croce CM: Role of chromosome translocations in human neoplasia. Cell 49:155–156, 1987
8. Fukuhara S, Hinuma Y, Gotoh Y, Uchino H: Chromosome aberrations in T lymphocytes carrying adult T-cell leukemia-associated antigens (ATLA) from healthy adults. Blood 61:205–207, 1983
9. Miyamoto K, Tomita N, Ishii A, et al: Chromosome abnormalities of leukemia cells in adult patients with T-cell leukemia. J Natl Cancer Inst 73:353–362, 1984
10. Sanada I, Tanaka R, Kumagai E, et al: Chromosomal aberrations in adult T cell leukemia: Relationship to the clinical severity. Blood 65:649–654, 1985
11. Fujita K, Fukuhara S, Nasu K, et al: Recurrent chromosome abnormalities in adult T-cell lymphomas of peripheral T-cell origin. Int J Cancer 37:517–524, 1986
12. Sadamori N, Nishino K, Kusano M, et al: Significance of chromosome 14 anomaly at band 14q11 in Japanese patients with adult T-cell leukemia. Cancer 58:2244–2250, 1986
13. Kaneko Y, Abe R, Sampi K, Sakurai M: An analysis of chromosome findings in non-Hodgkin's lymphomas. Cancer Genet Cytogenet 5:107–121, 1982
14. Maseki N, Kaneko Y, Sakurai M, et al: Chromosome abnormalities in malignant lymphoma in patients from Saitama. Cancer Res 47:6767–6775, 1987.
15. Kristoffersson U, Heim S, Olsson H, et al: Relationship between cytogenetic findings and histopathology in non-Hodgkin lymphoma. Acta Pathol Microbiol Immunol Scand 95:1–5, 1987
16. Kadin ME, Berard CW, Nanba K, Wakasa H; Lymphoproliferative diseases in Japan and western countries: Proceedings of the United States-Japan Seminar, September 6 and 7, 1982, in Seattle, Washington. Hum Pathol 14:745–772, 1983
17. The Non-Hodgkin's Lymphoma Pathologic Classification Project. National Cancer Institute sponsored study of classifications of non-Hodgkin's lymphomas. Summary and description of a working formulation for clinical usage. Cancer 49:2112–2135, 1982
18. Suchi T, Tajima K, Nanba K, et al: Some problems on the histopathological diagnosis of non-Hodgkin's malignant lymphoma. A proposal of a new type. Acta Pathol Jpn 29:755–776, 1979
19. Kaneko Y, Larson RA, Variakojis D, et al: Nonrandom chromosome abnormalities in angioimmunoblastic lymphadenopathy. Blood 60:877–887, 1982
20. Kaneko Y, Rowley JD, Variakojis D, et al: Prognostic implications of karyotype and morphology in patients with non-Hodgkin's lymphoma. Int J Cancer 32:683–692, 1983
21. Hecht F, Morgan R, Kaiser-McCaw Hecht B, Smith SD: Common region on chromosome 14 in T-cell leukemia and lymphoma. Science 226:1445–1447, 1984
22. Mecucci C, Michaux JL, Tricot G, et al: Rearrangements of the short arm of chromosome No. 6 in T-cell lymphomas. Leukemia Res 9:1139–1148, 1985
23. Maseki N, Kaneko Y, Sakurai M: Interstitial deletion of the short arm of chromosome 6 as a new cytogenetic marker of T-cell lymphoma. Jpn J Cancer Res (Gann) 77:334–337, 1986
24. Fifth International Workshop on Chromosomes in Leukemia-Lymphoma. Correlation of chromosome abnormalities with histologic and immunologic characteristics in non-Hodgkin's lymphoma and adult T cell leukemia-lymphoma. Blood 70:1554–1564, 1987

9

Flow Cytometry in the Diagnosis and Classification of Non-Hodgkin's Lymphoma

Raul C. Braylan

Abstract

Highly informative but inherently subjective morphologic observations of individual cells can now be complemented by the rapid and quantitative analysis performed by flow cytometry. Although tissue architecture cannot be preserved, the relative ease with which single cell suspensions can be obtained from lymphoma tissues and the availability of large number of suitable biological probes, makes flow cytometry an important tool in the study of these neoplasms.

The diagnosis and classification of lymphomas, currently based on microscopic observations, can be greatly aided by more quantitative analytical methodologies. Non-Hodgkin's lymphomas are extremely variable tumors, both clinically and in their histologic and cytologic expressions. Numerous attempts have been made over the years to classify these tumors into morphologically homogeneous groups, so that meaningful clinical and biologic correlations could be established. However, despite the advances that have taken place recently in this regard, difficulties still remain. Many cellular and tissue changes are difficult to quantify and interpret reproducibly, and important structural and functional cellular components cannot be visualized by conventional microscopy.

Modern techniques are now complementing morphologic observations. Monoclonal antibodies and immunohistology are providing relevant biological information and will very likely become indispensable tools in the diagnosis and classification of lymphomas.[1] The flow cytometer is adding a new dimension. This instrument has the capacity to quantify simultaneously multiple elements in individual cells rapidly and accurately. Many biological and clinical relevant cellular parameters such as size, surface, cytoplasmic and nuclear antigens, DNA and RNA content, and proliferative capacity can be easily measured by flow cytometry. This capability may be applied advantageously to the characterization of lymphoid neoplasia.

THE FLOW CYTOMETER

The flow cytometer may be regarded as a complex microscope with the capacity of examining very rapidly, single cells flowing in a liquid medium. Cells stained with fluorescent labels that bind specifically to relevant cellular components flow at high speed in single file formation through an intense light. As they are illuminated, the cells emit scattered and fluorescent light signals. These optical signals are converted into electrical signals that are amplified and then digitized. They are further processed, stored, and expressed graphically by a computer. Some instruments are also capable of measuring electronic cell volume. The various parameters measured from each cell (i.e., one or more fluorescence signals, forward light scatter, right angle light scatter, electronic volume) can be analyzed independently or in a correlated manner. Results are expressed as histograms showing in relative units the distribution of the element(s) being studied.

FLOW CYTOMETRIC MEASUREMENTS

Lymphoid tissues are ideal for flow cytometric analysis since they can be relatively easily dispersed into single cell suspensions by simple mechanical force. Although a variety of measurements can be made on these tissues, in practice, the most common parameters analyzed are light scattering, immunofluorescence, and nucleic acid content.

Light Scattering

The intensity of the light scattered by a cell as it is illuminated by a light beam depends on certain physical properties of the cells such as size or granular content.[2] Cell size influences the light scattered in a forward direction along the axis of the light beam (forward light scatter). Thus, cells of different sizes can be easily recognized by forward light scatter analysis. Also, this measurement permits the recognition (and elimination from the analysis) of non-viable cells that emit low forward scatter signals,[3] and cell debris.

Immunofluorescence

Analysis of cell surface antigens by immunofluorescence is the most common application of flow cytometry. This analysis has been facilitated by the availability of monoclonal antibodies against a variety of differentiation-related and functionally important molecules. Flow cytometric measurement of immunofluorescence is unique in that it provides quantitative information on the fluorescence intensity emitted by each cell. This information is not only useful in determining the fraction of labeled cells, but it also allows the analysis of antigen distribution both in homogeneous as well as in heterogeneous cell populations. Another distinctive feature of flow cytometry is that two or more antibodies can be used simultaneously to label different antigens on individual cells. This is accomplished by using either a single light source and two or more fluorochromes that emit fluorescence at separable wavelengths, or two light sources with different excitation wavelengths (e.g., two lasers).

Nucleic Acid Content

The use of fluorescent dyes that bind specifically and stoichiometrically to nucleic acids provides a simple means of measuring content of DNA and RNA in an individual cell. A variety of fluorochromes can be used to measure DNA. Intercalating fluorochromes, such as ethidium bromide or its derivative, propidium iodide, are commonly used. Propidium iodide is a popular dye that can be efficiently excited with argon ion lasers used in most commercial instruments. Specific DNA bind-

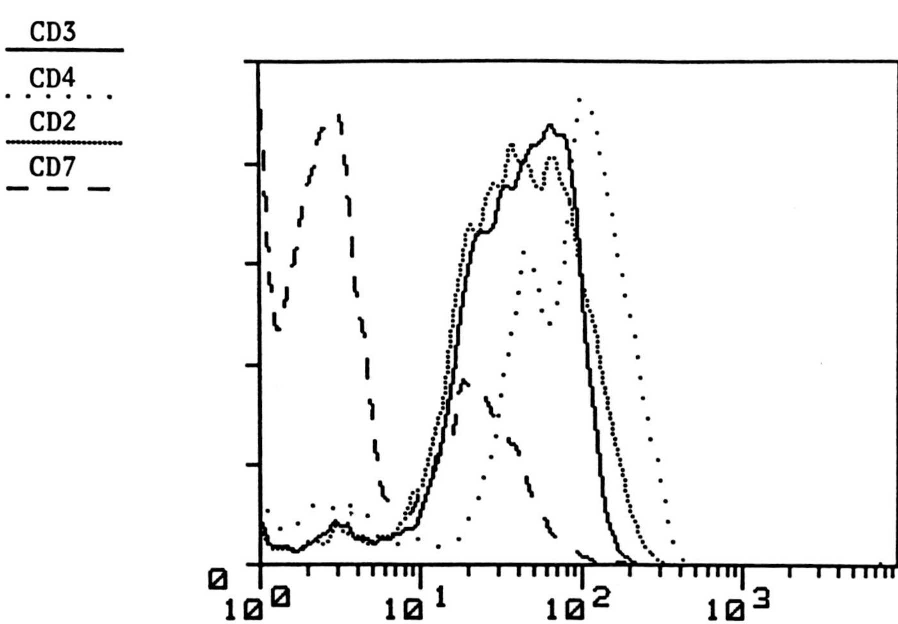

Fig. 9-1. Immunofluorescence analysis of cells obtained from a lymph node with adult T-cell lymphoma and exposed to several antibodies against T-cell antigens. The horizontal axis indicates relative fluorescence intensity. The vertical axis corresponds to the number of cells analyzed. Curves were normalized to facilitate comparisons. Negative (control) cells fall below channel 10. CD7 antigen is only expressed in a fraction of the cells (probably residual normal T-cells). CD4 is present in almost all cells but the distribution of fluorescence is abnormal (bimodal). The other antigens (CD2 and CD3) show normal distributions.

ing dyes such as 4,6-diamidino-phenylindole dihydrochloride (DAPI) can be excited by ultra-violet light and are useful with instruments equipped with mercury arc lamps as light source. DNA measurements are frequently performed because they allow the detection of cells with quantitative chromosomal abnormalities, and the calculation of the fraction of cells in the various phases of the cell cycle. DNA can be simultaneously measured in conjunction with other cellular elements. For example, acridine orange is used to analyze simultaneously DNA and RNA;[4] DNA and surface antigens can also be measured simultaneously by means of fluorescein labeled antibodies and propidium iodide.[5]

APPLICATIONS OF FLOW CYTOMETRIC ANALYSIS

Surface Antigen Expression

Surface antigen analysis has been widely applied to the diagnosis and classification of hemopoietic malignancies. The study of these antigens is usually performed on tissue sections where one can simultaneously observe antibody binding areas, and tissue and cell morphology. Immunohistology, however, does not permit a precise measurement of surface antigens. By quantifying antibody binding on single cells, flow cytometry provides additional valuable information. This information facilitates the detection and enumeration of cells with quantitative abnormalities in surface antigen expression, a phenomenon frequently observed among neoplastic lymphoid cells. For example, it has been observed that different types of B-cell lymphomas express varying amounts of surface associated antigens.[6] The level of expression of CD5 (an antigen normally expressed on T-cells) in chronic lymphocytic leukemia or small lymphocytic lymphomas is lower than the level exhibited by normal T-cells.[7] Figure 9-1 illustrates another example of a quantitative abnormality of surface antigen expression in a case of adult T-cell leukemia/lymphoma.

Normally, the distribution of CD4-bearing lymphocytes is unimodal. In this example, the neoplastic T lymphocytes express more CD4 antigens than those of normal T-cells that are also present in the sample resulting in a bimodal distribution. Also CD7, an antigen present on normal T-cells is absent in the majority of leukemic cells. This aberrant expression of T-cell-related antigens is highly suggestive of a T-cell neoplasia.[1]

Simultaneous analysis of two antibodies is helpful in the recognition of neoplastic cells that co-express antigens in an abnormal fashion. As mentioned above, most chronic lymphocytic leukemia (or small lymphocytic lymphoma) cells bear B-cell associated antigens and simultaneously express CD5.[7,8] Another example is hairy cell leukemia cells, which co-express B-cell and some monocyte associated antigens.[9] Lymphoblastic lymphoma cells often co-express CD4 and CD8 or early T-cell antigens,[1] a phenotype not seen in normal lymph nodes or blood. Multi-antigen analysis is also useful in the detection of neoplastic cells that fail to show antigens that are normally co-expressed. For example, discrepancies between the expression of mature B-cell antigens and surface immunoglobulin, is highly suggestive of a B-cell neoplasia.[1,10] Similarly, discrepancies between expression of surface immunoglobulin heavy and light chains may be seen in neoplastic B-cell populations.

Correlated multi-color analysis of different antigens on individual cells increases the sensitivity of detection of lymphoma cells. This is particularly applicable to B-cell lymphoproliferative disorders that are characterized by the expansion of B-cells bearing a single immunoglobulin light chain. The presence of these neoplastic cells alters the normal kappa to lambda ratio in lymphoid tissues,[11] blood,[12] or bone marrow.[13] The simultaneous use of pan-B and anti-immunoglobulin light chain antibodies allows enumerating light chain-bearing cells within the B-cell compartment only, thus eliminating large numbers of irrelevant cells from the analysis. In our hands, this technique permits the detection of less than 5% circulating lymphoma cells in peripheral blood. It has recently been shown that this approach detects neoplastic cells at a level below 3% in the bone marrow.[13]

Abnormal DNA Content (Aneuploidy)

Total cellular DNA content can be easily and rapidly measured by flow cytometry. The abnormal gain or loss of chromosomes frequently observed in tumors results in quantitative abnormalities of DNA content, which can often be detected by flow cytometry.[14] These abnormalities have been designated as "flow aneuploidy." Although aneuploidy has been reported in lymphoid hyperplasia in patients with acquired immune deficiency syndrome,[15] in practice, this abnormality is not observed in reactive processes and its presence is highly suggestive of neoplastic transformation. Ploidy changes have been associated with prognosis in many neoplasms. In lymphomas, aneuploidy is more frequent and more pronounced in intermediate and high-grade lymphomas than in low-grade lymphomas.[16–18] With few exceptions,[19,20] the prognostic impact of aneuploidy within uniform groups of non-Hodgkin's lymphomas has not been determined.

Cell Cycle Fractions

As cells traverse the cell cycle they increase their DNA content. Thus, the fraction of cells in the various phases of the cell cycle can be determine by simply measuring DNA content in individual cells. Flow cytometry has facilitated this analysis since the measurements are precise and are made on a large number of cells in a relatively short time.[21] Although immunological and genetic changes in lymphomas have been the focus of intense study, growth kinetics, which are directly responsible for many of the clinical manifestations of these tumors, have received little attention. Numerous studies utilizing tritiated thymidine uptake,[22,23] DNA quantitation by flow cytometry[4,16–18,24–29] and, more recently, immunohistology with an antibody (Ki67) against a cell cycle dependent nuclear protein,[30] repeatedly and consistently demon-

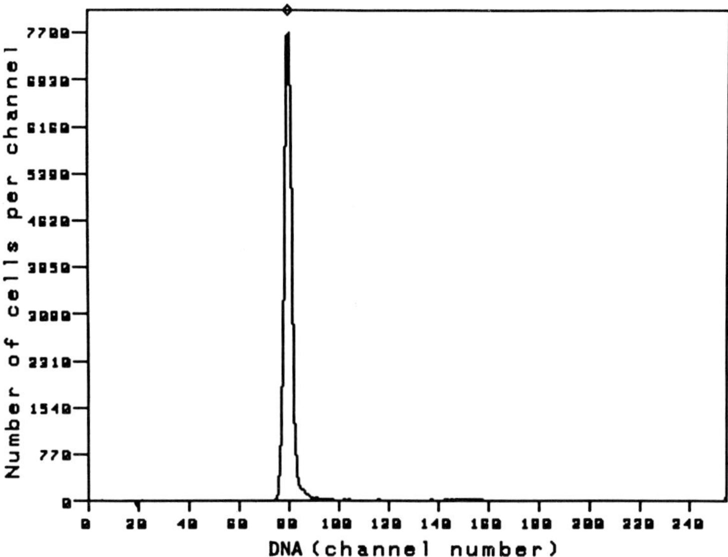

Fig. 9-2. Typical DNA content distribution of a low-grade lymphoma (small cleaved cell type). The horizontal axis indicates fluorescence intensity from DNA stained cells (propidium iodide/ribonuclease). The large peak is unimodal and corresponds to diploid cells in G1. The area to the right of G1 (cells in DNA synthesis (S), G2 and mitosis) contains very few cells.

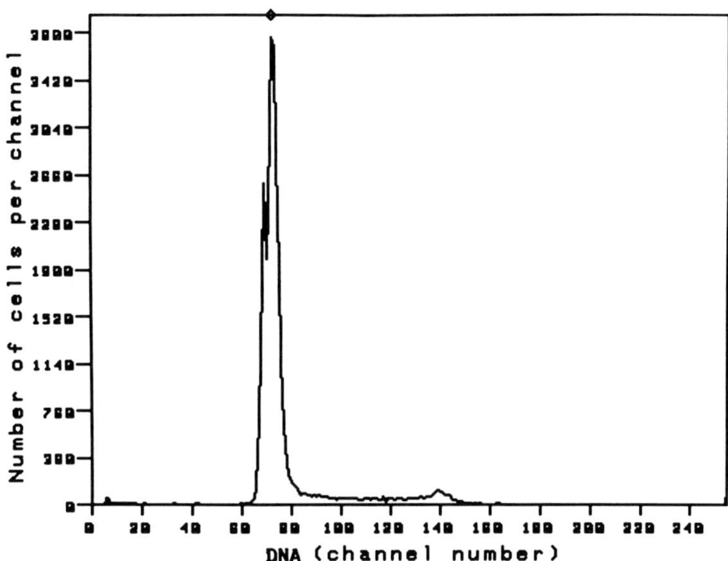

Fig. 9-3. Typical DNA content distribution of a diffuse large cell lymphoma (B-cell type). In contrast to the case in Fig. 9-2, the G1 peak is bimodal due to the presence of diploid normal cells and neoplastic hyperdiploid cells. S, G2 and mitotic cells (to the right of the G1 peaks) are relatively abundant.

strated a correlation between the proliferative fraction and histologic grade of non-Hodgkin's lymphomas. Thus, low-grade lymphomas contain fewer number of cycling cells than intermediate and high grade lymphomas (Figs. 9-2 and 9-3). These findings confirm previous in vivo (Review in 23) and in vitro[31] observations demonstrating a correlation between fraction of cells in DNA synthesis and tumor doubling time. Not surprisingly, patient survival studies also suggested a correlation with proliferative fraction.[4,17,19,32–34] Interestingly, the proliferative fraction may have prognostic value within histologically uniform lymphomas. In a series of patients with diffuse large cell lymphomas treated in a similar manner, a recent study using nuclei extracted from paraffin-embedded histologic material showed a better survival for patients whose tumors contained a low number of cycling cells.[19] Obviously, these observations need to be confirmed in controlled prospective clinical trials. It is important to emphasize that the marked heterogeneity of diffuse large cell lymphomas observed both morphologically and clinically, is also noted by flow cytometry. Analysis of cell size,[23,24] surface antigen expression,[35–37] RNA,[4] ploidy, and cell cycle fractions[16] have shown marked variability in these tumors. For cell cycle fractions, this variability is observed even when normal cells in the samples are excluded from the analysis.[16] Accurate measurements of these parameters may provide the means to classify this heterogeneous group of lymphomas in a reproducible manner, a task that unfortunately has not been possible by conventional microscopy.

MORPHOLOGIC CORRELATIONS

In comparison to histology, flow cytometric analysis offers unique advantages, but suffers from some significant limitations.This analysis requires the tissues to be dissociated into monodispersed cell suspensions, which destroys tissue architecture. Potentially, selective cell loss may occur. Furthermore, a direct observation of the morphology of cells being

TABLE 9-1
Flow Cytometric Analysis of Lymph Nodes

Histologic diagnosis	Immunologic phenotype	Ploidy	S-phase	Predominant cell size
Non-neoplastic	Polyclonal	Normal	Low or intermediate	Small
Hodgkin's	Polyclonal CD_4 predominates in many cases	Usually normal Occasionally aneuploid	Low	Small
Small lymphocytic lymphoma	Monoclonal B-cell (faint SIg fluoresc.) CD5 (+)	Usually normal	Low	Small
Follicular lymphoma	Monoclonal B-cell (intense SIg fluoresc.) Often CD10 (+)	Usually normal or near diploid. Occasionally tetraploid	Low	Variable
Diffuse mixed cell lymphoma	Variable*	Usually aneuploid	Intermediate	Small & large
Diffuse large cell lymphoma	Variable*	Usually aneuploid	Intermediate	Large
Lymphoblastic lymphoma	Early T-cell	Normal or aneuploid	High	Intermediate
Small non-cleaved lymphoma	Monoclonal B-cell CD10 (+)	Frequently aneuploid	Very high	Intermediate
Cutaneous T-cell lymphoma	Mature T-cell	Frequently aneuploid	Variable	Variable

*Some of these tumors display mature T-cell phenotypes and often lack one or more pan T-cell antigens. They are designated as "peripheral T-cell lymphomas."

analyzed is very difficult. However, the combined analysis of cell size, surface antigens, and DNA content by flow cytometry provides in most instances sufficient information to diagnose and classify non-Hodgkin's lymphomas into the major histologic categories. Table 9-1 illustrates typical flow cytometric observations in the various types of lymphoid tumors. This scheme is by no means perfect but serves as the basis for future developments. With growing availability of probes for biologically relevant cell constituents the applications of flow cytometry will undoubtedly increase. Speed, sensitivity, precision, automation, and the capacity for data storage and transmission make this technique a unique and powerful analytical tool, which is expected to play an important role in the diagnosis and classification of lymphomas.

REFERENCES

1. Picker LJ, Weiss LM, Medeiros LJ, et al: Immunophenotypic criteria for the diagnosis of non-Hodgkin's lymphoma. Am J Pathol 128:181–201, 1987
2. Salzman GC, Crowell JM, Martin JC, et al: Cell classification of laser light scattering: Identification and separation of unstained leukocytes. Acta Cytol 19:374–377, 1975
3. Loken MR, Herzenberg LA: Analysis of cell populations with a fluorescence activated cell sorter. Ann NY Acad Sci 254:163–171, 1975
4. Andreeff M, Hansen H, Cirrincione C, et al: Prognostic value of DNA/RNA flow cytometry of B-cell non-Hodgkin's lymphoma: Development of laboratory model and correlation with four taxonomic systems. Annls NY Acad Scien 468:368–386, 1986
5. Braylan RC, Benson NA, Nourse VA, Kruth HS: Correlated analysis of cellular DNA, membrane and light scatter of human lymphoid cells. Cytometry 2:337–343, 1982
6. Cossman J, Neckers LM, Hsu S, et al: Low-grade lymphomas. Expression of developmentally regulated B-cell antigens. Am J Pathol 115:117–124, 1984
7. Wormsley SB, Collins ML, Royston I: Comparative density of the human T-cell antigen of T65 on normal peripheral blood T-cells and chronic lymphocytic leukemia cells. Blood 57:657–662, 1981
8. Spier CM, Grogan TM, Fielder K, et al: Immunophenotypes in "well-differentiated" lymphoproliferative disorders with emphasis on small lymphocytic lymphoma. Hum Pathol 17:1126–1136, 1986
9. Kristensen JS, Ellegaard J, Hokland P: A two-color flow cytometry assay for detection of hairy cells using monoclonal antibodies. Blood 70:1063–1068, 1987
10. Gregg EO, Al-Saffar N, Jones DB, et al: Immunoglobulin negative follicle center cell lymphoma. Br J Cancer 50:735–744, 1984
11. Weinberg DS, Pinkus GS, Ault KA: Cytofluorometric detection of B cell clonal excess: A new approach to the diagnosis of B cell lymphomas. Blood 63:1080–1087, 1984
12. Ault KA: Detection of small numbers of monoclonal B lymphocytes in the blood of patients with lymphoma. N Engl J Med 300:1401–1405, 1979
13. Leemhuis T, Srour E, Hanks S, et al: Detection of infiltration of bone marrow by B-cell lymphoma using two-color fluorescence clonal-excess analysis. Blood 70:217a, 1987
14. Barlogie B, Rabar MN, Schumann J, Flow cytometry in clinical cancer research. Cancer Res 43:3982–3997, 1983
15. Srigley J, Butler JJ, Osborne BM, et al: Nucleic acid cytometry of homosexual-associated lymphoproliferative disease. Am J Pathol 123:563–569, 1986
16. Braylan RC, Benson NA, Nourse VA: Cellular DNA of human neoplastic B-cells measured by flow cytometry. Cancer Res 44:5010–5016, 1984
17. Christensson B, Tribukait B, Linder I, et al: Cell proliferation and DNA content in non-Hodgkin's lymphoma: Flow cytometry in relation to lymphoma classification. Cancer 58:1295–1304, 1986
18. Diamond LW, Nathwani BN, Rappaport H: Flow cytometry in the diagnosis and classification of malignant lymphoma and leukemia. Cancer 50:1122–1135, 1982
19. Bauer KD, Merkel DE, Winter JN, et al: Prognostic implications of ploidy and proliferative activity in diffuse large cell lymphomas. Cancer Res 46:3173–3178, 1986
20. Bunn PA, Jr, Whang-Peng J, Carney DN, et al: DNA content analysis by flow cytometry and cytogenetic analysis in mycosis fungoides and Sézary syndrome. J Clin Invest 65:1440–1448, 1980
21. Crissman HA, Tobey RA: Cell-cycle analysis in 20 minutes. Science 184:1297–1298, 1974
22. Meyer JS, Higa E: S-phase fractions of cells in lymph nodes and malignant lymphomas. Arch Pathol Lab Med 103:93–97, 1979
23. Hansen H, Koziner B, Clarkson B: Marker and kinetic studies in the non-Hodgkin's lymphomas. Am J Med 71:107–123, 1981
24. Braylan RC, Fowlkes BJ, Jaffe ES, et al: Cell volumes and DNA distributions of normal and neoplastic human lymphoid cells. Cancer 41:201–209, 1978
25. Costa A, Mazzini G, Del Bino G, Silverstrini R: DNA content and kinetic characteristics of non-Hodgkin's lymphoma. Cytometry 2:185–188, 1981
26. Juneja SK, Cooper IA, Hodgson GS, et al: DNA ploidy patterns and cytokinetics of non-Hodgkin's lymphoma. J Clin pathol 39:987–992, 1986
27. Scarffe JH, Crowther D: The pre-treatment proliferative activity of non-Hodgkin's lymphoma cells. Cancer 17:99–108, 1981
28. Shackney SE, Levine AM, Fisher RI, et al: The biology of tumor growth in the non-Hodgkin's lymphomas. J Clin Invest 73:1201–1214, 1984

29. Srigley J, Barlogie B, Butler JJ, et al: Heterogeneity of non-Hodgkin's lymphoma probed by nucleic acid cytometry. Blood 65:1090–1096, 1985
30. Gerdes L, Dallenbach F, Lennert K, et al: Growth fractions in malignant non-Hodgkin's lymphomas (NHL) as determined in situ with the monoclonal antibody Ki67. Hematol Oncol 2:365–369, 1984
31. Lang S, Diehl V: Proliferation kinetics of malignant non-Hodgkin's lymphomas related to histopathology of lymph node biopsies. Virch Archiv A Path Anat and Histol 389:397–407, 1980
32. Braylan RC, Diamond LW, Powell ML, Harty-Golder B: Percentage of cells in the S-phase of the cell cycle in human lymphoma determined by flow cytometry. Cytometry 1:171–174, 180
33. Costa A, Bonadonna G, Villa E, et al: Labeling index as a prognostic marker in non-Hodgkin's lymphomas. J Natl Cancer Inst 66:1–5, 1981
34. Roos G, Dige U, Lenner Per, et al: Prognostic significance of DNA-analysis by flow cytometry in non-Hodgkin's lymphoma. Hematological Oncology 3:233–241, 1985
35. Cossman J, Jaffe ES, Fisher RI: Immunologic phenotypes of diffuse, aggressive, non-Hodgkin's lymphomas. Cancer 54:1310–1317, 1984
36. Doggett RS, Wood GS, Horning S, et al: The immunologic characterization of 95 nodal and extranodal diffuse large cell lymphomas in 89 patients. Am J Pathol 115:245–252, 1984
37. Freedman AS, Boyd AW, Anderson KC, et al: Immunologic heterogeneity of diffuse large cell lymphoma. Blood 65:630–637, 1985

10

The PATHFINDER Project: Computer-Aided Diagnosis of Lymph Node Diseases

Bharat N. Nathwani
David Heckerman
Eric Horvitz
Lawrence Fagan

Abstract

In the PATHFINDER research project, the authors are attempting to construct a useful computerized diagnostic system for hematopathology. This research addresses fundamental problems of knowledge representation, reasoning strategies, user modeling, explanation of diagnostic strategies, and user acceptance. We have built a prototype expert system, called PATHFINDER, which arrived at diagnoses on 50 malignant and 30 benign diseases of the lymph nodes on the basis of approximately 500 different histopathologic findings. The program uses the method of sequential diagnosis; it can generate a differential diagnosis on the basis of a small number of findings and then recommend additional features that are useful for narrowing of the differential diagnosis in subsequent steps. It also provides explanations for its recommendations. A highlight of our research is the involvement of four hematopathology experts (Drs. Berard, Burke, Dorfman, and Nathwani) in the construction of the knowledge base for the PATHFINDER system.

These experts plan to develop PATHFINDER further so that it not only can become a regularly used diagnostic tool for pathologists who have different levels of training and experience, but so that it can also serve as a powerful teaching system. This expert system will provide a unique integrated knowledge base for diseases of lymph nodes, giving the practicing pathologist immediate access to accurate morphologic classification and diagnostic criteria, while at the same time providing guidance as to whether additional tests (immunologic, cytogenetic, cell-kinetic, and immunogenetic) are likely to be informative. The authors will monitor their progress through iterative testing of the reasoning strategies and the knowledge.

The PATHFINDER project is devoted to the development of a computer-based expert system that will assist pathologists to make accurate diagnoses of diseases of lymph nodes. This project was begun in September 1983. This expert system for lymph node pathology is designed to address fundamental problems of knowledge representation, reasoning strategies, user modeling, explanation of diagnostic strategies, and user acceptance. The successful application of such a system in hematopathology would be expected to have a beneficial impact on the development of computer-based medical decision aids for other areas of surgical pathology and for other medical specialties as well. The authors believe that a working system will be of considerable benefit in the field of lymph node pathology. We believe that a working system will improve the reproducibility and reliability of diagnoses of lymphoma. This, in turn, may facilitate the standardization of diagnoses in clinical trials, and it is expected to assist oncologists in the institution of appropriate therapy at community hospitals.

TABLE 10-1A
Diseases of Lymph Nodes

Name	Number
Benign Diseases	29
Hodgkin's Disease	12
Non-Hodgkin's Lymphoma	
Follicular	8
Diffuse	28
Metastatic Diseases	17
Total	94

TABLE 10-1B
Types of Features

Histologic
Laboratory
Clinical
Immunologic
Cytogenetic
Cell Kinetic
Gene Rearrangement

CURRENT STATUS OF THE PATHFINDER SYSTEM:

Overview of the Current System

The PATHFINDER system is the result of a 4-year concentrated effort to build a system that efficiently and accurately reasons about lymph node diseases.[1,2] The expert system is written in the computer language Portable Standard Lisp (PSL) and runs on the HP9836 Lisp computer.

At its current stage, the system reasons about 55 malignant and 29 benign diseases of lymph nodes, constructing plausible differential diagnoses by considering evidence about the status of approximately 160 morphologic features in lymph node tissue (Tables 10-1 and 10-2).

In PATHFINDER, each *feature* is modified (divided) into a set of 3–5 mutually exhaustive and exclusive lists of values. For example, the feature "pseudofollicularity" can take on any one of four values (modifiers): *absent, slight, moderate,* or *prominent.* A given feature is reported by the selection of a value that reflects the severity of the feature. A particular feature and its value are referred to as a *feature-value.*

PATHFINDER builds an initial differential diagnosis on the basis of the first set of feature-values input to the system. It then uses one of several hypothesis-directed evidence acquisition strategies in an attempt to narrow the list of diseases under consideration most efficiently into a single diagnosis. It does this by recommending features that are most useful for narrowing of the differential diagnosis.

Over the last year and a half, many facets of the PATHFINDER system have been developed and tested. In addition to doing fundamental work on refinement of the knowledge base and the development of reasoning strategies, the PATHFINDER team has developed and tested capabilities for explaining recom-

TABLE 10-2
Histopathologic Features Considered by the PATHFINDER System

Feature Category	Number of features in Category
Follicular	22
Architectural	11
Other Low Power	13
Inflammatory Components	28
S-R Cells and Variants	18
Large Lymphoid Cells	12
Medium Sized Lymphoid Cells	12
Small lymphoid Cells	12
Miscellaneous	6
Special Stains	28
Total	162

mendations, for user customization, for efficient knowledge base modification, and for system evaluation. The team has also tended carefully to issues related to the human interface, such as implementing of efficient entry techniques and providing help to users.

Consensus Knowledge Structure

A crucial step in the construction of the current system was obtaining a consensus among four experts about the optimal structure of the knowledge base, (i.e., the diseases, features, and feature-values that PATHFINDER should consider).

Computer Methods Used in the System:

Reasoning Methodology

Two symbolic reasoning approaches were considered in the initial stages of the design for PATHFINDER: the INTERNIST-1 hypothetico-deductive approach[3] and the MYCIN rule-based production system approach.[4] Early informal "process tracing"[5] involving discussions with experts and observation of expert diagnostic protocols suggested that the diagnosis of lymph node abnormalities often involves refinement of iterative hypothesis. The hypothesis-directed model of physician problem-solving that is explicit in INTERNIST-1 attracted attention as a potentially useful means of simulating diagnostic strategies in pathology. INTERNIST-1 is an expert system for internal medicine, which was initiated at the University of Pittsburgh 10 years ago.[3] It is the core of a continuing research program called QMR.[6]

PATHFINDER and INTERNIST-1 are based on the method of *sequential diagnosis*. With this approach, a set of salient disease manifestations (histologic features) is first presented to the program. A list of plausible disease hypotheses (a differential diagnosis) is then formulated (by the program) based on these features, and recommendations are made by the program (i.e., questions are selected) that are most likely to help the user narrow the number of diseases in the differential diagnosis. After the user answers these recommendations (questions), a new (revised) differential diagnosis (set of hypotheses) is formulated, and the process is repeated until a definitive diagnosis is reached.

The method of sequential diagnosis is hypothesis-directed in that the questions are selected according to strategies, or *modes,* that consider a current list of differential diagnoses. The method of sequential diagnosis is an advancement over older probability-based programs that require all relevant findings in a patient case at one time for arriving at a diagnosis. As there are often hundreds of possible clinical findings to be considered, the nonsequential approach has been regarded as less suitable for application in a clinical setting than are systems based on the method of sequential diagnosis.[7]

Reasoning Under Uncertainty

In most areas of medicine, the relationships between manifestations of diseases and the diseases themselves are rarely categorical. Usually, a given piece of evidence only provides partial support for or against a disease. This is especially true in the domain of lymph node pathology. The ability to represent and process such uncertainty accurately is crucial for the success of PATHFINDER. Most medical expert systems represent uncertainty by assigning to each disease hypothesis a numerical score based on the evidence entered into the program. Many different methods for the scoring of diseases have been used in such systems. We experimented with two popular methods: (1) the Dempster-Shafer theory of uncertainty and (2) probability theory. After gaining experience with both methods, and through careful theoretical considerations, we decided to concentrate on the probabilistic approach.

Probability theory provides the most highly developed method for reasoning under uncertainty. Unlike other schemes for managing uncertainty, it is based on widely accepted axioms. Expert systems in which probabilistic methods are used for inferential reasoning draw from a rich and consistent set of tools that have been developed over the last three centuries.

A central theorem of probability theory was first formulated by Bayes in the seventeenth century. Bayes' theorem is a simple equality derived from the definition of conditional probability. It defines how the probability assigned to a hypothesis should be updated in the light of new evidence.

Algorithms Used in the System

A central feature of sequential diagnosis systems is the ability to pose questions (i.e., make recommendations) that direct the user to collect useful information about additional histologic features. PATHFINDER's hypothesis-directed strategies for selecting questions that can minimize uncertainty in the differential diagnosis will now be described.

The present PATHFINDER system dynamically applies several different modes (strategies) for question selection, depending on the number and types of disease on the current differential diagnosis list. These methods are called *focus* mode, *entropy-discriminate mode, group-discriminate mode, pursual mode,* and *confirmation mode.* The authors will describe these modes, the heuristics used in the decision to apply them, and the motivation for their development.

Focus Mode

Focus mode considers all of the diseases included in the differential diagnosis. The mode selects questions about the status of those features that will tend to prune away completely those diseases remaining on the differential diagnosis list after values for these features are reported. The mode operates by calculating the number of diseases that are pruned from the differential diagnosis when the user reports a value for a particular feature. The mode then selects (recommends) those features that yield the largest number of diseases expected to be pruned.

Entropy-Discriminate Mode

In focus mode, the utility of a question (recommendation) is solely a function of the number of diseases removed from the differential diagnosis. The resulting change in the number of diseases included in the differential diagnosis reflects a change in the uncertainty of that diagnosis. *Entropy-discriminate mode* makes use of a more general notion of uncertainty that is used in information theory.[8] In this mode, a quantity called *entropy* is used as the measure of certainty. This mode selects questions that maximize the expected value of a measure of certainty what is reflected in the entire differential diagnosis.

Group-Discriminate Mode

Preliminary testing showed that the rationale for questions (recommendations) selected by the powerful entropy-discriminate mode was often not easily understood. Although these questions yielded information providing the best discrimination among the diseases in the differential diagnosis, the authors found that they were not natural questions (features) to be recommended for the problem-solving protocol followed by the human experts.

Thus, entropy-discriminate mode selects questions (features) that best discriminate among all diseases in a differential diagnosis. However, we found that experts reason about small numbers of diagnostic *categories*. For example, if there are benign and malignant diseases in a differential diagnosis, pathologists often deem most appropriate those questions that best discriminate between the benign and malignant groups, rather than questions that might best discriminate among all of the diseases. Alternatively, if there are only primary malignant and metastatic diseases in the differential diagnosis, the pathologist will attempt to discriminate between the primary malignancy and the metastatic categories. Therefore, questions are found (recommendations of features) that discriminate among various natural groupings of diseases on the differential diagnosis to be more readily understandable than is a question that could best discriminate among all of the diseases.

The diagnostic strategy, in which the group-discriminate mode is used, can be described most easily in terms of traversal of a strategic hierarchy of disease categories. This hierarchy is a binary tree of disease groups that can be used for grouping of the differential diagnoses at various levels of refinement. In several previous studies of medical problem-solving, similar decision trees have been identified in other medical domains.

The existence of such a categorical reasoning strategy led to the formulation of the *group-discriminate mode*. For a given differential diagnosis, the group-discriminate mode identifies the most specific grouping of diseases possible and then selects questions (features) that best discriminate among the diseases in a group.

Pursual Mode

The pursual mode was initially abandoned by us in favor of entropy-discriminate mode. The entropy discriminate mode, which considers the entire differential diagnosis, usually produced more acceptable questions than did the early implementation of pursual mode, which only considers the leading disease. However, after informal testing, they found that the entropy-discriminate mode was slow in the ''end game.'' That is, when the leading disease in the differential diagnosis was much more likely than any other disease in this diagnosis, entropy-discriminate mode often did not select the features that could most quickly establish the diagnosis.

With this problem in mind, the authors implemented a pursual mode that seeks to clinch the leading diagnosis. The mode is basically a hybrid made up of the group-discriminate mode and focus mode.

Confirmation Mode

In addition to designing the pursual mode, a confirmation mode was designed. This new mode is similar to the pursual mode in that questions are asked when a single disease is being considered as the diagnosis. Confirmation mode differs from pursual mode in that the questions are marked when (features) selected as being ''important'' to the disease under consideration. For example, the presence of Sternberg-Reed cells is an important feature of Hodgkin's disease. If a diagnosis of Hodgkin's disease is to be concluded by the program and if Sternberg-Reed cells have not been evaluated, PATHFINDER will ask the user to evaluate this feature.

The confirmation mode uses expert knowledge as a safeguard that counters the tendency of the method of sequential diagnosis to focus the differential diagnosis. One objective in both the traditional medical review of systems and the PATHFINDER confirmation mode is to ensure that the conclusions reached are not completely off target. A confirmation strategy addresses those cases in which a preponderance of unimportant information leads an INTERNIST-like expert system to an inaccurate diagnosis.

Heuristics Used for Narrowing of Differential Diagnoses

In reasoning about a case, PATHFINDER first attempts to classify diseases in the differential diagnosis into two groups, doing so at the most specific level of the strategic hierarchy for diagnosis of lymph node diseases. If two disease groups can be ascertained, the group-discriminate mode is applied to the differential diagnosis. If there are two or more diseases in the differential diagnosis and all of these diseases can be classified in a group at one leaf of the strategic hierarchy, the entropy-discriminate mode is applied. If, at any time, the probability of the leading disease exceeds a preset threshold (currently set at .9), the pursual mode is invoked. Finally, if a single disease remains on the differential, the confirmation mode is applied. If the disease remains the same at the completion of confirmation mode, this disease is concluded to be the one diagnosed.

Explanation Strategies

A very important aspect of the acceptability of an expert system is a clear explanation of its reasoning processes. This has been suggested in surveys of potential users of medical advice systems.[9,10] Unfortunately, explanation systems for frame-based systems like PATHFINDER are uncommon. For example, INTERNIST-1 only informs the user about the current question-generating strategy in progress; specific reasons as to why a particular finding is being requested are absent.

We have experimented with several question justification (explanation) schemes. They first implemented a free text system that evaluated the questions selected in terms of their discriminating power, tedium, reliability, and cost. Early versions of PATHFINDER simply reported that a question was ''good'' or ''very good'' for discriminating among diseases in the differential diagnosis based on their computed utility. It was decided later to offer the system user more specific information about the discriminatory capabilities of a question (recommendation). The present version of PATHFINDER has a graphic display of information about the relative impact of alternative responses on a particular differential diagnosis.

Figure 10-1 depicts the justification offered by PATHFINDER when two diseases or disease groups are being considered. In this sample case, the feature karyorrhexis has been recommended by the system as having the

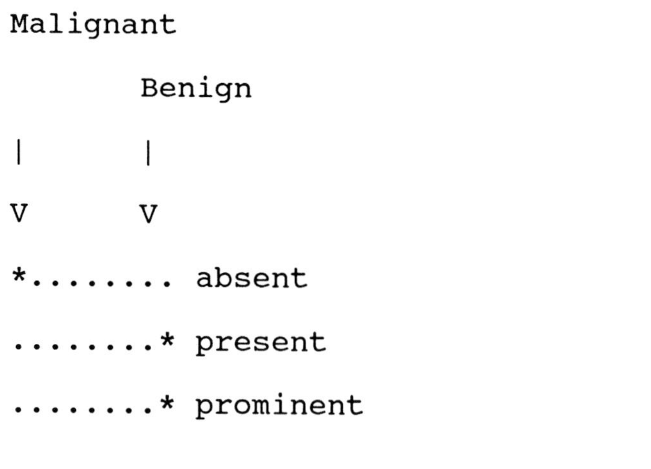

Fig. 10-1. Explanation of recommendation is represented graphically.

capacity to narrow a particular differential diagnosis (not shown) containing a number of benign and malignant diseases. The positions of a set of asterisks indicate the degree to which each group of diseases is favored by each possible feature-value. For example, the values *present* and *prominent* strongly support diseases in the differential diagnosis that are in the benign group, whereas the value absent strongly supports the malignant-disease hypothesis. This graphic justification format has been extremely useful in providing insight into the impact of questions (recommendations) on a differential diagnosis, and in facilitating the refinement of the knowledge base.

REFERENCES

1. Horvitz EJ, Heckerman DE, Nathwani BN, Fagan LM: Diagnostic strategies in the hypothesis-directed Pathfinder system. Proc 1st Conf AIA, IEEE Comp Soc, 1984, 630–636.
2. Horvitz E, Heckerman D, Nathwani BN, Fagan L: The use of a heuristic problem-solving hierarchy to facilitate the explanation of hypothesis-directed reasoning. MEDINFO 1986.
3. Miller RA, Pople HE, Myers JD: Internist-1, an experimental computer-based diagnostic consultant for general internal medicine. N Engl J Med 307:468–476, 1982
4. Shortliffe EH: Computer-based medical consultations: MYCIN, New York, American Elsevier, 1976
5. Elstein AS, Shulman LS, Sprafka SA: Medical problem solving: An analysis of clinical reasoning. Cambridge, Massachusetts, Harvard University Press, 1978
6. Pople H: ''Heuristic methods for imposing structure on ill-structured problems: The structuring of medical diagnostic,'' in Szolovits P (ed): Artificial Intelligence in Medicine, Westview Press, pp 119–190, 1982
7. Gorry GA, Barnett GO: Experience with a model of sequential diagnosis Computers and Biomedical Research. Vol 1:719–762, 1984
8. Shannon CE, Weaver W: The Mathematical Theory of Communication. Urbana, Illinois, University of Illinois Press, 1949
9. Neches R, Swartout W, More J: Explainable (and Maintainable) Expert Systems. Proceedings of the Ninth IJCAL, 1985
10. Swartout W: XPLAIN: A system for creating and explaining expert consulting systems. Artificial Intelligence 21:285, 1983. (Also available as ISI/RS-83–4)

Part II

T-Cell Lymphomas

11

An Approach to the Classification of Post-Thymic T-Cell Malignancies

Elaine S. Jaffe

Abstract

The classification of post-thymic or mature T-cell neoplasms has lagged behind that of the B-cell lymphomas, in part due to the relative infrequency of these lesions. In fact, most existing classification schemes for the non-Hodgkin's lymphomas are not readily applicable to the mature T-cell lymphomas. This review discusses the author's approach to the classification of post-thymic T-cell lymphomas and delineates several distinct clinicopathologic entities.

The post-thymic T-cell lymphomas are clinically heterogeneous and range in behavior from low to high-grade. The term peripheral T-cell lymphoma (PTL) has been used generically to describe those non-Hodgkin's lymphomas with a mature T-cell phenotype. Most PTL are clinically aggressive and fall into the Working Formulation categories of diffuse, mixed, small, and large cell type, and diffuse large cell immunoblastic. Adult T-cell leukemia/lymphoma is a distinct entity closely linked to the human retrovirus HTLV-I. The angiocentric immunoproliferative lesions (AIL) are emerging as still another category of T-cell malignancy. A pathologic grading scheme for the AIL has been proposed that is demonstrated to be clinically useful in predicting the behavior of these lesions.

The concept that hematopoietic neoplasms can be related phenotypically and functionally to their normal counterparts in the immune system has greatly improved our understanding of this clinically and morphologically complex group of malignancies. Post-thymic T-cell malignancies represent those lymphomas and leukemias in which the neoplastic cells express antigens normally encountered on mature T-cell lymphocytes.[1] The cells usually express CD4 or CD8 but not both. The neoplastic cells frequently exhibit an abnormal phenotype in that they express some, but not all, pan T-cell antigens.[1,2] Phenotypic markers cannot be used to demonstrate clonality, which can be shown through molecular genetic analysis for rearrangements of the T-cell receptor genes. Terminal trans-

TABLE 11-1
Classification of Post-Thymic T-Cell Malignancies

I. T-cell chronic lymphocytic leukemia
  helper
  suppressor or T γ lymphoproliferative disease
II. T-cell prolymphocytic leukemia
III. Mycosis fungoides/Sezary syndrome
IV. Peripheral T-cell lymphomas
  Morphologic variants include:
    Node-based T-cell lymphoma
    T-zone lymphoma
    AILD-like T-cell lymphoma
    Lymphoepitheloid cell (Lennert's) lymphoma
    Multilobated T-cell lymphoma
V. Adult T-cell leukemia/lymphoma
  (HTLV-I-associated disease)
VI. AIL including angiocentric lymphomas
  (Lymphomatoid granulomatosis)
  (Polymorphic reticulosis)

ferase activity is negative in mature T-cell neoplasms.

Neoplasms of mature T-cell origin include a spectrum from low-grade to high-grade lymphoid malignancies listed in Table 11-1. This review will focus on those T-cell malignancies with predominantly lymphomatous rather than leukemic manifestations. The peripheral T-cell lymphomas (PTL) and adult T-cell leukemia/lymphoma (ATL) are clinically aggressive, while the angiocentric immunoproliferative lesions represent a spectrum from low-grade to high grade lymphoproliferative disorders.

PERIPHERAL T-CELL LYMPHOMAS

The PTL represent a spectrum of cytologic subtypes in the Rappaport scheme and the Working Formulation. These lesions are all diffuse and in the Working Formulation are classified predominantly as mixed-small and large cell (DMCT) and large cell immunoblastic (LC-IBL) subtypes.[1] Approximately 10%–15% of PTL are composed of small atypical lymphoid cells. These lesions are difficult to classify in the Working Formulation.

Those lymphomas classified as DMCT often have an inflammatory background composed of eosinophils, histiocytes, and plasma cells. This polymorphous cellular composition may lead to difficulty in the distinction from Hodgkin's disease. The presence of cytologic atypia in the background lymphocytes argues against a diagnosis of Hodgkin's disease. Phenotypic markers are also useful in this differential diagnosis.[3,4]

A prominence of post-capillary venules is another feature often noted in PTL. Histologically, it may be difficult to distinguish PTL from angioimmunoblastic lymphadenopathy (AILD). The majority of the infiltrating cells in AILD are T-cells. They have a mature T-cell phenotype, usually with a predominance of CD4- over CD8-positive cells. The T-cells exhibit an activated phenotype in that they express IL-2 receptors, transferrin receptors, and HLA-DR. There are few B-lymphocytes, but frequent plasma cells that are polyclonal. In 3 of 6 biopsy specimens diagnosed histologically as AILD, a reduction of CD7 expression was noted when compared with other mature T-cell antigens such as CD2 and CD3.[5] In 2 cases of AILD showing progression to malignant lymphoma, the predominant cells had markers consistent with peripheral T-cell lymphoma. In one of 2 cases, the infiltrating cells lacked the CD7 antigen but were CD3 positive. One lymphoma studied by Southern blot analysis demonstrated a clonal rearrangement of the T-cell receptor, beta chain gene, as well as immunoglobulin gene rearrangements involving both heavy and light chain alleles.[6]

While many PTL have characteristic histologic features, these features are not specific and can also be encountered in diffuse lymphomas of B-cell type. Many such B-cell lymphomas contain numerically predominant T lymphocytes and have been referred to as B-cell lymphomas with T-cell predominance.[7] In many cases, this process occurs in patients with a prior diagnosis of follicular lymphoma. The inflammatory background seen in these cases may be a consequence of lymphokine production by infiltrating normal activated T lymphocytes and may represent a beneficial host response.

PTL classified in the Working Formulation as large cell, immunoblastic usually lack a prominent inflammatory background and demonstrate marked nuclear pleomorphism. Although polylobated nuclei are described in some cases, polylobated nuclear forms have also been reported in some high grade B-cell lymphomas. In B-cell tumors, the nuclear pleomorphism appears to be an exaggeration of the irregularity seen in large cleaved follicular center cells.

Clinically, most patients with PTL present with generalized lymphadenopathy. In the NCI series, most patients had Stage IV disease by virtue of involvement of the skin, liver, peripheral blood, lungs or pleura.[1] Skin involvement, when present, is usually dermal in location and spares the epidermis, readily permitting a distinction from mycosis fungoides. It is of interest to note that risk of peripheral blood involement is closely associated with cutaneous involvement and that no patient had peripheral blood involvement in the absence of skin disease. PTL is within the spectrum of diffuse aggressive lymphomas and should be approached accordingly. In the NCI series, patients with PTL were equally likely to attain a complete remission as patients with diffuse aggressive B-cell lymphomas, and survival was also comparable.[8]

ADULT T-CELL LEUKEMIA/ LYMPHOMA

ATL is a unique clinicopathologic entity associated with the human retrovirus HTLV-I. ATL is characterized by a broad range of morphologic expressions. The most specific feature is the presence of markedly pleomorphic lymphoid cells in the peripheral blood. Although not all patients present with peripheral blood involvement, a leukemic phase develops in the vast majority of cases at some time during the clinical course. The histopathology seen in lymph nodes is diverse, but histologic subtype does not appear to influence prognosis.[9] A common feature in lymph nodes is a leukemic pattern of infiltration. Other frequent sites of involvement include skin, liver, lungs, gastrointestinal tract, and cerebrospinal fluid. The disease is usually aggressive with a median survival of less than one year.

Angiocentric Immunoproliferative Lesions

The angiocentric immunoproliferative lesions (AIL) include lesions previously reported as polymorphic reticulosis and lymphomatoid granulomatosis. The AIL and angiocentric lymphomas have been proposed to represent a single clinicopathologic entity with varying degrees of clinical aggressiveness.[10] A recent study conducted at the NIH clinically and pathologically evaluated 23 patients with AIL. Pathologic subclassification was performed without knowledge of the clinical outcome and divided the cases into three histologic grades. Grade I lesions (9 cases) had little or no cytologic atypia. Grade II lesions (6 cases) maintained an inflammatory background, but the lymphoid cells, which were predominantly small, demonstrated significant cytologic atypia. Grade III (8 cases) was considered equivalent to angiocentric lymphoma. An inflammatory background was absent, and there was conspicuous cytologic atypia in both small and large lymphoid cells.

The results of this study support the concept that AIL and angiocentric lymphoma represent a single clinicopathologic entity with varying degrees of clinical aggressiveness. Moreover, they demonstrate that histologic criteria are useful in the subclassification of AIL and can be predictive of clinical course. The most important prognostic indicator for long-term survival was achieving an initial complete remission. Moreover, both patients with low-grade and high-grade disease appear capable of achieving a complete remission that is durable if appropriately treated.

Five of 9 patients with Grade I lesions and 3 of 6 with Grade II are alive with no evidence of disease after initial conservative therapy with cyclophosphamide and prednisone. However, of the 7 patients with Grade I and II lesions that progressed to angiocentric lymphoma, only one achieved a complete remission when treated for lymphoma. While the risk of progression to lymphoma appears relatively low in Grade I lesions (3 of 9), the risk appears greater in Grade II lesions (4 of 6). Moreover, the time to progression is considerably shorter in the Grade II patients: median 12 months as opposed to a median of 23 months. A more aggressive therapeutic approach with combination chemotherapy or radiation therapy appears warranted for patients presenting with Grade II lesions.

The survival for patients presenting with angiocentric lymphoma was excellent in this study. Seven of 8 patients are alive with no evidence of disease. While 2 of the 7 achieved a complete remission with only cyclophosphamide and prednisone, 5 of the 7 received aggressive treatment that included combination chemotherapy. In 2, consolidative radiation therapy was necessary to achieve a complete remission for persistent localized disease after chemotherapy. Only the one patient who failed to achieve an initial complete remission has died of his disease.

The clinical behavior of the AIL, including angiocentric lymphoma, appears analogous in many respects to the follicular center cell lymphomas of the B-cell system.[11] Follicular lymphomas of low histologic grade present with an indolent clinical course, and patients may survive for many years with or without aggressive therapy. However, if histologic progression occurs to a diffuse lymphoma of mixed or large cell type, the disease is associated with a more aggressive clinical course. Paradoxically, the high-grade follicular center cell lymphomas appear to be more responsive to aggressive combination chemotherapy. Patients who achieve an initial complete remission and sustain that remission for more than 2 years are frequently cured of their disease.

Those Group I and Group II patients that progress after having achieved a complete or partial remission on cyclophosphamide and prednisone have a poor prognosis and are unlikely to achieve a complete remission with more aggressive therapy. This situation is also analogous to that observed in the low-grade follicular lymphomas where initial conservative chemotherapy may compromise the ability of these patients to achieve a complete remission when they progress histologically.[12]

This study demonstrated that histologic grading is of value in the subclassification of AIL. Grade I lesions have a polymorphous cellular composition without any cytologic atypia. The histologic features of Grade I lesions appear comparable in many respects to the benign lymphocytic angiitis and granulomatosis (BLAG) of Saldana et al.[13] Lesions with this histologic appearance appear cytologically benign and respond to conservative management with cyclophosphamide and prednisone. Grade II and Grade III lesions appear more closely related and are more suggestive of malignancy on cytologic and histologic grounds. Cytologic atypia is more prominent and necrosis secondary to profound vascular involvement more readily observed. Grade II lesions are distinguished from Grade III lesions by their more polymorphous cellular appearance. However, in other respects they are similar. This author believes that Grade II and Grade III lesions are probably both malignant lymphoid proliferations. It is well recognized that the peripheral T-cell lymphomas commonly have an inflammatory background of plasma cells, eosinophils, and histiocytes.[1] Thus, the polymorphous cellular composition of the Grade II lesions does not rule out a neoplastic character. Whether or not Grade II and III lesions should be separated in the future cannot be entirely resolved from this study. Clinically, they appear quite comparable; in fact, the conservative therapy that patients with Grade II lesions received in this study may have contributed to a relatively poor survival for this group (50%). However, the immunophenotypic studies support the concept of separating Grade II and Grade III lesions. Grade II lesions failed to demonstrate phenotypic abnormalities, whereas they were present in the one Grade III case included in this study.

Additional evidence supporting the concept that the AIL represent a single clinicopathologic entity comes from the immunophenotypic studies. The proliferating cells had mature T-cell characteristics in all cases studied. A predominance of CD4-positive or "helper" T cells was usually observed. The immunophenotypic studies are not helpful in resolving whether or not AIL are neoplastic at onset. In contrast to the B-cell system, where kappa and lambda can serve as markers of clonality, there are no easily available phenotypic markers for clonality in the T-cell system. A common feature observed in the peripheral T-cell lymphomas is abnormalities of antigenic phenotype.[1,2] Many peripheral T-cell lymphomas fail to express one or more of the usual pan T-cell antigens. The one Grade III lesion included in this study did demonstrate abnormalities of antigenic phenotype, comparable to that seen in T-cell lymphomas. However, the results for the Grade I and Grade II lesions fail to provide supportive evidence for malignancy. Of the 5 Grade I and Grade II lesions studied, no phenotypic abnormalities were demonstrated, and an admixture of both CD4- and CD8-positive cells was seen in biopsy specimens. The peripheral T-cell lymphomas frequently demonstrate a CD4+, CD− or CD4−, CD8+ phenotype.

Molecular genetic analysis performed in one Grade III lesion provided additional supportive evidence for its malignant nature. It demonstrated rearrangement of the T-cell receptor beta chain gene, a clonal marker seen in most T-cell malignancies.[14] Unfortunately, no Grade I or Grade II lesions were available for molecular genetic analysis in this study. Future studies of these lesions should enable determination as to whether or not Grade I and Grade II lesions are clonal at presentation. Clonality would be strong presumptive evidence of malignancy in this clinical situation. Moreover, clonality may be a useful tool in determining which patients require initial aggressive therapy for Grade I and Grade II lesions.

REFERENCES

1. Jaffe ES: Pathologic and clinical spectrum of post-thymic T-cell malignancies. Cancer Invest, 2:413–426, 1984
2. Weiss LM, Crabtree GS, Rouse RV, Warnke RA: Morphologic and immunologic characterization of 50 peripheral T cell lymphomas. Am J Pathol, 118:316–324, 1985
3. Hsu SM, Jaffe ES: Leu M1 and peanut agglutinin stain the neoplastic cells of Hodgkin's disease. Am J Clin Pathol, 82:29–32, 1984
4. Hsu SM, Yang K, Jaffe ES: Phenotypic expression of Hodgkin's and Reed-Sternberg cells in Hodgkin's disease. Am J Pathol, 118:209–217, 1985
5. Jaffe ES: Morphologic features and immunoarchitecture, In Steinberg A (moderator), Angioimmunoblastic Lymphadenopathy with Dysproteinemia. Ann Intern Med 108:575–584, 1988
6. Lipford EH, Smith HR, Pittaluga S, et al: Cloanlity of angioimmunoblastic lymphadenopathy and implications for its evolution to malignant lymphoma. J Clin Invest 79:637–642, 1987
7. Jaffe ES, Longo DL, Cossman J, et al: Diffuse B cell lymphomas with T cell predominance in patients with follicular lymphoma or "pseudo T cell lymphoma." Lab Invest 50:27A–28A, 1984
8. Cossman J, Jaffe ES, Fisher RI: Immunologic phenotypes of diffuse, aggressive, non-Hodgkin's lymphomas. Correlation with clinical features. Cancer 54:1310–1317, 1984
9. Jaffe ES, Blattner WA, Blayney DW, et al: The pathologic spectrum of adult T-cell leukemia/lymphoma in the United States. Human T-cell leukemia/lymphoma virus-associated lymphoid malignancies. Am J Surg Pathol, 8:263–275, 1984
10. Jaffe ES, Lipford EH, Jr, Margolick JB, et al: Lymphomatoid granulomatosis and angiocentric lymphoma: A spectrum of post-thymic T-cell proliferations. Sem Resp Med 10:167–172, 1989
11. Jaffe ES: Relationship of classification to biologic behavior of non-Hodgkin's lymphoma. Sem Oncol, 13:3–9, 1986 (No. 4, Suppl. 5)
12. Jaffe ES: Follicular lymphomas: Possibility that they are benign tumors of the lymphoid system. (Guest Editorial) J Natl Cancer Inst 70:401–403, 1983
13. Saldana MJ, Patchefsky AS, Israel H, Atkinson GW, Jr: Pulmonary angiitis and granulomatosis. The relationship between histological features, organ involvement and response to treatment. Hum Pathol 8:391–409, 1977
14. Flug F, Pellici PG, Bonetti F, et al: T-cell receptor gene rearrangements as markers of lineage and clonality in T-cell neoplasms. Proc Natl Acad Sci 82:3460–3464, 1985

12

The Classification of T-Cell Leukemias

E. Matutes
V. Brito-Babapulle
L. Foroni
K. Yamaguchi
C. Dearden
A. Gates
D. Catovsky

Abstract

T-cell leukemias are a heterogeneous group of disorders that reflect the morphologic, phenotypic, and functional diversity of the T lymphocytes at different stages of their differentiation pathway. Because of the overlap of some of these features in the various diseases, a multiparameter analysis is necessary for their precise characterization. The authors propose a disease classification that takes into account: (1) the membrane phenotype of the neoplastic cells; (2) the morphological appearance of these cells under light and electron microscopy; (3) clinical and pathological features of the disease and its epidemiological clustering; (4) the HTLV-I status as assessed by serologic, immunologic and molecular probes; (5) karyotypic abnormalities when specific to particular disorders; and (6) evidence of clonality by demonstration of the rearrangement of the T-cell receptor (TCR) β, γ, and δ chain genes. Based on the expression of the enzyme terminal deoxynucleotidyl transferase (TdT) and membrane antigens, the T-cell malignancies can be classified in: thymic (TdT+) and post-thymic (TdT−) proliferations. Within the post-thymic group, at least five disease entities can be recognized: T-prolymphocytic leukemia (T-PLL), adult T-cell leukemia lymphoma (ATLL), Sezary syndrome (SS), T-chronic lymphocytic leukemia (T-CLL) and peripheral T-cell non-Hodgkin's lymphoma (T-NHL).

T lymphoid malignancies constitute a broad spectrum of diseases that result from the neoplastic expansion of cells commited to the T-cell lineage. During the early 1970s, the availability of heterologous anti-human cell sera, rosetting tests, and the enzyme terminal transferasc (TdT) allowed to delineate the B and T lineages of lymphoid

TABLE 12-1
Two Major Groups of T-Cell Malignancies

Disease	Age, onset	Clinical features	Morphology	TdT
Thymic (T-ALL; T-LbLy)	children and young adults	Acute course. Mediastinal mass, bone marrow, and peripheral blood involvement	Blasts	+
Post-thymic (see Table 12-2)	adults	Subacute/chronic course Spleen, lymph nodes, liver, skin, and peripheral blood involvement	Non-blastic lymphoid cells	−

differentiation, and to demonstrate the T-cell nature of some disorders. This has been lately confirmed by immunophenotypic studies with monoclonal antibodies (McAb), which detect membrane antigens on T lymphocytes[1] and molecular analysis showing rearrangement of the TCR genes.[2] These approaches have also disclosed the heterogenity of the T lymphoproliferative disorders that can be classified in two major groups according to clinical and biological characteristics: thymic (immature) and post-thymic (mature) (Table 12-1).[3] The presence of TdT distinguishes these two groups since TdT is exclusively expressed by lymphoblasts from the thymic disorders and not in post-thymic cells.

THYMIC MALIGNANCIES

These are proliferations of T-lymphoblasts that affect mainly children and young adults of the male sex with an acute clinical course (Table 12-1). An anterior mediastinal mass and a high white blood cell (WBC) count (often more than $100 \times 10^9/1$) are common.[4] Two disease entities with overlapping features can be recognised: T-acute lymphoblastic leukemia (T-ALL) and T-lymphoblastic lymphoma (T-LbLy). It is considered that T-ALL and T-LbLy may be different clinico-biological manifestations of the same disease, with T-ALL being the leukemic form of T-LbLy and the latter the tumoral expression of T-ALL.

Light microscopy analysis reveals that T-lymphoblasts correspond to L1 or L2 blasts of the FAB classification and show a regular or, more often, convoluted nucleus, fine reticular chromatin and a strong paranuclear acid phosphatase reaction.[5]

Although the diagnosis of these leukemias can be suspected by clinical and cytochemical features, immunological studies are essential to establish the thymic nature of the cells. T-lymphoblasts are, as a rule, TdT+, CD7+, and almost always HLA-Dr negative. The p 40 glycoprotein recognized by the CD7 group of McAb (eg 3A1, WT1, Leu-9, OKT16) is the earliest and most consistently expressed membrane antigen in the thymic proliferations. However, because blasts from a proportion (c.30%) of acute myeloid leukemias may be CD7+, the myeloid nature of the blasts should be always excluded, particularly in cases with a very immature T-cell phenotype (pre-T-ALL). Other T-cell McAb: CD5, CD2/E-rosette, CD1, CD4, and CD8 may also be positive with varying frequency. The antigen identified by CD3, which is part of TCR complex, appears early in the cytoplasm of early thymic cells and only later in the membrane.[6] Thus the demonstration of CD3 on fixed cells may also be used for diagnostic purposes.

POST-THYMIC MALIGNANCIES

These represent clonal expansions of mature, immunocompetent lymphoid cells and

TABLE 12-2
Post-Thymic T-Cell Malignancies

Disease	No. of cases
T-prolymphocytic-leukemia (T-PLL)	50
Adult T-cell leukemia lymphoma (ATLL)	25
Sezary syndrome (SS)	22
T-chronic lymphocytic leukemia (T-CLL)	23
T-cell non-Hodgkin's lymphoma (T-NHL)	5

include conditions that are characterized by a number of clinical, cytomorphologic, and immunologic features. Because some of these features are common to several of these disorders, for instance the expression of the antigen recognized by McAb of the CD4 group (see below), a multidisciplinary approach is often required for their precise classification. The clinical and laboratory features of 125 cases of post-thymic leukemias (Table 12-2) seen at the Royal Postgraduate Medical School, London over the past few years will be summarized here.

T-Prolymphocytic Leukemia (T-PLL)

PLL is a clinico-morphologic condition described by Galton et al.[7] in 15 patients as a distinct disorder. T-PLL is a rare disease and represents at least 20% of all PLL cases.[8] Clinically, T-PLL patients present with splenomegaly (77%), hepatomegaly (45%) lymphadenopathy (56%), and a high WBC count (median: $226 \times 10^9/1$; range 28–1000). Skin lesions may be present (24%), but these are not seen as erythroderma; serous effusions (ascitis/pleural) are documented in a minority (15%). The clinical course is usually aggressive and response to chemotherapy is poor; the median survival for this group was 7 months (Fig 12-1).

Morphologically, T-prolymphocytes appear under light microscopy as mature medium-sized lymphoid cells with a prominent, single nucleolus and scanty cytoplasm devoid of granules (Fig 12-2). In over half of the T-PLL cases, the nucleus is irregular and this, in addition to the presence of a deeply basophilic and often bleby cytoplasm, permits one to suspect a possible diagnosis of T-PLL. The nuclear irregularities of T-prolymphocytes are overall less pronounced than those of the Sezary and ATLL cells; however, a varying proportion of cells from the irregular T-PLL types may show a cerebriform or multilobed nucleus when seen under the electron microscope, which may create problems of differential diagnosis with Sezary syndrome (SS) and ATLL. The homogeneity of the morphological picture, the prominency of the nucleoli and the peripheral distribution of the nuclear heterochromatin in addition to clinical and immunologic data help to support the diagnosis of T-PLL. T prolymphocytes with a regular nucleus resemble B-prolymphocytes. Ultrastructural analysis has enabled the authors to identify some atypical T-PLL cases of small cell variant in which the nucleolus, a key feature for the diagnosis of T-PLL, could be visualized more clearly by electron microscope[9] (Figs. 12-3 and 12-4). This group of patients correspond to c.25% of T-PLL cases and their clinical and laboratory features are otherwise similar to those of the typical T-PLL.

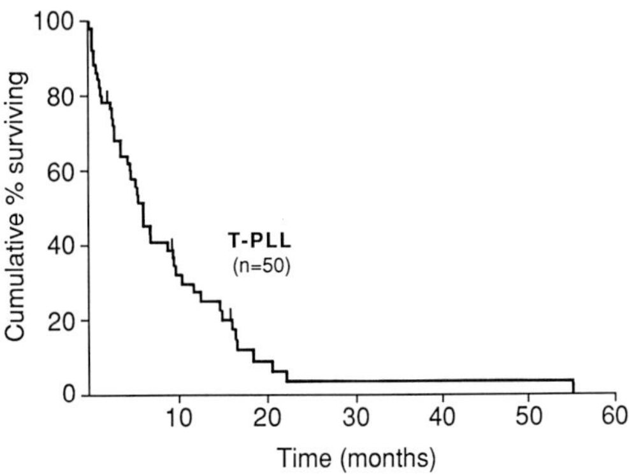

Fig. 12-1. Kaplan-Meier actuarial survival of the Matutes et al series of patients with T-cell prolymphocytic leukemia.

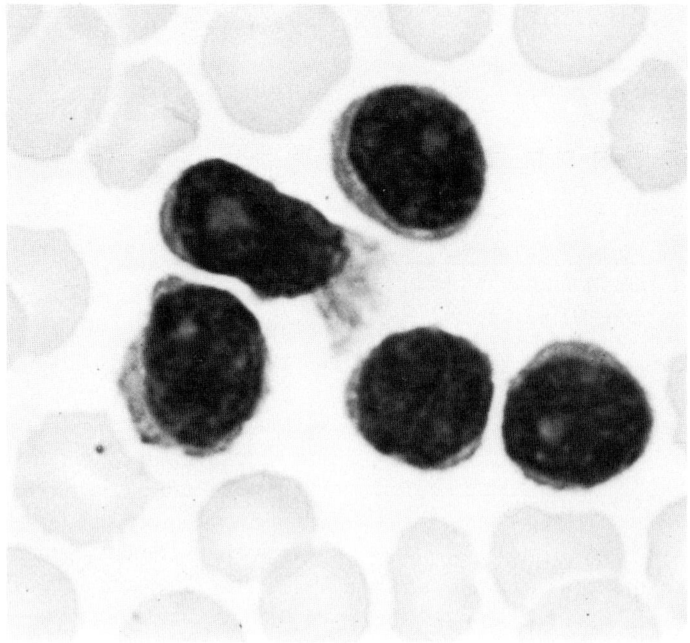

Fig. 12-2. Peripheral blood film of a case of T-cell PLL; note conspicuous nucleoli in each cell (× 1,400).

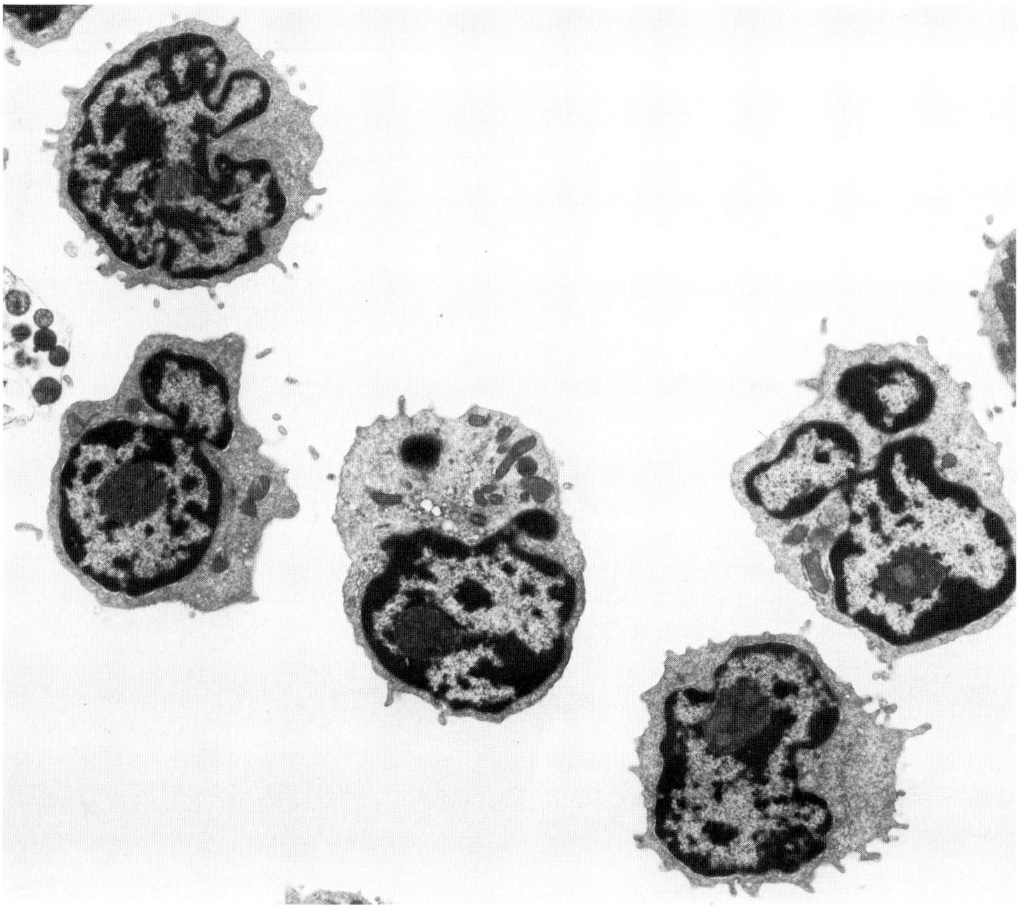

Fig. 12-3. Electron microscopy of prolymphocytes from a case of small cell variant of T-PLL. Note irregular nuclear outline, peripheral heterochromatin, and prominent nucleoli (× 8,000).

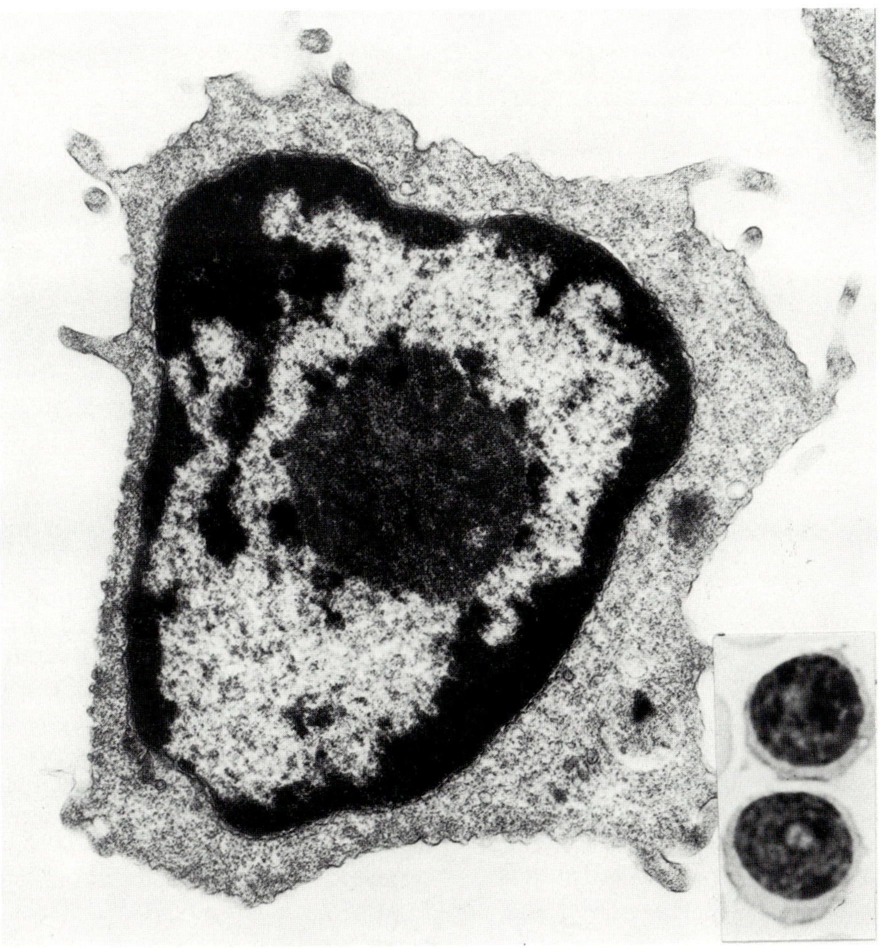

Fig. 12-4. Prolymphocyte from another case of small cell variant of T-PLL (× 24000); inset: peripheral blood film from this case (× 1400).

Phenotypical analysis of T-PLL demonstrates that this disease corresponds mainly to a proliferation of CD4+ CD8− cells. Other phenotypes observed are the coexpression of CD4+ CD8+ cells, CD4− CD8+, and rarely CD4− CD8− (Table 12-3). T-prolymphocytes are reactive with most pan-T markers: CD5,CD2/E-rosette, OKT17, and CD3-cytoplasmic or membrane, and characteristically, show strong expression of CD7[9] that, in contrast, is often absent from cells of other postthymic malignancies.

Cytogenetic analyses of 35 cases of mature T-cell leukemia, which included 16 T-PLL, has demonstrated that 10 of the 16 T-PLL had inv(14) (q11;q32).[10] It is likely that inv(14)(q11;q32) in T-PLL may bring together the TCR α chain gene and an oncogenic sequence such as akt-1[11] or a putative oncogene tcl-1.[12] Another karyotypic abnormality common in T-PLL was a trisomy for 8q resulting from an i(8q) or t(8;8)(p12;q11), found in 10 out of 16 cases. Because inv(14) is rare among other T cell disorders[10,13–15] including ATLL, this abnormality appears to be characteristic of T-PLL.[10]

TABLE 12-3
Immunophenotypic Features in Post-Thymic Malignancies (TdT-, CD1-; mean % of positive cases)

Marker	T-PLL	ATLL	SS	T-CLL	T-NHL
CD3	74	80	87	100	40
CD5	100	83	92	60	50
CD7	93	21	35	50	80
CD2/E-rosettes	96	71	94	100	100
CD4+ CD8−	67	90	67	9	20
CD4+ CD8+	18	0	11	4	40
CD4− CD8+	11	0	5	87	20
CD4− CD8−	2	10	17	0	20
CD25	27	85	20	0	33

Adult T-cell Leukemia Lymphoma (ATLL)

The 25 patients with ATLL were black and from Caribbean or African descent, except one which was a white female born in Iran. All patients had been residents in the United Kingdom for a number of years. In 6 patients (24%), the disease was confined to the lymphnodes without obvious peripheral blood or bone marrow involvement and were considered to have a lymphoma form of ATLL. The remaining 19 patients presented with the various leukemic forms of ATLL: acute (15), chronic (1), and smouldering (3): 2 of the 3 patients with smouldering ATLL evolved later into acute ATLL. The most common clinical manifestations were: lymphadenopathy (87.5%), hepatosplenomegaly (50%), skin lesions (40%), hypercalcemia (68%), and a raised WBC count (median 31 × 10^9/1; range 6–197). Other less common features were: osteolytic lesions (17%), central nervous system involvement (8%), and opportunistic infections. Infestation by *Strongyloides stercoralis* preceded or complicated the clinical course in three patients. Overall, the distribution of the clinical forms and hematologic features on the authors' group of ATLL were similar to those of a series of 187 Japanese patients (mean: 56 years).[16] The median survival of ATLL patients was very short (Fig. 12-5), similar to the series reported from Japan, and not very different either from the survival of T-PLL patients (Fig. 12-1).

Morphologically, ATLL is characterized by a heterogeneous picture reflected in the cell size, degree of chromatin condensation, and nuclear shape. The predominant cell type is a 'polylobed' lymphocyte with several nuclear foldings resembling the flower petals. The nucleus of this lymphocyte is seen at ultrastructural level as integrated by several independent fragments (multi- or polyfragmented). A minority of cells (median 5%) in the peripheral blood show features of immunoblasts: large in size, immature nucleus integrated by euchromatin, one or several nucleoli and numerous ribosomes and polysomes in the cytoplasm. Immunoblasts may constitute the predominant cell type in the lymph node.

Membrane marker studies show that most ATLL cases correspond to CD4+ CD8− proliferations and rarely, the cells lacked reactivity with these two McAb (CD4− CD8− phenotype) (Table 12-3). In one CD4+ ATLL case, the cells from the lymph node showed a CD4+ CD8+ phenotype. Interleukin 2 (IL-2) receptors demonstrated by the McAb anti-Tac (CD25) were expressed in resting cells or after 24-48 hours culture without lectin stimulation from most ATLL cases. In contrast to T-PLL, CD7, but not other pan-T markers, was usually negative in ATLL cells. Despite that ATLL cells are CD4+, functional studies have shown that they act as suppressors of the B cell differentiation in a pokeweed mitogen culture system.[17,18] This suggests that ATLL results from the leukemic transformation of a distinct CD4+ T cell subset able to mediate directly or indirectly suppressor activity. There are still controversial views as to whether ATLL cells are suppressors by themselves[19] or mediate this function by acting upon a subpopulation of CD8+ suppressor cells-inducers of suppressors.[20]

It is now widely accepted that ATLL, first described by Takatsuki et al[21] in Japan and later by Catovsky et al[22] in the U.K., is a distinct disease entity etiologically related to the human T-cell leukemia lymphoma virus (HTLV-I).[23] HTLV-I can be detected by either serologic, immunologic and ultrastructural studies in almost 100% of ATLL cases. The etiological role of HTLV-I in ATLL has now been definitively proven by molecular analysis showing monoclonal integration of the HTLV-I proviral DNA sequences in the leukemic cells of ATLL.[24]

In Matutes et al's group of patients, the presence of HTLV-I was demonstrated in cells from 20 out of 21 cases investigated while serologic and immunological-ultrastructural studies for HTLV-I yielded negative results in cells from 35 post-thymic T-cell leukemias other than ATLL, which included: 16 T-PLL, 11 SS, 6 T-CLL, and 2 peripheral T-cell non-Hodgkin's lymphoma. Therefore, the detection of HTLV-I represents an important key diagnostic feature of this disease.

Cytogenetic analysis in 2 cases showed: (1) trisomy or partial trisomy 7 (2 cases) and trisomy 3 (1 case), both abnormalities frequently demonstrated in ATLL;[13,14] (2) a 6q− with breakpoint q21 (1 case) abnormality reported also in ATLL.[13,14] As these abnormalities were also found in cells from patients with other T-cell disorders (2 SS and 2

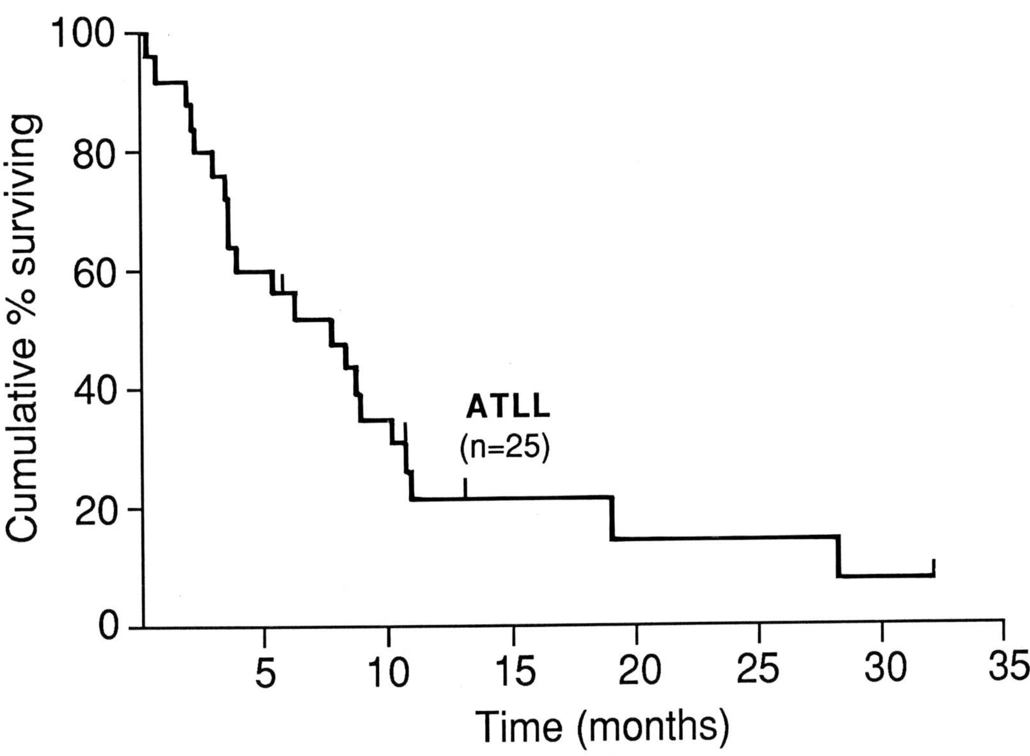

Fig. 12-5. Kaplan-Meier actuarial survival of the Matutes et al series of Caribbean ATLL patients.

T-PLL), they cannot be considered as specific of ATLL. Although a 14q+ was found in one ATLL case,[25] the breakpoint was 14q22 and not 14q32 as reported in some Japanese cases.[14]

Sezary Syndrome (SS)

SS and mycosis fungoides (MF) are the most representative clinical entities within the spectrum of cutaneous T-cell lymphomas. Both are characterized by a typical clinical feature: generalized erythroderma in SS and plaques/tumors in MF and by the proliferation of lymphoid cells with a distinct morphology designated cerebriform cells. The histologic pattern of skin infiltration is also characteristic and very similar in SS and MF; the abnormal cells infiltrate the upper dermis and show a tendency to involve the epidermis. In Matutes et al's series of patients, involvement of tissues other than skin was seen as lymphadenopathy (50%) and hepatomegaly (25%).

The identification of the neoplastic cells as lymphocytes with a cerebriform nucleus is the key diagnostic element of SS/MF. In the authors' experience, light microscopy examination allowed the diagnosis of SS to be established with certainty in 40% of cases. In a number of cases, however, the precise characterization of the neoplastic cells required ultrastructural examination; therefore, electron microscopy, seems to be essential for the identification of Sezary cells, particularly in those cases with the small cell variant of SS.[26] This finding is not surprising since the nuclear identations of Sezary cells are markedly narrow and deep and such degree of overlap in the nuclear foldings makes difficult their visualization under light microscopy. A semiquantitative analysis by measuring the ratio between the length of the longest nuclear indentation and the maximal nuclear diameter (I/N) shows that this ratio is greater than 0.66 in at least 30% of cells from 95% of SS cases. This analysis is also of value to distinguish Sezary cells from ATLL cells in which the I/N is usually less than 0.66 and, in contrast, the latter cells have great number ($\geq$ 2) of nuclear lobes. Similarly, the assessment of the nuclear contour index (NCI) has proven to be of value for the early diagnosis of SS and MF.[27]

Membrane marker analysis shows that SS usually corresponds, as ATLL and T-PLL, to a CD4+ CD8− post-thymic proliferation (Table 12-3). Subtle differences between Sezary cells and T-prolymphocytes and ATLL cells, in particular the expression of CD7 in T prolymphocytes and IL-2 receptors in ATLL cells, usually absent in SS, may help to distinguish them. Such phenotypic differences in addition to the distinct morphology would substantiate that these T-cell leukemias arise from distinct CD4+ T cell subpopulations as it has been suggested by studies carried out in normal blood T lymphocytes.[28] In addition, functional studies demonstrate that Sezary cells often have a helper activity on a B-cell differentiation system and rarely are suppressors as ATLL cells are.[19]

Matutes et al also studied 3 patients with a post-thymic leukemia in whom skin involvement was not apparent and the most relevant feature was a leukemic picture with lymphoid cells similar or identical to Sezary cells. These cases have been designated by us Sezary cell leukemia. Morphologically the cells were either identical to the small Sezary cells (1 case), corresponded to a mixture of large cerebriform Sezary cells and multilobed cells (1 case), or were typical Sezary cells coexisting with T prolymphocytes (1 case). Cells from none of these patients had the common phenotype seen in SS. They were: CD4− CD8+; CD4+/− CD8+/−; and CD4− CD8−. Although designated as Sezary cell leukemia, it is likely that identification of a larger number of cases with similar features together with further functional and ultrastructural studies may allow the recognition of this leukemic process as a distinct post-thymic disease entity.

T-Chronic Lymphocytic Leukemia (T-CLL) or Large Granular Lymphocyte Leukemia

The term T-CLL, first used by Brouet et al[29] refers to a disorder with a relatively benign clinical course and persistent lymphocytosis ($>5 \times 10^9/l$) without apparent evidence of it being secondary or reactive (e.g., to a viral infection). Cytopenias, usually neutropenia, and involvement of other lymphoid tissues (chiefly spleen) may be present. A previous history of rheumatoid arthritis has been documented with a high frequency in the series reported by Newland et al.[30]

The common and most characteristic feature of T-CLL is the morphologic aspect of the T lymphocytes that are seen at light microscopy as lymphocytes with abundant cytoplasm containing azurophilic granules and for this denominated large granular lymphocytes (LGL). Ultrastructural analysis reveals that T-CLL cells have a nucleus integrated mainly by heterochromatin, no visible or small nucleolus and abundant cytoplasm containing a markedly developed Golgi zone with microtubules, microvesicles, and scattered granules of variable size and density. A special structure integrated by bundles of microtubules packed wall to wall and designated parallel tubular array (PTA) is consistently found in T-CLL cells. This structure is not unique to T-CLL but is also found in normal Tγ (Fcγ +) lymphocytes.[31] PTA were identified in all but one of the T-CLL cases studied but were not seen in cells from over 100 cases of T-cell leukemia other than T-CLL, except for 3 ATLL (HTLV-I+) cases in which c.20% of cells had PTA. The only T-CLL case without PTA corresponded to a case with an unusual phenotype: CD4+,CD8−,CD11b+, CD16+.[32]

Immunophenotypic analysis shows that T-CLL is a disorder of T (Fc γ +) lymphocytes that usually display the CD8+, CD4− phenotype. Other T cell antigens expressed in subpopulations of normal LGL and recognized by the McAb Leu-7, CD11b, and CD16 may be found in T-CLL with varying frequency. In the 23 T-CLL cases studied, cells from most of them displayed the CD8+ CD4− phenotype; Leu-7 was positive in 53%, but reactivity with the McAb clustered under CD11b and CD16 was seen in only 2 cases. Thus, CD8+, CD4−, Leu7+/− CD11b−, CD16− may be considered the common phenotype of T-CLL. In a minority of cases, rare phenotypes: CD4+ CD8− (2 cases) were seen. In one of these cases, the McAb Leu-7 was also positive and in the other, CD11b and CD16 were expressed. In fact the different phenotypes seen in T-CLL reflect the heterogeneity demonstrable in the subsets of LGL seen in normal blood.[33] Although the clinical course of this group of T-CLL patients was overall benign and chronic, it should be noted that in 4 out of 5 cases with uncommon phenotypes, the disease had a more aggressive course.

One aspect of interest relates to the clonality of T-CLL. Over the past few years it has been argued as to whether T-CLL is a truly neoplastic proliferation or, rather, if it represents a reactive or secondary expansion of a discrete subset of LGL. The demonstration of clonality by cytogenetic analysis[25,34–36] in some patients and more recently by molecular analysis showing clonal rearrangement of the TCR β chain gene in most of these cases supports the view that this disease is indeed monoclonal in nature. In the group of patients studied by us, clonal chromosome abnormalities were observed in 4 out of 8 cases investigated in which mitoses were obtained. No abnormality specific for T-CLL was demonstrated.[25] Rearrangement of the β and γ chain genes of the TCR was found in 10 out of 12 cases investigated.[40] These included 4 cases with an uncommon membrane phenotype (3 of them with an aggressive clinical course) but also cases with common phenotypes and benign/indolent clinical course. Interestingly, one of the 2 cases in whom the TCR/β chain gene was in germ line configuration, the γ chain gene was rearranged suggesting that the leukemia resulted from the neoplastic expansion of a minor T lymphoid subset, which carries the γ/δ rather than the α/β TCR.[40] This has been recently confirmed in one of them by the demonstration of rearrangement of the δ chain gene of the TCR (L. Foroni, in preparation). The other case in which the T cell receptor β chain gene was in germ line showed a polyclonal pattern of the TCR γ chain gene as do normal T cells. This case corresponded to a patient who presented with an aggressive form of peripheral T-cell lymphoma with a leukemic picture of CD8+, CD4− LGL with karyotypic abnormalities, t(8;14)(q24;q32) similar to those of Burkitt lymphoma.[41] Because monoclonality could not be established by molecular probes, it is possible that the chromosome abnormality arose prior to the TCR γ gene rearrangement.

Peripheral T-cell Non-Hodgkin's Lymphoma (T-NHL)

This term has been applied to all non-lymphoblastic (TdT−) T-cell lymphomas other than cutaneous T-cell lymphoma.[42] The main clinical features are: hepatosplenomegaly, lymph node enlargement and involvement of non-lymphoid tissues (e.g., lung). The peripheral blood and skin may be secondarily involved and the clinical course is usually aggressive.

Histologically, T-cell NHL correspond to a diffuse type of NHL. However, there is a great spectrum of cytologic subtypes according to the cell size and degree of morphologic differentiation. Large cells with features of immunoblasts are often present. Therefore, the designation of peripheral T-cell NHL would include a variety of entities such as the lymphoma form of ATLL, and thus, assessment of the HTLV-I status of the patient represents here too an important test to distinguish between the HTLV-I positive and negative T cell NHL.

Phenotypically, the lymphoid cells in T cell NHL have a mature/post-thymic phenotype and may correspond to either CD4+ or CD8+ proliferations. In the authors' experience, membrane markers associated to T-cell activation (HLA-Dr, CD25, CD38) are often expressed in those cases in which the predominant cell type is an immunoblast.

Treatment

The management of mature T-cell leukemias has been disappointing, particularly in those with an aggressive clinical course and poor survival as T-PLL and ATLL. The authors' experience with the adenosine deaminase inhibitor, 2′deoxycoformycin (DCF), used in low doses showed that responses in patients with post-thymic leukemias correlate with the membrane phenotype of the cells but not with the cytopathological diagnosis.[43] Our updated results (Table 12-4) showed that complete or partial responses were documented only in patients with a CD4+ CD8− phenotype while no responses were recorded in cases with a different phenotype. The only exception was ATLL where only one complete remission was seen out of six patients treated. If confirmed, these results would suggest the beginning of a more rational approach to the treatment of T-cell leukemias.

TABLE 12-4
Response to DCF in Post-Thymic T-Cell Leukemias

Penotype	No.	Responders*	No remission
CD4+, CD8−	15	10 (67%)	5
CD4+, CD8+	8	0	8
CD4−, CD8+	5	0	5
All cases	28	10 (36%)	18

* Partial and complete remission

REFERENCES

1. Reinherz EL, Haynes BF, Nadler LM, Bernstein ID; Leucocyte Typing II. Human T Lymphocytes, Vol. 1, New York, Springer-Verlag, 1986
2. Rabbitts TH, Stinson A, Forster A, et al: Heterogeneity of T-cell β-chain gene rearrangement in human leukaemias and lymphomas. EMBO Journal, 4:2217–2224, 1985
3. Catovsky D, Melo JV, Matutes E: Biological markers in lymphoproliferative disorders, in Bloomfield CD (ed): Chronic and Acute Leukemias in Adults, Boston, Martinus Nijhoff Publishers, 1985, 69–112
4. Greaves MF, Janossy G, Peto J, Kay H: Immunologically defined subclasses of acute lymphoblastic leukaemic in children: Their relationship to presentation features and prognosis. Brit J Haemat 48:179–197, 1981
5. Catovsky D, Galetto J, Okos A, et al: Cytochemical profile of B and T leukaemic lymphocytes with special reference to acute lymphoblastic leukaemia. J Clin Path 27:767–771, 1974
6. Campana D, Thompson JS, Amlot P, et al: The cytoplasmic expression of CD3 antigens in normal

and malignant cells of the T lymphoid lineage. J Immunol, 138:648–655, 1987
7. Galton DAG, Goldman JM, Wiltshaw J, et al: Prolymphocytic leukaemia. Brit J Haemat 27:7–23, 1974
8. Catovsky D, Linch DC, Beverley PCL: T cell disorders in haematological diseases. Clin in Haemat, 11:661–695, 1982
9. Matutes E, Garcia Talavera J, O'Brien M, Catovsky D: The morphologic spectrum of T-prolymphocytic leukaemia. Brit J Haemat, 64:111–124, 1986
10. Brito-Babapulle V, Pomfret M, Matutes E, Catovsky D: Cytogenetic studies on prolymphocytic leukemia. II. T-cell prolymphocytic leukemia. Blood 70:926–931, 1987
11. Testa JR, Huebner K, Croce CM, Stall S: AKT-1 gene, the human homologue of a retroviral oncogene, is located on chromosome 14 at band q32. Cytogenet Cell Genet, 40:761, 1985 (abstract).
12. Croce M, Isobe M, Palumbo A, et al: Gene for α chain of human T-cell receptor. Location on chromosome 14 region involved in T-cell neoplasms. Science 227:1044–1046, 1985
13. Rowley JD, Haven JM, Wong-Staal F, et al: Chromosome pattern in cells from patients positive for human T-cell leukemia/lymphoma virus, in Gallo RC, Essex ME, Gross L (eds): Human T-cell Leukemia/Lymphoma Virus, New York, Cold Spring Harbor Laboratory, 1984, 85–89
14. Miyamoto K, Tomita N, Ishii A, et al: Chromosome abnormalities in leukemia cells in adult patients with T-cell leukemia. J Natl Cancer Inst, 73:353–361, 1984
15. Fujita K, Fukuhara S, Nasu K, et al: Recurrent chromosome abnormalities in adult T-cell lymphomas of peripheral T-cell origin. Int J Cancer 37:517–524, 1986
16. Yamaguchi K, Matutes E, Catovsky D, et al: Strongyloides stercoralis as candidate cofactor for HTLV-I induced leukaemogenesis. Lancet 2:94–95, 1987
17. Yamada Y: Phenotypic and functional analysis of leukemic cells from 16 patients with adult-T-cell leukemia/lymphoma. Blood 61:192–199, 1983
18. Miedema F, Terpstra FG, Smit JW, et al: Functional properties of neoplastic T cells in adult T-cell lymphoma/leukemia patients from the Caribbean. Blood 63:477–481, 1984
19. Miedema F, Melief CJM: Immunobiology of the expanded T cells in T-cell leukemia and T-gamma lymphocytosis. Leuk Res, 10:469–474, 1986
20. Morimoto C, Matsuyama T, Oshige C, et al: Functional and phenotypic studies of Japanese adult T-cell leukemia cells. J Clin Invest 75:836–843, 1985
21. Takatsuki K, Uchiyama J, Sagawa K, Yodoi J: Adult T-cell leukaemia in Japan, in Seno S, Takaku F, Imino S (eds): Topics in Hematology, Excerpta Medica, Amsterdam, 1977, 73–77
22. Catovsky D, Greaves MF, Rose M, et al: Adult T cell lymphoma-leukaemia in blacks from the West Indies. Lancet 1:639–643, 1982
23. Gallo RC, Essex ME, Gross L: Human T-cell Leukemia/Lymphoma Virus. New York, Cold Spring Harbor Laboratory, 1984
24. Yoshida M, Seiki M, Yamaguchi K, Takatsuki K: Monoclonal integration of human T-cell leukemia provirus in all primary tumors of adult T-cell leukemia suggests causative role of human T-cell virus in the disease. Proc Natl Acad Sci, 81:2534–2537, 1984
25. Brito-Babapulle V, Matutes E, Parreira L, Catovsky D: Abnormalities of chromosome 7q and Tac expression in T cell leukemias. Blood 67:516–521, 1986
26. Lutzner MA, Emerit I, Durepaire R, et al: Cytogenetic, cytophotometric and ultrastructural study of large cerebriform cells of the Sezary Syndrome and description of a small cell variant. J Nat Cancer Inst, 50:1145–1162, 1973
27. Van der Loo EM, Van Vloten WA, Cornelisse CJ, et al: The relevance of morphometry in the differential diagnosis of cutaneous T cell lymphomas. Brit J Dermat 104:257–269, 1981
28. Matutes E, Robinson D, O'Brien M, et al: Candidate counterparts of Sezary cells and adult T-cell lymphoma-leukemia cells in normal peripheral blood. An ultrastructural study with the immunogold method and monoclonal antibodies. Leuk Res, 7:787–801, 1983
29. Brouet JC, Flandrin G, Sasportes M, et al: Chronic lymphocytic leukaemia of T cell origin. Immunological and clinical evaluation in eleven patients. Lancet 2:890–893, 1975
30. Newland AC, Catovsky D, Linch D, et al: Chronic T cell lymphocytosis: A review of 21 cases. Brit J Haemat 58:433–446, 1984
31. Payne CM, Glasser L: Evaluation of surface markers on normal human lymphocytes containing parallel tubular arrays: A quantitative ultrastructural study. Blood 57:567–573, 1981
32. Moss VE, Miedema F, Matutes E, et al: An unusual variant of T-CLL: Evidence of hitherto unrecognized T cell subset. Clin Exp Immunol, 63:303–311, 1985
33. Polli N, Matutes E, Robinson D, Catovsky D: Morphological heterogeneity of Leu7, Leu11 and OKM1 positive lymphocyte subsets: An ultrastructural study with the immunogold method. Clin Exp Immunol, 68:331–339, 1987
34. Brody JI, Burningham RA, Nowell PC, et al: Persistent lymphocytosis with chromosomal evidence of malignancy. Am J Med 58:547–552, 1975
35. Siegal FP, Rambotti P, Siegal M, et al: Helper cell function of leukemic Leu2a+ histamine receptor+ T gamma lymphocytes. J Immunol, 129:1775–1781, 1982
36. Loughran TP, Kadin ME, Starkebaum G, et al: Leukemia of large granular lymphocytes: Association with clonal chromosomal abnormalities and autoimmune neutropenia, thrombocytopenia and hemolytic anemia. Ann Int Med, 102:169–175, 1985
37. Knowles DM, Dalla-Favera R, Pelicci PG: T-cell receptor β-chain gene rearrangements. Lancet 2:159–160, 1985
38. Rambaldi A, Pelicci PG, Allavena P, et al: T-cell receptor β-chain gene rearrangement in lymphoproliferative disorders of large granular lymphocytes/natural killer cells. J Exp Med, 162:2156–2162, 1985
39. Foa R, Pelicci PG, Migone N, et al: Analysis of T-cell receptor beta chain (Tβ) gene rearrangements

demonstrates the monoclonal nature of T-cell chronic lymphoproliferative disorders. Blood 67:247–250, 1986
40. Foroni L, Matutes E, Foldi J, et al: T cell leukemias with rearrangement of the γ but not β T cell receptor genes. Blood 71:356–362, 1988
41. Brito-Babapulle V, Matutes E, Pomfret M, Catovsky D: A t(8;14)(q24;q32) in a T-lymphoma/leukemia of CD8+ large granular lymphocytes. Leukemia, 1:789–794, 1987
42. Jaffe ES: Pathologic and clinical spectrum of post-thymic T-cell malignancies. Cancer Invest 2:413–426, 1984
43. Dearden CE, Matutes E, Hoffbrand AV, et al: Membrane phenotype and response to deoxycoformycin in mature T-cell malignancies. Br Med J, 295:873–875, 1987

13

Surgical Pathology of Lymph Node Biopsy Specimens in Taiwan with an Update on Adult T-Cell Leukemia/ Lymphoma

Tseng-tong Kuo
Lee-Yung Shih

Abstract

A total of 665 consecutive lymph node biopsy specimens collected during a 2-year-period were investigated. They were histopathologically classified into 6 groups: metastatic disease, 221 cases (33.2%); malignant lymphoma, 121 cases (18.2%); granulomatous disease, 109 cases (16.4%), reactive hyperplasia 80 cases, (12.0%); necrotizing lymphadenitis, 38 cases (5.7%); and miscellaneous conditions, 96 cases (14.5%). The important observations made were the highly prevalent metastatic nasopharyngeal carcinoma and mycobacterial infection and increased number of T-cell lymphomas and necrotizing lymphadenitis. Among miscellaneous conditions, polyvinylpyrrolidone (PVP) storage disease and nodal involvement by Kimura's disease were emphasized for their regional importance. The nodal pathologic findings reflected the regional disease pattern.

In the group of malignant lymphoma, Hodgkin's disease and follicular lymphoma were lower in frequency than diffuse lymphoma. A large proportion of non-Hodgkin's lymphoma (43.5%) was high-grade in malignancy. The male to female ratio was 1.5:1, and their median ages were 42 years and 46 years, respectively. Increased rate of T-cell lymphomas as compared to that of the Western countries was revealed but the prevalence rate of B-cell lymphoma (54.5%) was still higher than that of T-cell lymphoma (29.7%).

From 1983 to 1987, 11 adult T-cell leukemia/lymphoma (ATL) patients were identified in Taiwan. Cutaneous eruptions were observed in 5 patients. One patient presented with unusual follicular type of cutaneous involvement. the histopathologic types did not correlate with the clinical types. HTLV-I proviral DNA was demonstrated in 2 patients studied. ATL patients occurred only sporadically in Taiwan. Kuo's and Shih's previous seroepidemiological survey also concluded that Taiwan is not an endemic area for HTLV-I infection.

Diagnostic lymph node biopsy for pathologic study is an important clinical procedure in unveiling primary or secondary nodal diseases. Analysis of the pathologic changes of the lymph nodes provides data for understanding the regional disease pattern of geographic importance. Kuo and Shih studied consecutive lymph node biopsy specimens for understanding the nodal disease patterns in Taiwan and for comparative geographic study. In addition, a recent investigation of adult T-cell leukemia/lymphoma (ATL) including a seroepidemiological study in Taiwan[1–3] is summarized and updated.

The study conducted by Kuo and Shih was based on a total of 665 consecutive lymph node biopsy specimens collected during a 2-year-period from 1985 to 1986 at Chang Gung Memorial Hospital in Taiwan, which represented approximately 1% of their surgical specimens. Lymphoid marker study using the avidin-biotin complex method[4] with various monoclonal antibodies was performed on non-Hodgkin's lymphomas.

PATHOLOGIC CHANGE OF THE LYMPH NODES

The lymph nodes were classified according to their pathologic change into 5 major groups and a miscellaneous group to include all other conditions. Their prevalence rates and the median age and sex distribution of each group are summarized in Table 13-1. Malignant conditions were seen in the older age group. The male to female ratio of the entire series was 1.2:1.

Approximately one half of the cases were due to primary or secondary malignant diseases. Metastatic tumors formed the largest group and accounted for one-third of the cases. Among them, a high proportion of metastatic nasopharyngeal carcinoma was noted, which reflected the fact that nasopharyngeal carcinoma is highly prevalent in Taiwan.[5,6] Malignant lymphoma accounted for 18% and will be analyzed in detail.

A significant number of lymph nodes showed granulomatous inflammation. Most

TABLE 13-1

Classification of Lymph Nodal Diseases in Taiwan

	Total		Male		Female	
	No.	Median Age	No.	Median Age	No.	Median Age
Metastatic Disease	221 (33.2%)	51Y	127	53Y	94	48Y
Malignant Lymphoma	121 (18.2%)	46Y	73	42Y	48	46Y
Granulomatous Lymphadenitis	109 (16.4%)	31Y	52	37Y	57	29Y
Reactive Hyperplasia	80 (12.0%)	28Y	45	28Y	35	29Y
Necrotizing Lymphadenitis	38 (5.7%)	28Y	12	25Y	26	30Y
Miscellaneous Conditions	96 (14.5%)	34Y	58	34Y	38	36Y
	665		367		298	

of them were found to be due to mycobacterial infection. No data on culture and identification were available. It is suspected that some of those cases were caused by atypica mycobacterial infection as reported recently by Benjamin.[7]

Kikuchi's necrotizing lymphadenitis[8–12] was not uncommonly observed in Taiwan. One of them was initially misdiagnosed as malignant lymphoma. From 1983 until 1985, Kuo and Shih collected and studied 21 cases. The clinical features were similar to that of the Japanese series.[8, 9, 12] Lymphoid marker study was performed on 6 cases. Both CD4- and CD8- positive cells in various proportions were found in the lesions along with histiocytes. The result was similar to the findings of Asano et al[12] and Kikuchi et al.[13]

The more important conditions observed in the miscellaneous group are listed in Table 13-2. Among them, the polyvinylpyrrolidone (PVP) storage disease[14,15] and Kimura's disease[16–18] are of particular regional interest. PVP, a plasma expander, was used in Taiwan until late 1970s.[15] The presence of PVP-containing histiocytes in the lymph nodes should not be mistaken for a metastatic signet-ring cell carcinoma.[15] Kimura's disease is an angiolymphoid proliferative disorder affecting primarily the subcutaneous soft tissue,[16–18] and typically presenting as a huge tumorous swelling of the preauricular, postauricular, or submandibular areas, but sometimes it involves inguinal region or the upper extremity. Kuo and Shih had the opportunity to examine several cases of lymph nodes adjacent to the soft tissue tumors, which proved to be Kimura's disease. The lymph nodes showed prominent germinal centers and heavy interfollicular eosinophilic infiltrates with many branching blood vessels, but their endothelial cells were not vacuolated or "histiocytoid" as seen in the angiolymphoid hyperplasia with eosinophilia.[19] Eosinophilic microabscesses were sometimes observed. Frequently, the pericapsular soft tissues showed similar findings. Although this nodal picture is not entirely specific, it should alert pathologists to the possibility of Kimura's disease involving the lymph nodes. On several occasions, the possibility of Kimura's disease was suspected upon examination of lymph node biopsy specimens and led to that diagnosis by finding typical changes of Kimura's disease in the adjacent subcutaneous soft tissues, subsequently removed. In the Kuo and Shih series, the regional lymph nodes were almost always involved by the Kimura's disease. Similar observation was made by Kung et al.[18]

TABLE 13-2
The Miscellaneous Group of Lymph Nodal Disease

Dermatopathic Lymphadenopathy	19
Toxoplasma Lymphadenitis	18
Kimura's Disease	8
PVP Storage Disease	3
Castleman's Disease	3
Others	45
Total	96

PVP : Polyvinylpyrrolidone

MALIGNANT LYMPHOMA IN TAIWAN

The entire series consisted of 73 males and 48 females. The median age was 46 years (42 years for males and 46 years for females).

Hodgkin's disease accounted for 16.5% (20 cases) and non-Hodgkin's lymphoma for 83.5% (101 cases). Among the Hodgkin's disease, 9 cases were classified as mixed cellularity (45%), 7 cases as nodular sclerosis (35%), 2 cases as lymphocyte predominance (10%), and 2 cases as lymphocyte depletion (10%). Immunophenotyping of non-Hodgkin's lymphoma cases revealed 55 cases (54.5%) of B-cell lymphomas, 30 cases (29.7%) of T-cell lymphoma, and 16 cases (15.8%) of undetermined type. The histopathologic classification performed according to the revised working formulation[20] revealed 15 cases (17.7%) of low-grade lymphomas, 33 cases (38.8%) of intermediate grade lymphomas, and 37 cases (43.5%) of high-grade lymphomas as shown in Table 13-3.

TABLE 13-3
Histopathologic Types of Non-Hodgkin's Lymphoma

Histologic Type	No.	Total
Small lymphocytic	4	
Follicular small cleaved	2	
Follicular mixed	3	
Follicular large	6	15 (17.7%)
Diffuse medium	17	
Diffuse mixed	5	
Diffuse large	11	33 (38.8%)
Immunoblastic	25	
Lymphoblastic	9	
Small non-cleaved	3	37 (43.5%)

ADULT T-CELL LEUKEMIA/ LYMPHOMA IN TAIWAN

From 1983 to 1987, Kuo and Shih identified 11 ATL patients, 5 which were first reported from Taiwan in 1985.[1,2] The clinicopathologic features of the ATL patients are summarized in Table 13-4. There were 7 male patients and 4 female patients. Their ages ranged from 28 to 60 years with a median of 41 years. Eight patients of acute or acute crisis type all expired with a median survival time of 6 months. Three cases of smoldering type are still surviving for 7, 36, and 48 months, respectively. Five patients presented with cutaneous eruptions. The clinicopathologic features of the skin lesions are summarized in Table 13-5. The vesicular eruption of hands and feet of Case 2, which simulated pompholex, was reported previously.[1] The follicular eruptions encountered in Case 5 (Figs. 13-1 and 13-2) have not been described before.

All 11 patients proved to have serum anti-HTLV-I associated antibody by indirect immunofluorescence test on the MT-1 cell line.[21] Using the Southern blot hybridization method,[22] HTLV-I proviral DNA was demonstrated in the leukemic cells of 2 ATL patients.[23] Therefore, the occurrence of ATL patients in Taiwan has been definitely confirmed.

A previous seroepidemiological survey of

TABLE 13-4
ATL Patients in Taiwan (1983–1987)

Case No.	Age	Sex	Birth Place	Presentation	Clinical Type	Histologic Type	Outcome (Survival)
1	39	F	Ilan	Skin rashes	Acute	Pleomorphic	Died (6M)
2	60	F	Ilan	Skin rashes	Acute crisis	Medium-sized cell	Died (10M)
3	41	M	Ilan	Dyspnea, consciousness disturbance	Acute	NA	Died (6M)
4	56	M	Taichong	Dyspnea	Acute	NA	Died (2M)
5	34	M	Taipei	Dyspnea, backache	Acute	NA	Died (12M)
6	37	M	Pengfu	Diarrhea	Acute	Medium-sized cell	Died (0.5M)
7	48	M	Taipei	Dyspnea, consciousness disturbance	Acute	Pleomorphic	Died (7M)
8	42	F	Ilan	Skin rashes	Acute	Medium-sized cell	Died (2M)
9	52	F	Ilan	Skin rashes	Smoldering	Medium-sized cell	Alive ($36M^+$)
10	31	M	Taoyuan	Lymphadenopathy	Smoldering	Pleomorphic	Alive ($7M^+$)
11	28	M	Taipei	Skin rashes	Smoldering	Pleomorphic	Alive ($48M^+$)

NA: not available

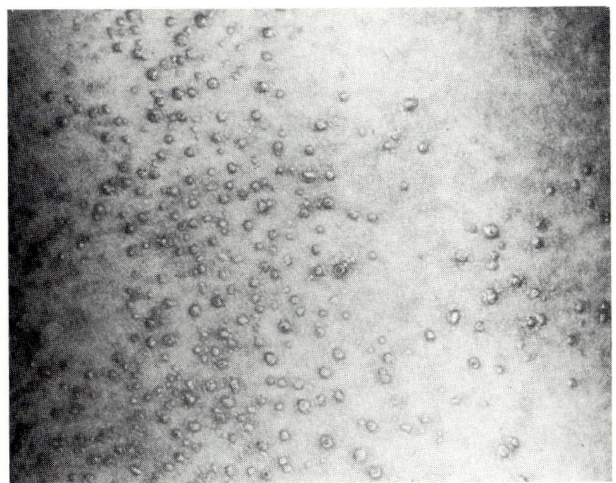

Fig. 13-1. Follicular eruptions in a patient of adult T-cell leukemia/lymphoma.

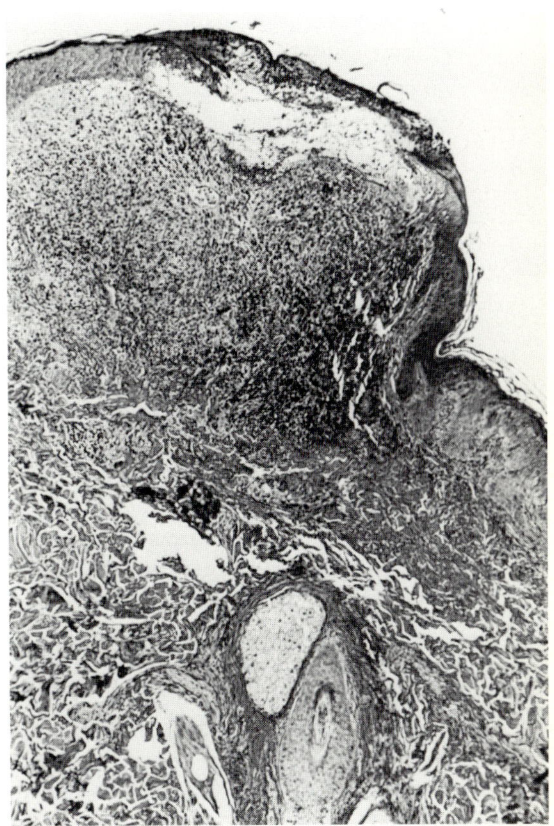

Fig. 13-2. Photomicrograph of a follicular eruption shown in Figure 13-1. The malignant lymphoid infiltrates form a papule around a hair follicle.

TABLE 13-5
Cutaneous Findings of ATL Patients

Case No.	Gross Appearance	Microscopic Appearance			
				Epidermotropsin	
		Type	Pattern	Diffuse	Pautrier Microabscess
1	Papules/nodules/ plaques	Pleomorphic	Perivascular, periadnexal	−	−
2	Vesicles/tumors	Medium-sized cell	Diffsue, perivascular	−	+
3	Plaques	Pleomorphic	Perivascular	+	+
4	Nodules/plaques	Medium-sized cell	Diffuse, perivascular	+	−
5	Follicular	Pleomorphic	Follicular	+	−

anti-HTLV-I associated antibody revealed a 0.43% positive rate or 0.90% for individuals 40 years or older in Taiwan.[3] This prevalence rate is similar to that of the ATL non-endemic areas in Japan.[24]

DISCUSSION

The study conducted by Kuo and Shih of consecutive lymph node biopsy specimens revealed the nodal disease pattern in Taiwan, which can be used for comparative geographic pathologic study. A high proportion of nasopharyngeal carcinoma was found among the metastatic diseases. Further analysis of the primary sites of this group will reveal the pattern of prevalent cancers in Taiwan.

Kuo and Shih also experienced a significant number of Kikuchi's necrotizing lymphadenitis,[8–12] which is apparently more prevalent among Oriental individuals. The etiology of this disease remains to be investigated. One important aspect of this disease is the possible misdiagnosis of this entity as a malignant lymphoma or vice versa.

Among the miscellaneous nodal diseases, the PVP storage disease observed represents a disease of regional problem. We call attention to the frequent involvement of regional lymph nodes by Kimura's disease,[16–18] which has been neglected in the literature. The authors agree with Kung et al[18] that Kimura's disease is a distinct entity, which differs from angiolymphoid hyperplasia with eosinophilia clinically and histopathologically.

The group of malignant lymphoma revealed that Hodgkin's disease and follicular lymphoma were also less commonly seen in Taiwan as reported from other Asian countries,[25–29] which were in sharp contrast to that of the American series.[30] Among the Hodgkin's diseases, the mixed cellularity type was the most predominant type in Taiwan. This observation was similar to previous reports from other Asian countries,[25,29,31] but differed from that of the American series,[30] in which the nodular sclerosis type was by far the most common type.

Kuo and Shih's immunophenotypic studies of the non-Hodgkin's lymphomas revealed that T-cell lymphomas were more frequently seen in Taiwan than that of Western countries,[32,33] but B-cell lymphomas were still more prevalent than T-cell lymphomas in Taiwan. The authors' observeration was at variance with the previous report by Su et al[34] from Taiwan in which only limited B-cell markers were used, and thus, some B-cell lymphomas were probably failed to be recognized. The rates of B- and T-cell lymphomas in Taiwan were close to that of ATL non-endemic areas in Japan.[28]

A large proportion of the non-Hodgkin's lymphomas in our region tended to be higher grade in malignancy. In contrast, only 2.2% of the M.D. Anderson Hospital series were high grade lymphomas.[35]

ATL patients occurred only sporadically in Taiwan. Its occurrence rate was similar to that of the ATL non-endemic areas in Japan.[24] Our seroepidemiologic survey also concluded that Taiwan is not an endemic area for HTLV-I infection.

ACKNOWLEDGMENT

This work was supported in part by the Chang Gung Memorial Hospital Research Fund No. 115 and No. 217 and by NSC 77-0412-B182-10 of the National Science Council of the Republic of China. Drs. T. Eimoto, M. Kikuchi, Y. Maeda, and H. Sato collaborated in the study of ATL. Ms. Shiu-Ming Cheng typed the manuscript.

REFERENCES

1. Chan HL, Su IJ, Kuo T, et al: Cutaneous manifestations of adult T-cell leukemia/lymphoma. Report of three different forms. J Am Acad Dermatol 13:213–219, 1985
2. Su IJ, Chan HL, Kuo T et al: Adult T-cell leukemia/lymphoma in Taiwan. A clinocopathologic observation. Cancer 56:2217–2220, 1985
3. Kuo T, Chan HL, Su IJ, et al: Serological survey of antibodies to the adult T-cell leukemia virus-associated antigen (HILV-A) in Taiwan. Int J Cancer 36:345–348, 1985

4. Hsu SM, Raine L, Fanger H: The use of anti-avidin antibody and avidin-biotin-peroxidase complex in immunoperoxidase technics. Am J Clin Pathol 75:816–821, 1981
5. Yeh S, Cowdry EV: Incidence of malignant tumors in Chinese, especially in Formosa. Cancer 7:425–436, 1954
6. Belamaric J: Malignant tumors in Chinese. A report based on biopsy and autopsy material from Chinese in Hong Kong. Int J Cancer 4:560–573, 1969
7. Benjamin DR: Granulomatous lymphadenitis in children. Arch Pathol Lab Med 111:750–753, 1987
8. Kikuchi M: Lymphadenitis showing focal reticulum cell hyperplasia with nuclear debris and phagocytes. A clinicopathological study. Acta Hematol Jpn 35:379–380, 1972 (in Japanese)
9. Fujimoto Y, Kojima Y, Yamaguchi K: Cervical subacute necrotizing lymphadenitis. Naika 30:920–927 (in Japanese)
10. Pileri S, Kikuchi M, Helbron K, Lennert K: Histiocytic necrotizing lymphadenitis without granulocytic infiltration. Virch Arch Pathol Anat 395:257–271, 1982
11. Turner RR, Martin J, Dorfman RF: Necrotizing lymphadenitis: A study of 30 cases. Am J Surg Pathol 7:115–123, 1983
12. Asano S, Kanno H, Tominaga K, et al: Necrotizing lymphadenitis. Electron microscopical and immunohistochemical study. Acta Pathol Jpn 37:1071–1084, 1987
13. Kikuchi M, Takeshita M, Tashiro K, et al: Immunohistological study of histiocytic necrotizing lymphadenitis. Virch Arch Pathol Anat 409:299–311, 1986
14. Reske-Nielsen E, Bojsen-Moller M, Vetner M, et al: Polyvinylpyrrolidone-storage disease. Light microscopical, ultrastructural and chemical verification. Acta Path Microbiol Scand (Sect. A) 84:397–405, 1976
15. Kuo T, Hsueh S: Mucicarminophilic histiocytosis. A polyvinylpyrrolidone (PVP) storage disease simulating signet-ring cell carcinoma. Am J Surg Pathol 8:419–428, 1984
16. Kimura T, Yoshimura S, Ishikawa E: On the unusual granulation combined with hyperplastic changes of lymphatic tissues. Trans Soc Pathol Jpn 37:179–180, 1948 (in Japanese)
17. Kawada A, Takahashi H, Anzai J: Eosinophilic lymphofolliculosis of the skin (Kimura's disease). Nippon Hifuka Gakkai Zasshi 76:117–134, 1966
18. Kung ITM, Gibson JB, Bannatyne PM: Kimura's disease: A clinico-pathological study of 21 cases and its distinction from angiolymphoid hyperplasia with eosinophilia. Pathol 16:39–44, 1984
19. Rosai J, Gold J, Landy R: The histiocytoid hemangiomas: A unifying concept embracing several previously described entities of skin, soft tissue, large vessels, bone and heart. Human Pathol 10:707–730, 1979
20. Nanba K, Yamamoto H, Kamada N, et al: Agreement rates and American-Japanese pathologist's comparability of a Modified Working Formulation for non-Hodgkin's lymphomas. An analysis of the cases collected for the fifth international workshop on chromosomes in leukemia-lymphoma. Cancer 59:1463–1469, 1987
21. Hinuma Y, Nagata K, Hanaoka M, et al: Adult T-cell leukemia: Antigen in an ATL cell line and detection of antibodies to the antigen in human sera. Proc Natl Acad Sci 78:6476–6480, 1981
22. Southern EM: Detection of specific sequences among DNA fragments separated by gel electrophoresis. J Mol Biol 98:503–517, 1975
23. Kuo T, Sato H, Dunn P, et al: Presence of HTLV-1 proviral DNA in patients with adult T cell leukemia/lymphoma in Taiwan. Cancer 62:702–704, 1988
24. The T- and B- cell Malignant Study Group. Statisfical analysis of clinico-pathological, virological and epidemiological data on lymphoid malignancies with special reference to adult T-cell leukemia/lymphoma. A report of the second nationwide study of Japan. Jpn J Clin Oncol 15:517–535, 1985
25. Ho FCS, Todd D, Loke SL, et al: Clinicopathological features of malignant lymphomas in 294 Hong Kong Chinese patients, retrospective study covering an eight-year period. Int J Cancer 34:143–148, 1984
26. The nationwide lymphoma pathology cooperative group (Directed by Prof. Sui-Yu Gu). A retrospective histological study of 9,009 cases of malignant lymphoma in China using the NLPCG classification. Jpn J Clin Oncol 15:645–651, 1985
27. Nanba K, Berard CW, Itagaki T, et al: Is reticulum cell sarcoma really frequent in Japan? An analysis of 331 cases of lymph-node biopsies (1962–1972). J Jpn Soc RES 13:96, 1973 (in Japanese)
28. Tajima K, Suchi T, Koike K: Malignant lymphoma—Immunological characters and histological features. J Jpn Soc RES 19:333–345, 1979 (in Japanese)
29. Chi JG, Shiu SS, Ahn GH, Lee SK: Malignant lymphomas in Korea. Jpn J Clin Oncol 15:653–659, 1985
30. Kim H, Zelman RJ, Fox MA, et al: Pathology panel for lymphoma clinical studies: A comprehensive analysis of cases accumulated since its inception. J Natl Cancer Instit 68:43–67, 1982
31. Teijima S, Watanabe S: Hodgkin's disease in Japan. Study of 110 cases from National Cancer Center Hospital. J Jpn Soc Res. 19:345–355, 1979 (in Japanese)
32. Lukes R. Collins RD: Lukes-Collins Classification and its significance. Cancer Treat Rep 61:971–979, 1977
33. Lennert K: Histopathology of Non-Hodgkin's lymphomas. (Based on the Kiel classification), New York, Springer-Verlag, 1981, 15
34. Su IJ, Shih LY, Kadin ME, et al: Pathologic and immunologic characterization of malignant lymphoma in Taiwan: With special reference to retrovirus-associated adult T-cell lymphoma/leukemia. Am J Clin Pathol 84:715–723, 1985
35. Newell GR, Cabanillas FG, Hagemeister FJ Butler JJ: Incidence of lymphoma in the US classified by the Working Formulation. Cancer 59:857–861, 1987

14

Immunohistopathology of Adult T-Cell Leukemia/Lymphoma

Masayoshi Tokunaga
Takahiro Tokudome
Kazuhisa Hasui
Eiichi Sato

Abstract

The reactivity of monoclonal antibodies, including newly developed ones, was examined in fresh frozen sections of 50 cases with adult T-cell leukemia/lymphoma.

The majority of ATL cells uniformly expressed CD3 and CD4, but there was some other marker expression for T-cells. There was occasional Leu-M1 and Ki-1 expression of the tumor cells.

In 74% of ATLL, intensive IL-2R positivity was shown. Among these, 25% expressed interleukin-2(IL-2) revealed by the monoclonal antibody DMS-3. The findings suggest that there is autocrine growth of the ATLL cells in the lymph node.

The monoclonal antibody FTF-148 showed positive reaction on the cellular surface and the Golgi area. This antibody marked positive reaction in the giant cells and in the large cells of ATL. This antibody is thought to be useful for the differential diagnosis of cutaneous lesion of ATLL.

Adult T-cell leukemia/lymphoma(ATL) is a unique well known T-cell neoplasia characterized by the endemic occurrence and by the surface markers of peripheral T-cells[1] such as T3+, T4+, T8-T11+, and by the expression of IL-2 receptor.[2]

The sera of ATL patients are positive for anti HTLV-1 antibodies,[3] and ATL cells contain the proviral DNA of HTLV-1.[4] Morphologic characteristics of ATL are the presence of cells with deeply indented nuclei having a nick name of flower cell in the peripheral blood, and a pleomorphic histology of lymph nodes involved.[5] The pleomorphic type in the Japanese Lymphoma Study Group classification is a core histologic pattern of this lymphoma, with characteristic giant cells as a hallmark.[6,7]

By use of fresh frozen sections of lymph nodes and tonsils from 50 patients of ATL, immuunocytological characteristics of ATL cells, including findings with some newly developed monoclonal antibodies are described here. All of these patients were anti HTLV-1 antibody positive.

IMMUNOHISTOCHEMISTRY OF T-CELL MARKERS

Immunohistologically, the tumor cells showed at least one of the pan T-cell markers such as Leu-4(BECTON DICKINSON), OKT-3, or OKT-11(ORTHO). Figure 14-1 shows positive Leu-4 on the surface of lymphoma cells. Out of 50 ATL cases, 47 cases showed surface markers of Leu-4 and OKT-11, but one case was negative for Leu-4 and 2 negative for OKT-11. Thirty-seven of the 50 cases showed T4+, T8−, (Table 14-1), but 3 were T4−, T8+; 8 were positive for both; and two were negative for both (Table 14-1). There was no obvious relationship among the immunologic phenotypes, histologic types, and clinical findings, though the numbers of cases examined were small.[8]

Recently, some monoclonal antibodies available on paraffin sections have been introduced, such as MT-1(Bio Science Products) and UCHL-1(Dako). These pan-T cell antibodies are useful for the diagnosis ATL when the biopsy specimen were fixed in the formalin. In the authors' series, however, only about one-third cases of ATL showed intensive positivity. Others were either weakly positive or negative. Mx-panB(KYOWA) or LN series (TECHNICLONE) for B-cell were negative in all cases.

OTHER MONOCLONAL ANTIBODIES

Tumor cells of these ATL were positive for some other monoclonal antibodies such as Leu-8, Tq-1, HLA-DR, OK-NK, Leu-7,

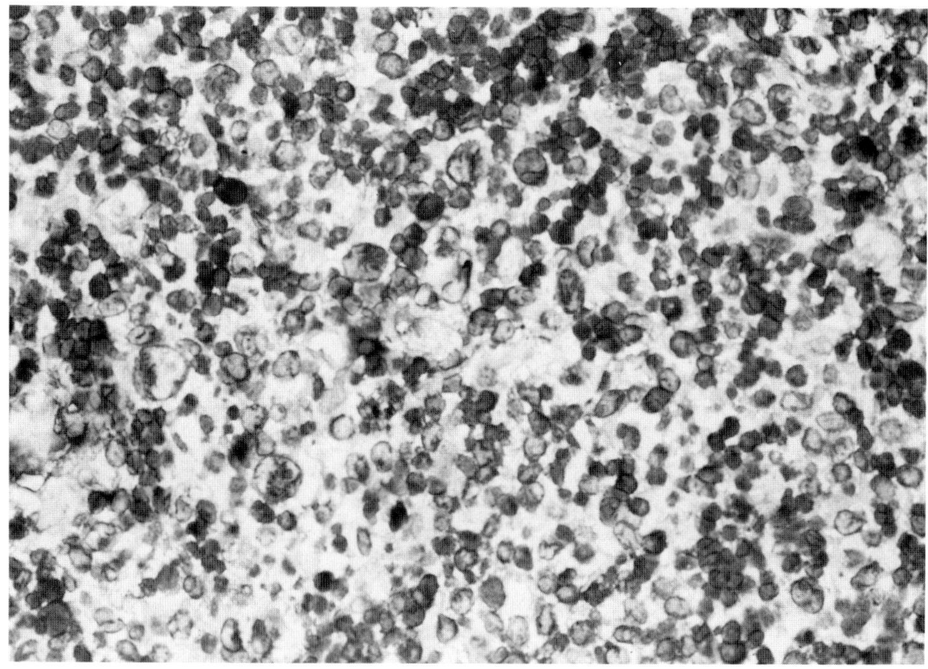

Fig. 14-1. Pleomorphic lymphoma of ATL showing membranous staining for OKT4 (Alkaline phosphatase labeled avidin method × 300).

TABLE 14-1
Histological Types and T-Cell Markers of ATL

	T4+T8−	T4−T8+	T4+T8+	T4−T8−	Total
Medium	6	0	2	0	8
Mixed	12	1	0	0	13
Large	4	0	0	1	5
Pleomorphic	15	2	6	1	24
Total	37	3	8	2	50

Leu-M1, and Ki-1(DAKO) (Fig. 14-2). The positive rate for Tq-1 was as high as 74%. This high rate was comparable to that of T4. This is probably related to the suppressor function of the tumor cells. 80% of the ATL cases were HLA-DR positive, suggesting the activated T-cell nature of the ATL. The antibodies for natural killer cells such as OK-NK and Leu-7 showed occasional expression on the ATL cases. Leu-M1 is a momoclonal antibody for the granulocytes. This antigen is also expressed in the Reed-Sternberg cells of Hodgkin's disease and in some kind of carcinoma cells.[9,10] Leu-M1 was observed on ATL cells in 6% of the cases. Ki-1 is a monoclonal antibody for Reed-Sternberg cell. It is well known that this antigen is expressed on a special kind of lymphoma called Ki-1 lymphoma. There were 8% positive cases among ATL in this study. The Ki-1 positive cases were histologically not uniform including 2 pleomorphic types, one medium cell type, and one large cell type.

Ki-67 positive cells were observed predominantly in the lymph nodes, but the positive rates varied among cases ranging from 65% to 99% of the tumor cells with an average positive rate of 86%. Ki-67 positive cells were

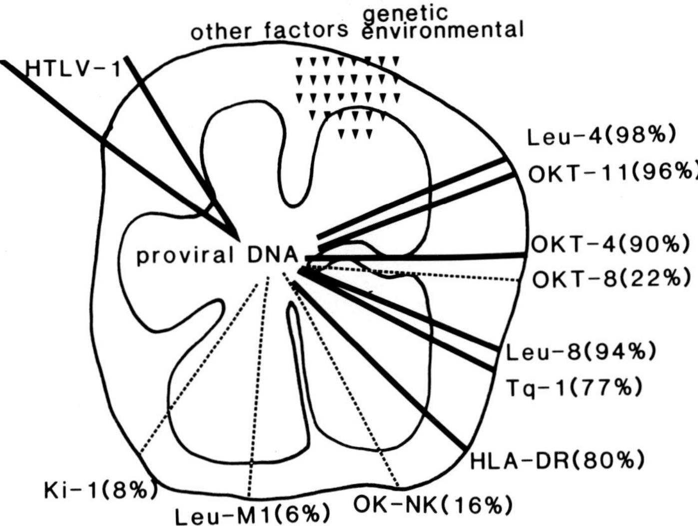

Fig. 14-2. ATL cell may develop in the cells infected by HTLV-1 under other genetical or environmental influences, and show heterogeneous phenotypic expression.

also observed in the circulating routes such as the lymphatics and sinuses. An early cutaneous lesion of ATL showed very low positivity, but once it formed a tumorous lesion, many of the tumor cells become Ki-67 positive.

BACKGROUND REACTIVE CELLS OF ATL

There were many kinds of reactive cells in the background of the lymph nodes with ATL (Fig. 14-3). B-cells were clustering occasionally with compressed residual follicle centers. Langerhans cells, natural killer cells, and histiocytes were also found. The degree of involvement by neoplastic cells varied according to their number but there were usually less than 10 in each high-power-field of lymphomas.

Interleukin-2 and Interleukin-2 Receptor

It is well known that leukemic cells in ATL express an IL-2 receptor spontaneously and continuously.[2,11] This abnormal IL-2 receptor expression in ATL is thought to be closely associated with HTLV-1 infection and may play an important role in the neoplastic growth of ATL cells.[11] In vitro studies have revealed that IL-2 stimulates the growth of activated T-cell clones for a prolonged time. If ATL cells produce IL-2, the autocrine growth mechanism of ATL cells can be triggered.[12]

The authors studied the IL-2 expression using the monoclonal antibodies DMS-1 and DMS-3 produced by Smith,[13] and for the IL-2 receptor expression using the monoclonal antibody of IL-2R (Fig. 14-4a). The DMS-3 binds I1-2 with a much greater efficiency than DMS-1, but the DMS-3 has proven to be far less effective in neturalizing biologic activity of the IL-2.[13]

Positive localization of DMS-3 was seen as an intracytoplasmic or a cellular surface staining (Fig. 14-4b). This antibody also reacted with some of the lymphocytes of the lymphadenitis and of B-cell lymphomas. The results of the examination of DMS-3 and IL-2 receptor are shown in Table 14-2. There were only 8 cases with positive lymphoma cells. These DMS-3 positive cases are listed

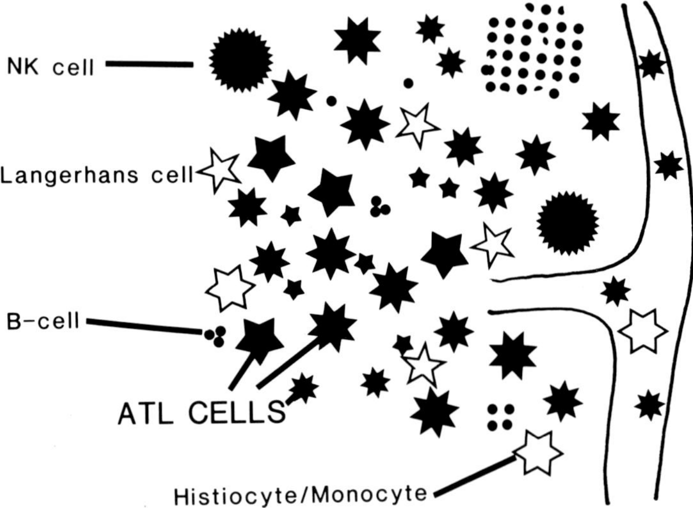

Fig. 14-3. Lymph node involved by ATL showing many kinds of background reactive cells.

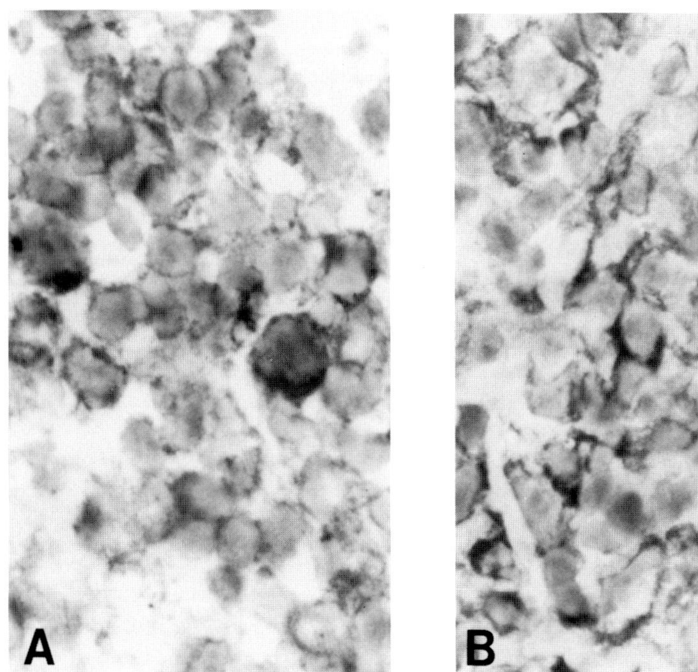

Fig. 14-4. ATL cells showing intensive positivity for interleukin 2 receptor (A) and interleukin 2 (DMS-3)(B) in the same lymph node. (A1-P labeled avidin method × 600).

TABLE 14-2
Expression of IL-2R and IL-2 (DMS-3)

IL-2R	IL-2 (DMS-3)			
	−	+	++	Total
−	6	5	0	11
+	9	14	8	31
Total	15	19	8	42

with other findings of marker study and histology in Table 14-3; No special histologic type were associated with DMS-3 positivity. Pan-T markers were all positive, but Cases 1–3 showed positivity for both OKT4 and OKT8, and Case 4 showed OKT4− and OKT8+. These 8 cases showed intense positivity for the IL-2 receptor in almost all of the tumor cells. These findings suggest that

TABLE 14-3
ATL Cases with Prominent Expression of IL-2(DMS-3)

No.	Age/Sex	Histological type	Leu-4	OKT4	OKT8	IL-2R	Other
1	58 M	Pleomorphic	+	+	+	+++	
2	67 F	Pleomorphic	+	+	+	+++	Leu-7
3	76 M	Pleomorphic	+	+	+	+++	OK-NK
4	48 F	Mixed	+	−	+	+++	
5	62 M	Mixed	+	+	−	+++	OK-NK
6	66 F	Mixed	+	+	−	+++	OK-NK
7	56 M	Mixed	+	+	−	+++	OK-NK
8	82 M	Mixed	+	+	−	+++	

there are tumor cells that produce IL-2 in the cytoplasm in about 20% of ATL cases, and consequently, possible autocrine growth mechanisms.

FTF-148 EXPRESSIN ON ATL

FTF-148 is a monoclonal antibody that reacts with an antigen expressed in HTLV-1 infected cells.[14] This antigen is thought to be a product of certain cellular genes activated by a transacting factor produced by HTLV-1 infection as described by Dr. Yujiro Namba elsewhere in this book.

The immunohistology of this FTF-148 showed a strong expression in the Golgi areas and on membranes of giant cells of ATL. (Fig. 14-5) FTF-148 was, however, also expressed in B-cell lymphomas and Hodgkin's disease. There was no positive cell in lymphadenitis cases except for a few cytoplasmic cross reactions. There is no positive reaction in the epithelial cells examined in 20 cases of carcinoma.

The results of FTF-148 reaction indicated that almost all of the lymph nodes of ATL contained positive cells. Giant cells of ATL showed an intense positive reaction (Fig. 14-5b). The positive reaction of FTF-148 did not always seem to be related to the HTLV-1 infection, because there were FTF148-negative cases in the group with positive anti HTLV-1 antibody and there were FTF148 positive lymphoma cases in the group with negative anti-HTLV-1 antibody. (Table 14-4).

Cutaneous lesions with atypical lymphocytic infiltration are the major diagnostic problem for those pathologists who live in the endemic area of ATL. The FTF-148 was positive in the cutaneous lesions of ATL, but negative in 6 non-ATL cutaneous T-cell lymphomas. These findings indicate that this antibody FTF-148 is useful for the differential diagnosis of ATL from other cutaneous le-

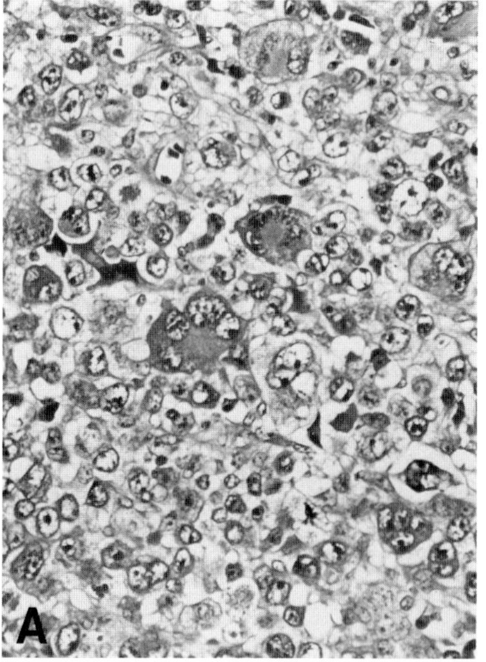

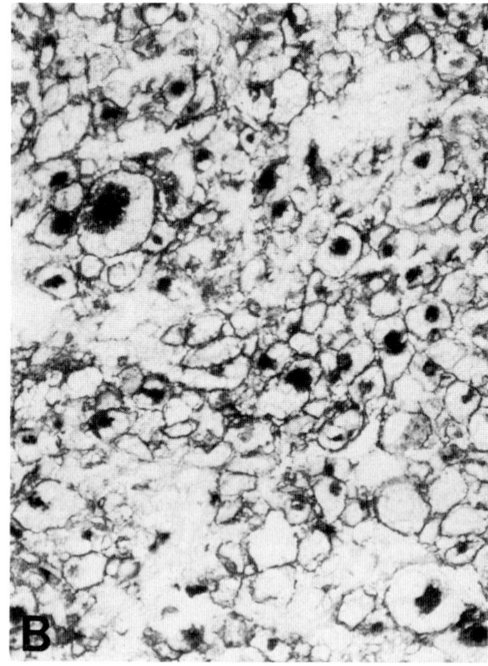

Fig. 14-5. ATL with numerous giant cells proliferation (A:H&E. × 300). Giant cells and large cells showing prominent positive staining for FTF-148 (B:ABC method. × 300).

TABLE 14-4
FTF-148 Expression in Lymphomas and Related Lesion

HTLV-1 antibody	FTF-148 +	FTF-148 −	Total
+	30[a]	3[b]	33
−	5[c]	6[d]	11
Total	35	9	44

[a] 27 cases of ATL and 3 cases of B-cell lymphoma
[b] 3 cases of ATL
[c] 3 cases of B-cell lymphoma and 2 cases of non-ATL T-cell lymphoma
[d] 6 cases of non-ATL cutaneous T-cell lymphoma

sions. It may make it possible to diagnose ATL in an early stage of smouldering and chronic cutaneous types.

PERCEPTIVES

ATL is thought to be a neoplastic process of peripheral T-cell lineage associated with HTLV-1 infection. Because HTLV-1 has no oncogene demonstrable by the recent virologic studies,[15] other genetic or environmental factors may be suspected to explain the neoplastic process. Viroepidermiologic studies suggest that ATL may occur in the HTLV-1 carriers infected vertically from the mother.[16] As in the other models of environmental carcinogenesis, the morphologic and immunologic expressions of tumor cells are heterogeneous.

But the characteristics of ATL are the pleomorphic cellular structure, and peripheral T-cell markers mostly with T4+ helper/inducer cell surface markers.

Interleukin 2(IL-2) is one of the T-cell growth factors. Some reports that peripheral blood and the cultured cells of ATL showed no IL-2 in the cells. Recently Arima reported 3 cases with IL-2 production in a short-term culture, and suggested that ATL cells in this group proliferate with autostimulation by IL-2.[12] Tokunaga et al found IL-2 expression in 20% of ATL cases in the immunohistologic study using the monoclonal antibody of DMS-3. The expression of DMS-3 and its relationship to other histologic and immunohistologic markers is interesting because these cases showed intense expression of IL-2R, suggesting autocrine mechanisms for the growth of ATL cells. Strong expression of IL-2 and IL-2R may have some correlation to the proliferation grade of neoplastic cells and clinical behavior.

In conclusion, our marker study disclosed that ATL cells can express many variable phenotypes such as helper inducer, suppressor, IL-2, as well as IL-2 receptor, even in a same cell.

REFERENCES

1. Uchiyama T, Yodoi J, Sagawa K, et al: Adult T-cell leukemia: Clinical and hematologic features of 16 cases. Blood 50:481–492, 1977
2. Hattori T, Uchiyama T, Toibana T, et al. Surface phenotype of Japanese adult T-cell leukemia cells characterized by monoclonal antibodies. Blood 58:645–647, 1891
3. Hinuma Y, Komoda H, Chosa T, et al: Antibodies to adult T-cell leukemia-virus-associated antigen-(ATLA) in sera from patients with ATL and controls in Japan: A nation-wide seroepidemiological study. Int J Cancer 29:31–635, 1982
4. Yamaguchi K, Seiki M, Yoshida M, et al: The detection of human T-cell leukemia virus proviral DNA and its applicastion for classification and diagnosis of T-cell malignancy. Blood 63:1235–1240, 1984
5. Hanoaka M, Sasaki M, Matsumoto H, et al: Adult T-cell leukemia: Histological classification and characteristics. Acta Pathol Jpn. 29:723–735, 1979
6. Suchi T, Tajima K, Nanba K, et al: Some problems on the histopathological diagnosis of non-Hodgkin's lymphoma- A proposal of a new type. Acta Pathol Jpn, 29:755–776, 1979
7. Kikuchi M, Mitsui T, Eimoto T, et al: Biopsy of adult T-cell leukemia: Adult T-cell leukemia and related disease. Jap. Sci. Soc. Press, Plenum Press, 1982, 37–50
8. Namba K, Aoki J, Sasaki N: A new enzyme immunohistochemical technique using alkaline phosphatase-laveled avidin and new fuchsin. Pathol and Clin Med 5:333–339, 1987 (in Japanese)
9. Swerdlow SH, Wright SA: The spectrum of Leu M1 staining in lymphoid and hematopoietic proliferations. Am J Clin Pathol, 85:283–288, 1986
10. Sheibani K, Battifora H, Burke JS, Rappaport H: Leu-M1 antigen in human neoplasms: An immunohistologic study of 400 cases. Am J Surg Pathol, 10:227–236, 1986

11. Uchiyama T, Hori T, Tsudo M, et al: Interleukin-2 receptor (Tac antigen) expressed on adult T-cell leukemia cells. J Clin Invest, 76:446–453, 1985
12. Arima N, Daitoku Y, Yamamoto Y, et al: Heterogeneity in response to interleukin 2 and interleukin 2 producing ability of adult T-cell leukemic cells. J Immunol 138:3069–3074, 1987
13. Smith KA, Favata MF, Oroszlan S: Production and characterization of monoclonal antibodies to human interleukin 2: Strategy and tactics. J Immunol, 131:1808–1815, 1983
14. Tsubai F, Namba Y, Kohno M, et al: A monoclonal antibody detecting a novel antigen expressed in the HTLV-1-infected cells. Blood 69:430–436, 1987
15. Seiki M, Hattori S, Hirayama Y, Yoshida M: Human adult T cell leukemia virus: complete nucleotide sequence of the provirus genome integrated in leukemia cell DNA. Proc Natl Acad Sci 80:3618–3622, 1982
16. Tajima K, Tominaga S, Suchi T. et al: Epidemiological analysis of the distribution of antibody to adult T-cell leukemia-virus-associated antigen: possible horizontal transmission of adult T-cell leukemia virus. Gann 73:893–901, 1982

15

Morphologic and Immunohistochemical Studies of Peripheral T-Cell Lymphoma Consisting of Clear Cells

Tsuyoshi Takami
Chen-Feng Qi
Akitsugu Ojima
Kokichi Kikuchi

Abstract

Nine cases of T-cell lymphoma with clusters of T-clear cells (TCCs) were studied morphologically and immunohistochemically comparing with 4 cases of diffuse lymphomas containing similar clear cells in appearance.

Histologically, it is confirmed that the clusters of TCCs are a significant landmark of certain T-cell lymphomas, though cells with abundant clear cytoplasm are rarely observed in some cell-lineages other than T-cell. All of the 9 cases showed phenotype of mature T-cells and 6 out of 9 cases had the surface-marker of helper/inducer T-cell (Th/i) subset ($CD3^+CD4^+CD8^-$) and of helper sublineage ($Leu8^-$ $2H4^-$ $4B4^+$). Moreover, because neither interleukin 2 (IL-2) nor gamma interferon (IFNγ) were detected by in situ immunohistochemistry, these TCCs were compatible with certain Th/i subset (TH2) determined by differing lymphokines productions.

It was confirmed that the combining of morphologic observations with the results of immunohistochemistry was valuable, not only for making precise diagnosis of malignant lymphomas, but also for understanding the histologic pictures.

Neoplastic T-lymphocytes with abundant "water clear" cytoplasm were first noticed by Lukes et al;[1] they categorized this type of lymphoma as T-immunoblastic lymphoma. Waldron et al[2] subsequently described peripheral T-cell lymphomas with abundant water clear cytoplasm. T-cell lymphomas with these morphologic characteristics have been classified as malignant lymphoma, large cell, immunoblastic, clear cell type in the Working Formulation.[3] Classification of peripheral T-cell lymphomas, however, is still controversial.[4] Shimoyama et al[5] proposed IBL-like T-cell lymphoma as a lymphoma of suppressor T-lymphocytes, and Watanabe et al[6] described histologic characteristics of "pale cell" clusters as a marker for differential diagnosis from immunoblastic lymphadenopathy (IBL).[7]

Their original description of "pale cell" was something different from transformed T-large cells with water clear cytoplasm by Lukes,[1,8] because the former cell was smaller and cytoplasm was not so water clear as the latter.

In this study, the main interest was to clarify the origin(s) of T-clear cell lymphoma in relationship to T-cell subsets. Takami et al wanted to know whether the histologic features correlated with the biological characteristics of lymphomas, as reflected by the production of lymphokines.

SELECTION OF T-CELL LYMPHOMA WITH CLEAR CELLS AND HISTOLOGIC VARIATION

Nine cases that showed clusters of TCCs were selected from the lymphoma files, 138 and 89 cases from the Department of Pathology in Sapporo Medical College and from Gifu University. Four other cases that showed diffuse proliferation of clear cells were also selected for comparison.

Histologic observations were made on hematoxylin and eosin (H & E) stains, periodic acid Schiff (PAS) reaction, and silver impregnation. Immunohistochemical staining with avidin-biotin-peroxidase complex (ABC) method were performed an acetone-fixed cryostat sections as well as routinely prepared paraffin sections by using commercially available mono-(MAb) and polyclonal antibodies as follows: Leu1, Leu2, Leu3, Leu4, Leu7, Leu8, Leu15, OKT3, OKT6, OKT9, OKT10, OKT11, OKI1(HLA-DR), 4B4-RD1(CDw29), MB1, MB2, MB3, MT1, LN3(HLA-DR), DAKO-UCHL1, DAKO-RSC-1(Ki-1), DAKO-PC(Ki-67), anti human DNA polymerase α (poly α) MAb, DMS-1(anti IL-2 MAb), anti IFN γ MAb (Kyowa Medex Co., Ltd.), monoclonal anti human immunoglobulin(Ig)G, IgM, IgD, κ, λ, and rabbit antisera against human IL-2 (Collaborative Res. Inc.), lysozyme(Lys), S-100 protein, α1-anti-chymotrypsin(ACT). Monoclonal antibodies, 2H4(CD45R) and anti Tac, were kind gifts of Drs. C. Morimoto (Harvard Medical School) and T. Uchiyama (Kyoto University), respectively, L-22[9] (reactive with B-CLL, small B-cells of primary follicles and mantle zone of secondary follicles) and L-26[10] (pan B-cell reactivity) were prepared in the authors' laboratory.

Retrospectively, the 9 T-clear cell cases were divided into 3 groups according to their morphologic pictures as summarized in Table 15-1. The common feature of these 3 groups was the existence of clusters of TCCs with PAS negative, abundant water-clear and well defined cytoplasms, medium to large nuclei, dispersed chromatins, 1–4 of small nucleoli. The first Group showed a unique histologic appearance, but Groups 2 and 3 were similar to previous descriptions of IBL[7] or angioimmunoblastic lymphadenopathy with dysproteinemia (AILD).[11]

The first Group (Cases 1,2) was characterized by large clusters of cohesively arranged TCCs buried in small dense, lymphocytes with active germinal centers (GCs) (2nd biopsy of Case 1, and Case 2). Silver impregnation demonstrated fine retinculin fibers surrounding TCCs clusters. Lymph node structures were relatively well preserved, and proliferation of blood vessels and amorphous eosinophilic material were obscure (Fig. 15-1A). Various cellular components other than lymphocytes were not conspicuous, but large aggregates of epithelioid cells were observed in Case 2. The TCCs had round and medium-

TABLE 15-1
Summary of Morphological and Immunohistochemical Findings of 13 Cases

case	age	sex	clear cell	admixture[‡]	eosinophilic material	increase of blood vessel
1.	59	F	cluster Th l[†]	small-B (GC)	−	obscure
2.	78	M	cluster Th s-m[†]	small-B (GC) Epi Eo	−	obscure
3.	47	F	cluster T* l	small-B GC	−	mild
4.	64	M	cluster T* l	small-B GC (B-IB, PC)	+	moderate
5.	72	F	cluster Th l	(small-B) (GC) (B-IB, PC)	+	moderate
6.	58	F	cluster Th l	various (small-B, B-IB, PC, Eo)	+	prominent
7.	77	F	cluster Th s-m	various (small-B, PC, Eo)	+	moderate
8.	80	F	(cluster) T* l	various (small-B, Mo, PC)	(+)	moderate
9.	56	M	(cluster) Th l	small-B (PC, B-IB)	+	prominent
10.	74	F	diffuse T* l	(PC)	−	mild
11.	59	F	diffuse Th m-l	(PC, Mo, PMN)	(+)	obscure
12.	65	M	diffuse B* l	GC	−	no
13.	67	M	diffuse B* m-l	small-B (GC)	−	obscure

* determined on paraffin sections (T: $MT1^+UCHL1^+L\text{-}26^-MB1^-MB2^-MB3^-$, B: $MT1^-UCKL1^-L\text{-}26^+MB1^+MB2^+MB3^+$)
[†] cell size (l: large, m: medium, s: small)
[‡] Epi: epithelioid cell, Eo: eosinophil, B-IB: B-immunoblast, PC: plasma cell, PMN: granulocyte

sized nuclei in Case 2 and in the first biopsy of Case 1, while they had larger nuclei with a few small nucleoli in the 2nd biopsy of Case 1 (Fig. 15-1B). Mitotic figures were rare in both cases.

The second Group (Cases 3, 4, 5) showed similar but smaller clusters of TCCs (Fig. 15-2), moderate proliferations of blood vessels with and without hypertrophic endothelium, and an admixture of non-lymphoid cells. Amorphous eosinophilic materials were scattered in subcapsular areas, and few burnt-out GCs occasionally with accumulations of PAS positive materials remained.

Group 3 (Cases 6, 7, 8, 9) were also characterized by small or incomplete clusters of TCCs, and the lymphocytes surrounding the TCCs were varied in size and had nuclear atypism. Proliferation of irregularly branched or hypertrophic blood vessels, an admixture of B-immunoblasts, plasma cells, and histiocytes were prominent. A few amorphous eosinophilic materials and burnt-out GCs with accumulated PAS-positive materials were occasionally present. The structures of lymph nodes were destroyed and were similar in appearance to IBL-like T-cell lymphoma[5] (Fig. 15-3).

The additional 4 cases selected for comparative study showed completely effaced lymph node structures by diffuse infiltration of lymphoma cells with pale to water clear cytoplasms and were discriminated from the former 3 groups. Cases 10 and 11 had medium to large TCCs, increased blood vessels and plasma cells, but admixtures of histiocytes and eosinophils were inconspicuous. Cases 12 and 13 showed preferential infiltration of subcapsular and interfollicular regions, and had remnants of GCs but with large, vesicular, round (Case 12) or cleaved (Case 13) nuclei and centrally located prominent nucleoli. Increase of blood vessels and polymorphous cellular components were not evident.

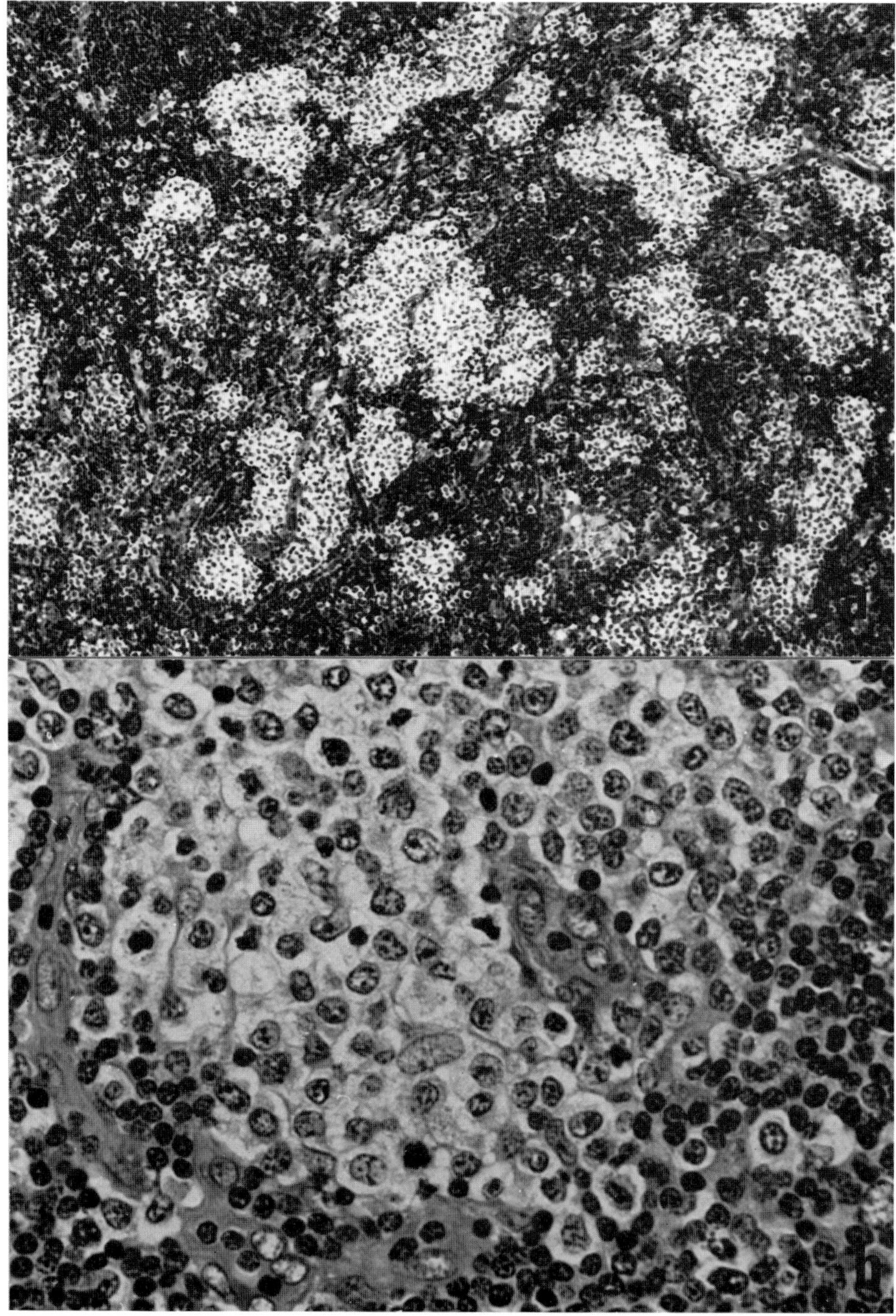

Fig. 15-1A & B. Histologic features of Case 1 (2nd biopsy) (H&E). The clusters of TCCs are buried in the small lymphocytes and make large clusters of TCCs (a, × 10). TCCs have abundant well demarcated, water clear cytoplasms and round nuclei with stippled chromatin and a few small nucleoli (b, × 132).

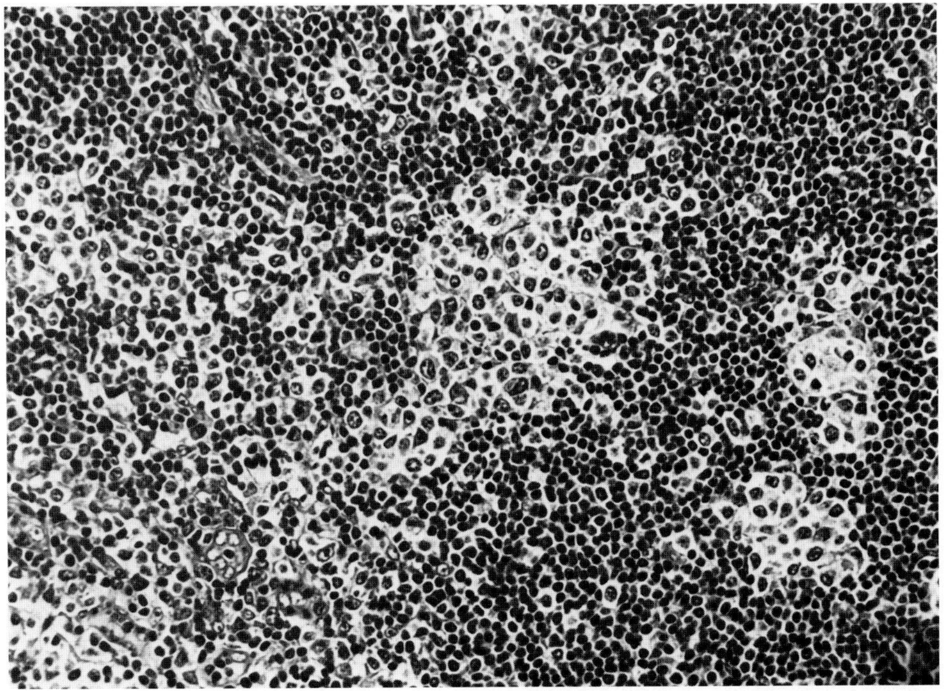

Fig. 15-2. Smaller and/or incomplete clusters of TCCs are characteristic of Group 2 (Case 3, H&E, × 25).

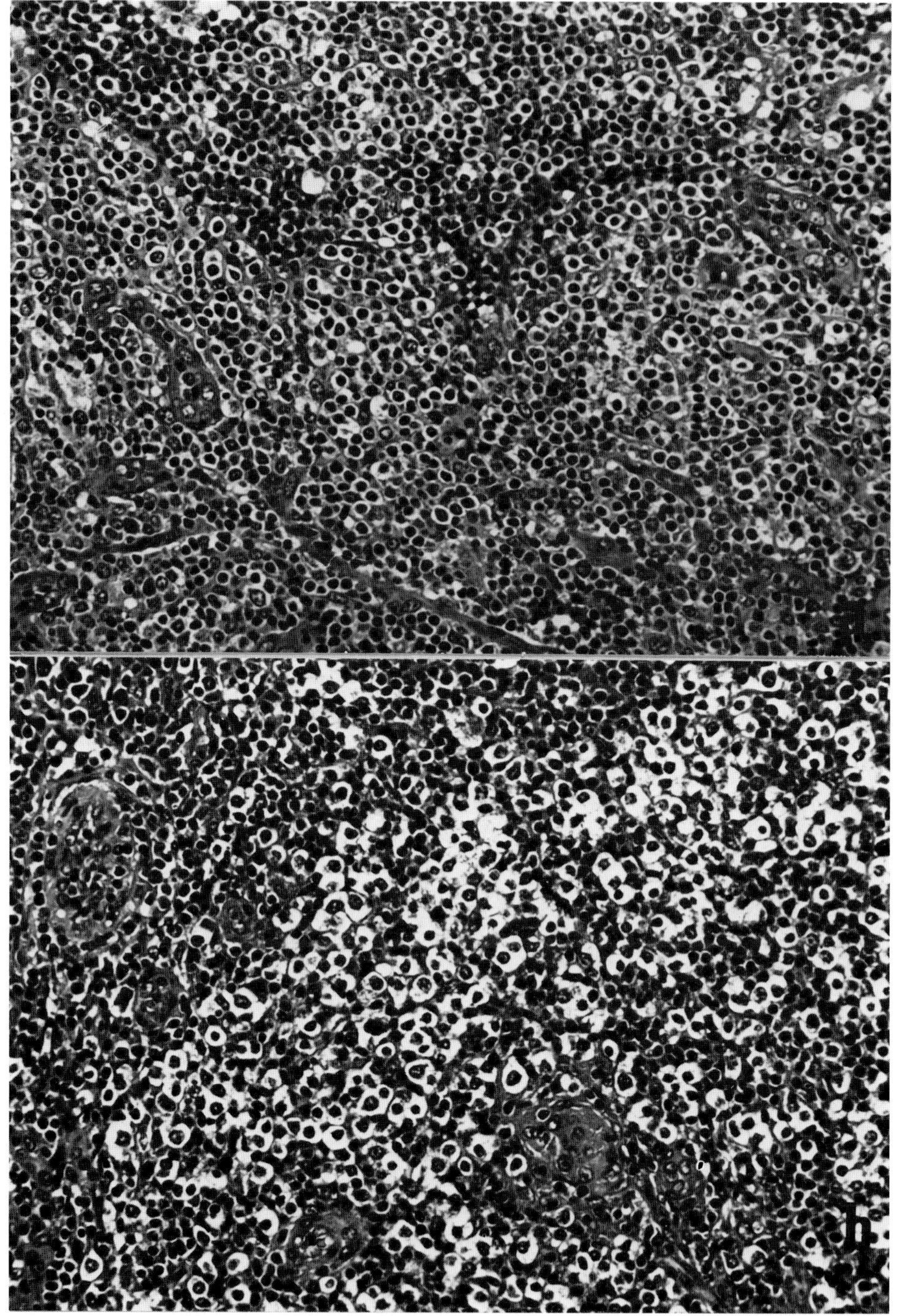

Fig. 15-3A & B. Morphologic features of Group 3 (H&E, × 25). TCCs have well demarcated cell borders, and increase of blood vessels was more prominent in Case 7 (a) than in Case 9 (b).

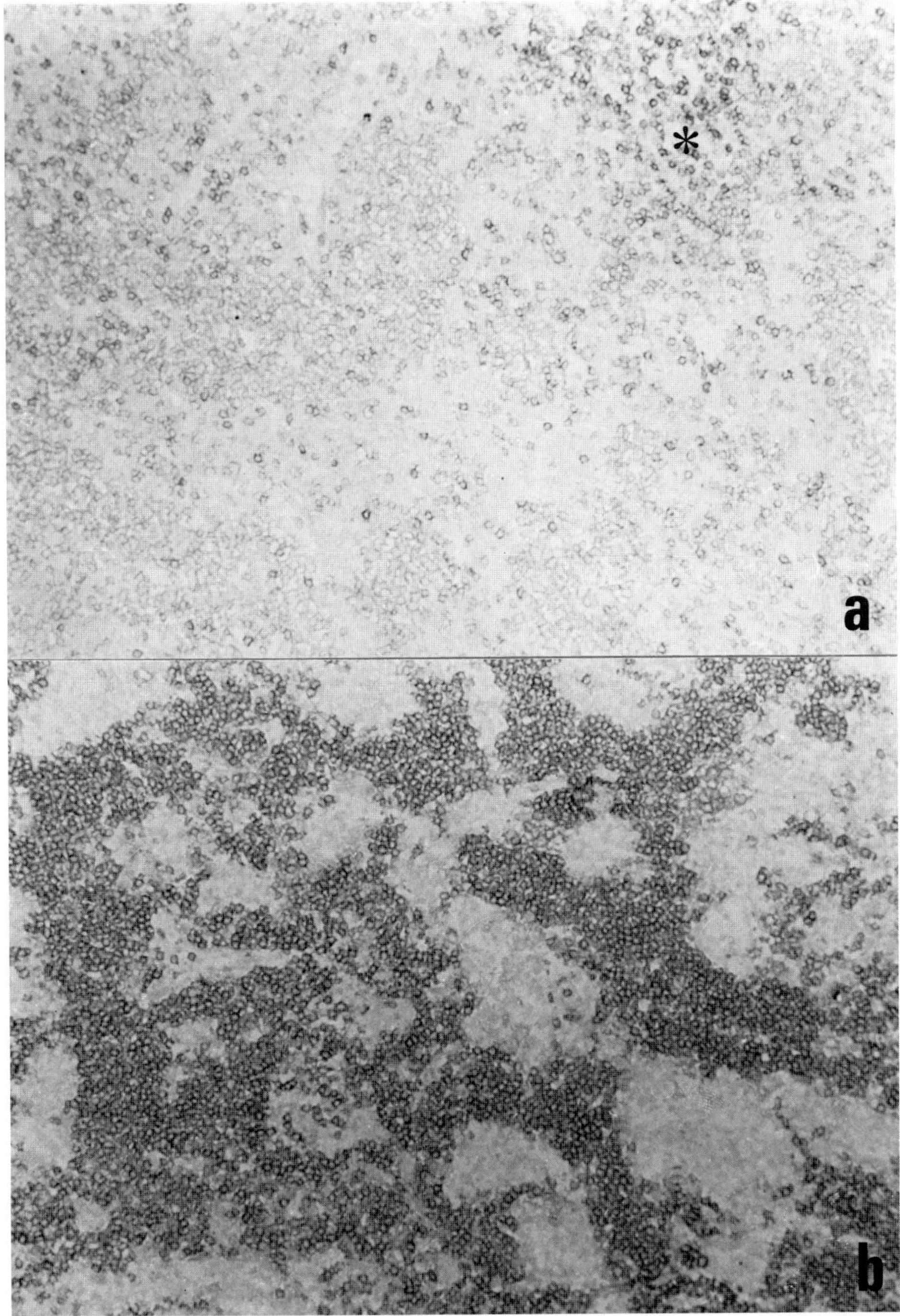

Fig. 15-4A & B. Immunochemistry of Case 1. (counter stain: methyl green, × 13.2) TCCs making clusters had the phenotype of Th/i, but staining intensities by Leu3, Leu4, OKT3, OKT11 were weaker than the small T-lymphocytes (*) as well as Leu1 (a). Most of the small lymphocytes surrounding the TCCs were polyclonal B-cells (b:L-26).

IMMUNOPHENOTYPING OF CLEAR CELLS

The immunophenotypic profiles of clear cells are summarized in Table 15-2. The clusters of clear cells in 3 groups, Cases 10 and 11 had the phenotype of T-cells, while Cases 12 and 13 were B-cell derived. Six cases having TCCs clusters, in which frozen tissues were available, revealed the phenotype of Th/i subset ($CD2^+CD3^+$ $CD5^+CD^+CD8^-$) (Fig. 15-4A). The majority of their TCCs had some activation associated antigens (OKT9, OKT10, HLA-DR) and markers of cell cycling (Ki-67, poly α), while neither Tac nor Ki-1 were expressed. TCCs of these 6 cases were $Leu8^-$, $2H4^-$, $4B4^+$, $IFN\gamma^-$, $IL\text{-}2^-$, and these phenotypes were compatible with a helper subset[12–14] and TH2 type[15] of Th/i. Segami et al[16] described such $Leu3^+$ $Leu8^-$ T-cells distributed in GCs of secondary follicles which may be their normal counterpart.

Most small lymphocytes surrounding TCCs in Groups 1 and 2 had the phenotype of small B-cells ($IgM^+IgD^+L\text{-}22^+L\text{-}26^+$) (Fig. 15-4B), and showed polyclonal proliferation as well as intermingled B-immunoblasts and plasma cells. In Group 3, many atypical lymphocytes around TCCs were confirmed to be T-cells, and B-cells were polyclonal as in former groups.

Chromosomal analysis of lymph node cells obtained from Cases 1, 5, and 9 disclosed a clonal abnormality in Case 1; 46, XX, −1, +der(1)t(1:?)(p36:?), and normal karyotypes in the latter cases. The abnormalities of 1p were significantly more frequent in T-cell rather than B-cell lymphomas, and the most frequent change was a translocation of an unknown chromosome segment to 1p36 as was Case 1.[17] The other abnormalities associated and correlated with T-cell lymphoma,[17] such as breaks in 6p, 14q11–13 abnormalities, trisomy 3 and 5, occurence of multiple clones, rearrangements in the long arms of chromosome 4, 7, and 15, were not observed.

Serum antibody against HTLV-I was negative in 7 cases of 3 groups, though cases 2 and 3 were not examined. In Case 2, antihistoplasma and toxoplasma antibodies in sera were within normal titers. None of 9 cases (Groups 1–3) had history of drug abuse nor any kind of medication prior to their development of lymphoma.

MEANING OF CLUSTERS OF TCCS

Takami et al concluded that the clusters of TCCs were a significant landmark of certain T-cell lymphomas, even though rare cases of B-cell lymphomas also had cells with abun-

TABLE 15-2
Summary of Marker Profile of T-Clear Cell

case	panT*	CD4*	CD8	2H4	4B4	Leu8	Leu15	HLA-DR	OKT9	OKT10	Tac	Ki-1	IFN_γ	IL-2
1.	+	+	−	−	+	−	−	(+)	++	+	−	−	−	−
2.	+	+	−	−	+	−	−	(+)	(+)	+	−	−	−	−
3.†								(+)‡						
4.†								(+)‡						
5.	+	+	−	−	+	−	−	(+)	+	+	−	−	−	−
6.	+	+	−	−	+	−	−	(+)	+	+	−	−	−	−
7.	+	+	−	−	+	−	−	(+)	+	+	−	−	−	−
8.†								(+)‡						
9.	+	+	−	−	+	−	−	(+)	+	+	−	−	−	−

* MAbs used were, pan T: Leu1, Leu4, OKT11, CD4: Leu3, CD8: Leu2
† $MTI^+UCHL1^+MB1^-MB2^-MB3^-L\text{-}26^-Igs^-Lys^-ACT^-S100^-$ on routine paraffin sections
‡ $LN3^+$ on paraffin sections

dant pale to clear cytoplasms (Cases 12 and 13). The so-called "clear cell" was first described by Suchi,[18] and lymphomas with clear cells were clarified to be of T-cell origin.[2,5,6,8,19] Shimoyama et al[5] and Watanabe[6] et al described pale cell, that was similar but somewhat different from TCCs, as a signficiant characteristic to discriminate IBL-like T-cell lymphoma from IBL and AILD. The terms "clear cell,"[4] "pale cell,"[5,6] and T-immunoblast[1] had been used to describe morphologically similar, but not exactly the same cells; however, their relationship and the position(s) in T-cell differentiation have not been fully understood.

Plasmacyatoid T-cell (PTC)[20,21] and "monocytoid" B lymphocyte (MBL)[22] also showed similar nest-like accumulations or clusters of proliferating cells as TCCs. Essentially, PTCs were composed of medium-sized cells with round nuclei, prominent nucleoli, relatively abundant, but faintly eosinophilic, cytoplasm. MBLs were distributed in subcapsular and parenchymal sinuses, and had medium-sized, oval, but mostly indented, nuclei, coarse chromatin, inconspicuous nucleoli, pale or clear cytoplasms with fine PAS-positive granules, and thus they were distinguishable from clusters of TCCs.

The polyclonal proliferation of small B-cells, B-immunoblasts, and plasma cells could be attributed to the functions of lymphoma cells, because pehnotypes of the authors' 6 cases were compatible to TH2 type of Th/i subset, which was originally distinguished by its helper functions in the immunoglobulin synthesis of B-cells from the other sublineage of Th/i subset (TH1), and now could be identified by differences in lymphokine production.[15,23] However, in this study Takami et al could demonstrate only the lack of production of IL-2 and IFNλ. The synthesis of other lymphokines that TH2-cells might produce has to be examined for further confirmation.

Although the 5 cases of Groups 1 and 2, especially cases 1 and 2, showed unique histologic pictures, it remains a controversial issue whether to reclassify them as a novel subtype of peripheral T-cell lymphoma. Peripheral T-cell lymphomas can show extremely diverse morphologic appearances,[4,24] and the same case can exhibit remarkable histologic changes over time.[25] Thus, to resolve this problem, more cases as well as long-term followup data are needed.

REFERENCE

1. Lukes RJ, Collins RD: A functional approach to the classification of malignant lymphoma. Recent Results Cancer Res 46:18–30, 1974
2. Waldron JA, Leech JH, Glick AD, et al: Malignant lymphoma of peripheral T-lymphocyte origin. Immunologic pathologic, and clinical features in six patients. Cancer 40:1604–1617, 1977
3. The non-Hodgkin's lymphoma pathologic classification project: National Cancer Institute sponsored study of classification of non-Hodgkin's lymphomas; Summary and description of a Working Formulation for clinical usage. Cancer 49:2112–2135, 1982
4. Suchi T, Lennert K, Tu LY, et al: Histopathology and immunohistochemistry of peripheral T-cell lymphomas: A proposal for their classification. J Clin Pathol 40:995–1015, 1987
5. Shimoyama M, Minato K, Saito H, et al: Immunoblastic lymphadenopathy (IBL)-like T-cell lymphoma. Jpn J Clin Oncol 9:347–356, 1979
6. Watanabe S, Shimosato Y, Shimoyama M, et al: Adult T-cell lymphoma with hypergammaglobulinemia. Cancer 46:2472–2483, 1980
7. Lukes RJ, Tindle BH: Immunoblastic lymphadenopathy. A hyperimmune entity resembling Hodgkin's disease. N Engl J Med 292:1–8, 1975
8. Lukes RJ, Tindle BH: Immunoblastic lymphadenopathy: A prelymphomatous state of immunoblastic sarcoma. Recent Results Cancer Res 64:241–246, 1978
9. Takami T, Ishii Y, Yuasa H, Kikuchi K: Three distinct antigen systems on human B cell subpopulations as defined by monoclonal antibodies. J Immunol 134:828–834, 1985
10. Ishi Y, Takami T, Yuasa H, et al: Two distinct antigen systems in human B lymphocytes: Identification of cell surface and intracellular antigens using monoclonal antibodies. Clin Exp Immunol 58:183–192, 1984
11. Frizzera G, Moran EM, Rappaport H: Angio-immunoblastic lymphadenopathy with dysproteinaemia. Lancet 1:1070–1073, 1974
12. Gatenby PA, Kansas GS, Xian CY, et al: Dissection of immunoregulatory subpopulations of T lymphocytes within the helper and suppressor sublineages in man. J Immunol 129:1997–2000, 1982
13. Morimoto C, Letvin NL, Distaso JA, et al: The isolation and characterization of the human suppressor inducer T cell subset. J Immunol 134:1508–1515, 1985

14. Morimoto C, Letvin NL, Boyd AW, et al: The isolation and characterization of the human helper inducer T cell subset. J Immunol 134:3762–3769, 1985
15. Mosman TR, Cherwinski H, Bond MW, et al: Two types of murine helper T-cell clone. I. Definition according to profiles of lymphokine activities and secreted proteins. J Immunol 136:2348–2357, 1986
16. Segami H, Abe M, Wakasa H: Peripheral T-cell lymphoma with helper T-cell phenotype ($Leu3a^+$ $Leu8^-$). Acta Pathol Jpn 38:591–603, 1988
17. Correlation of chromosome abnormalities with histologic and immunologic characteristics in non-Hodgkin's lymphoma and adult T-cell leukemia-lymphona. By the fifth international workshop on chromosomes in leukemia-lymphoma. Blood 70:1554–1564, 1987
18. Suchi T: Atypical lymph node hyperplasia with fatal outcome: A report on the histopathological, immunological and clinical investigation of the cases. Rec Adv RES Res 14:12–34, 1974
19. Said JW, Pinkus GS: Immunoblastic sarcoma of the T-cell type. An ultrastructural study of five cases. Am J Pathol 101:515–526, 1980
20. Lennert K, Kaiserling E, Müller-Hermelink HK: T-associated plasma cells. Lancet 1:1031–1032, 1975
21. Müller-Hermelink HK, Steinmann G, Stein H, Lennert K: Malignant lymphoma of plasmacytoid T-cells. Morphologic and immunologic studies characterizing a special type of T-cell. Am J Pathol 7:849–862, 1983
22. Sheibani K, Fritz RM, Winberg CD, et al: "Monocytoid" cells in reactive follicular hyperplasia with and without multifocal histiocytic reactions: An immunohistochemical study of 21 cases including suspected cases of toxoplasmic lymphadenitis. Am J Clin Pathol 81:453–458, 1984
23. Mosman TR, Coffman RL: Two types of mouse helper T-cell clone. Implications for immune regulation. Immunology Today 8:223–227, 1987
24. Knowles DM, Halper JP: Human T-cell malignancies. Correlative clinical, histopathologic, immunologic, and cytochemical analysis of 23 cases. Am J Pathol 106:187–203, 1982
25. Winberg CD, Sheibani K, Krance R, Rappaport H: Peripheral T-cell lymphoma: Immunologic and cell-kinetic observations associated with morphological progression. Blood 66:980–989, 1985

16

Immunoelectron Microscopic Studies on T-Cell Lymphomas

Mikihiro Shamoto

Abstract

Ultrastructural characteristics of T-cell lymphomas were studied using the immunoperoxidase technique. The majority of the peripheral T-cell lymphomas belonged to T4 types, and T8 types were minority. In these lymphomas, only the plasma membranes were positive for T4 or T8. However, their plasma membranes and the rough endoplasmic reticulum and perinuclear cisternae were positive for T3. All the cases of adult T-cell leukemias/lymphomas were T4 types, but some of the cases were T4/T8 types, namely the appearance of double-marker neoplastic cells having both T4 and T8 antigens or an admixture of T4 and T8 neoplastic cells were suggested. Tac antigen and FTF 148 antigen were rather specific for adult T-cell leukemias/lymphomas. The former was positive on the plasma membrane, the rough endoplasmic reticulum, Golgi cisternae, and perinuclear cisternae, while the latter was positive on the plasma membrane, particularly Golgi apparatus and sometimes the rough endoplasmic reticulum. All the mycosis fungoides cases were T4 types, and mycosis fungoides cells were negative for TAC and FTF 148. In the lymphoblastic type lymphomas, T3, T4, T6, and T8 positive cells were mixed at the various combinations.

The development of techniques for the production of monoclonal antibodies is very valuable, not only for accurate diagnosis, but also for the selection of the kind of treatment against lymphoid neoplasms.[1–3] It is no exaggeration to say that the prognosis of malignant lymphomas depends on the establishment of accurate diagnosis before treatment is commenced. There have been many studies relative to malignant lymphomas including many on T-cell tumors, in which monoclonal antibodies have been prepared.[4–6] However, the majority of these studies have been carried out at the light microscopic level. At the light microscopic level, there are serious doubts as to whether the localization of the positive reaction is truly only on the plasma membrane, in the cytoplasm, both on the plasma membrane and in the cytoplasm, or in the nucleus.

A method for the conjugation of peroxidase to antibody was first successfully adapted to electron microscopy by Nakane et al.[7] This method has since been improved by Leduc et al[8] and others.[9–12] With the improvement of immunoperoxidase methods, innumoelectron microscopic studies have also been performed. Immunoelectron microscopy can contribute to our studies by demonstrating positive localization beyond the resolution of the light microscope, and the ultrastructural localization of these antibodies can eventually be of great value for understanding of their biological significance.[13–16] Namely, the nature, and the process of the production of each antibody can be inferred by means of the characteristics of both immunoelectron microscopy and its biological features.

METHOD FOR IMMUNOELECTRON MICROSCOPY

Fifty cases of T-cell lymphomas were used for this study. The materials used were biopsy specimens of lymph nodes including adult T-cell leukemia/lymphoma(ATLL), and in some cases, mycosis fungoides (2 cases). In some of the cases of ATLL(7 cases), and all of the cases of mycosis fungoides(8 cases), sections were also prepared from skin biopsy specimens. The available antibodies used were as follows: OKT-3/Leu 4, OKT-4/Leu 3a, OKT-6, OKT-8, Tac, and FTF 148. FTF 148 antibody was prepared by Namba et al,[17] and it reacted with human T-cell leukemia virus I-infected cell lines. Biopsy specimens were fixed in periodate-lysine-paraformaldehyde and from these, frozen sections of 10 μ thickness were cut. The sections were placed on slides, and overlayed with the appropriately diluted monoclonal antibodies and incubated in a humidified chamber at room temperature for 2 hours. They were washed in 2–3 changes of cold PBS containing 10% sucrose for one hour at 4°C. Then they were incubated with biotinylated horse anti-mouse IgG for 2 hours, and in both an avidin-biotinylated peroxidase complex and a peroxidase mouse anti-peroxidase complex for 2 hours. Sections were rinsed in PBS after each of these incubations. They were fixed in 2% glutaraldehyde and then incubated with DAB hydrogen peroxide according to the method of Graham and Karnovsky,[18] and postfixed in 2% OsO4 for 1–2 hours. After dehydration in a graded series of alcohols, sections were embedded by the inverted gelatin capsule method.[19] Ultrathin sections were cut with a diamond knife on an LKB Ultratome, and both unstained sections and sections stained with uranyl acetate lead citrate were examined with Jeolco 100 CX electron microscope.

PERIPHERAL T-CELL LYMPHOMA WITH THE EXCEPTION OF ATLL AND MYCOSIS FUNGOIDES

The majority of the peripheral T-cell lymphomas were T4 positive (14/19 cases), although some cases were T8 positive (5/19 cases). Larger cells with irregularly shaped nuclei considered to be neoplastic, were positive either for and T4 and T8. However, in three cases of T4 type lymphomas, some of the T8 positive cells were also large and showed nuclear irregularity. Shamoto and colleagues concluded that these 3 cases were T4/T8 type lymphomas. This will be discussed later. Both the T4 and T8 types were only positive on the plasma membranes of the lymphoma cells (Figs. 16-1 and 16-2). Both T4 and T8 type lymphomas were, of course, positive for T3 (Fig. 16-3). Both the plasma membranes, and also the endoplasmic reticulum and perinuclear cisternae were positively stained with T3. It was therefore speculated that the T3 antigen may have been produced in the ribosomes and then have moved into the plasma membranes.

The nuclei of T4 type lymphomas were more irregular in outline than those of T8 type lymphomas. T8 type lymphoma cells possessed in their cytoplasm scattered dense bodies encircled by distinct membranes inter-

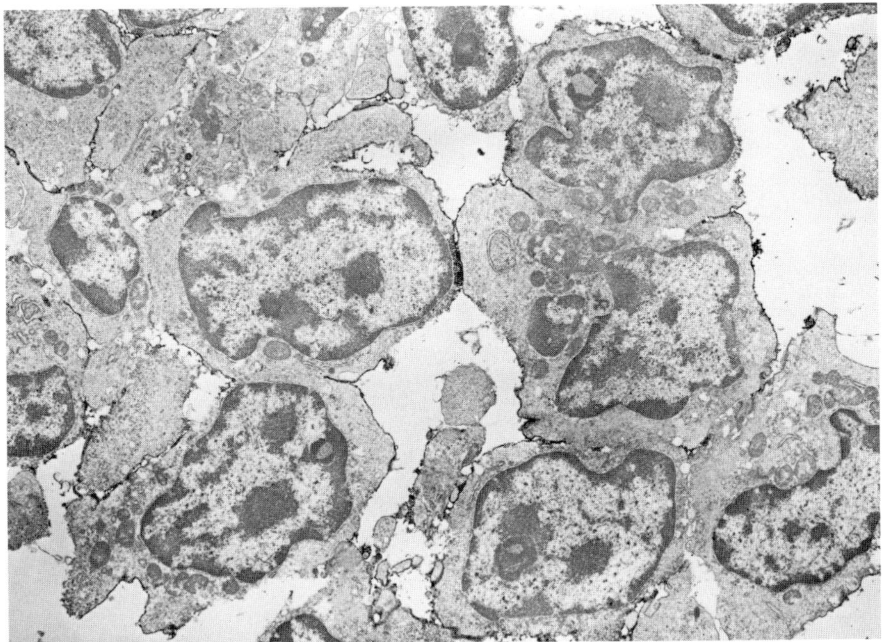

Fig. 16-1. A T4 type lymphoma. The cells express T4 antigen on the plasma membranes (× 4,300).

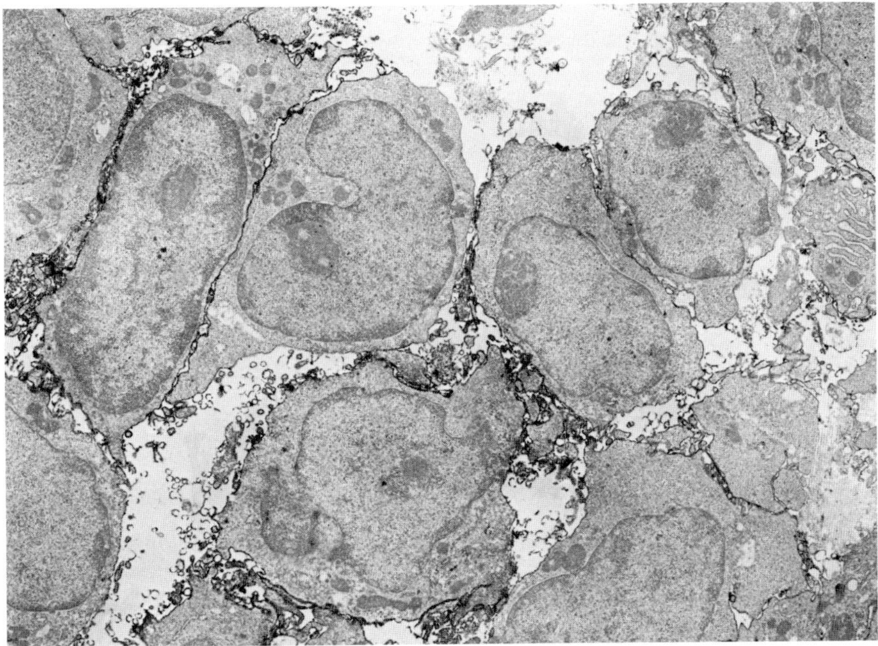

Fig. 16-2. A T8 typc lymphoma. The plasma membranes of neoplastic cells are positive with T8 (× 4,300).

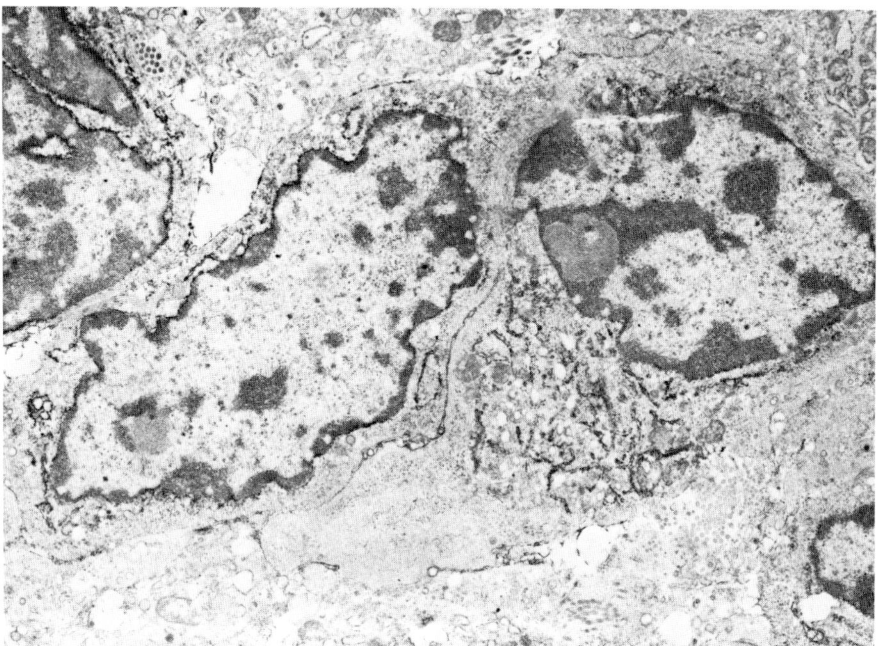

Fig. 16-3. A T4 type lymphoma. Not only are the plasma membranes positive with T3, but the rough endoplasmic reticulum and nuclear membranes are also positively stained with it (× 6,500).

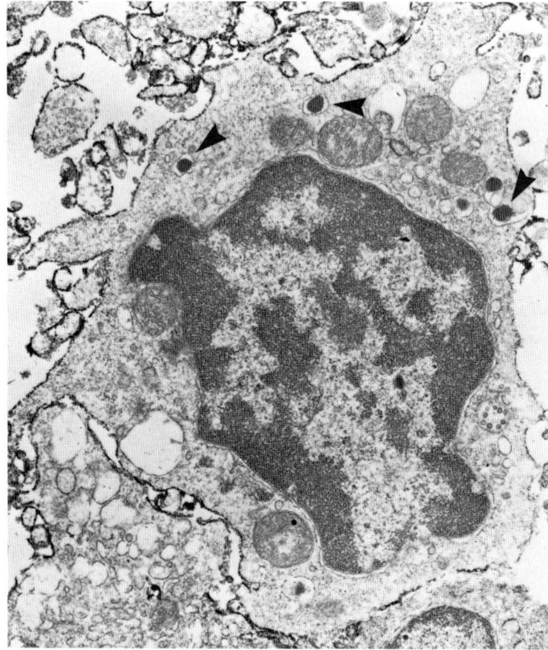

Fig. 16-4. A T8 type lymphoma. Dense bodies encircled by distinct membranes are found (arrows) (× 13,000).

spersed with narrow lucent zones (Fig. 16-4), and also clustered dense bodies that could serve as morphologic markers for T cells.[20] As has already been reported,[14,15] the lucent zones in these scattered dense bodies could not usually be observed in ordinary sections that were fixed with a mixture of glutaraldehyde and paraformaldehyde and postfixed in OsO4. This discrepancy may have been due to different fixatives. It is presumed that these scattered dense bodies are characteristic for T8 type lymphomas. On the other hand, T4 positive lymphoma cells had only clustered dense bodies.

In T4 type lymphomas, non-neoplastic T8 positive small cells were observed to a varying degree with the electron microscope. Similarly in the T8 type lymphomas, T4 positive cells, smaller and their nuclei less irregular than the neoplastic cells, were admixed.

ADULT T-CELL LEUKEMIA/ LYMPHOMA (ATLL)

All except one of the 20 cases of ATLL were T4 type lymphomas. The nuclei were markedly convoluted or indented in shape and the nuclear indentation of some cells pointed in only one direction. Figure 16-5A shows the scheme of an ATLL cell. The CDB means clustered dense bodies, TRS is tubuloreticular structures and NP shows the nuclear pocket. Shamoto and coworkers described[20,21] that CDB, NP, TRS, and sometimes test-tube and ring-shaped forms were peculiar for ATLL. Figure 16-5B shows a cerebriform cell that is characteristic of mycosis fungoides and/or ATLL.

Tac antigen was positive on the plasma membranes in some cells of the characteristic pleomorphic cells but negative in others. However, the greater part of the blastic cells were positive, not only on the plasma membranes, but also on the cisternae of the rough endoplasmic reticulum, Golgi cisternae, and perinuclear cisternae (Figure 16-6). It was previously reported[16] that when the plasma membranes were positive, it meant a membrane associated mature interleukin 2 receptor, and the positivity of rough endoplasmic reticulum, nuclear membranes, and Golgi complex was a precursor for an interleukin 2 receptor. All ATLL cells in the lymph nodes were positive for Tac. However, 2 of the 7 cases of skin biopsy specimens were negative for Tac. This appeared to be dependent on the fact that there were few infiltrating neoplastic cells, and the majority of the neoplastic cells were pleomorphic cells and blastic neoplastic cells were few in the skin.

In 2 cases, as has already been published,[14,15] the neoplastic cells were stained with both T4 and T8. The surface antigen

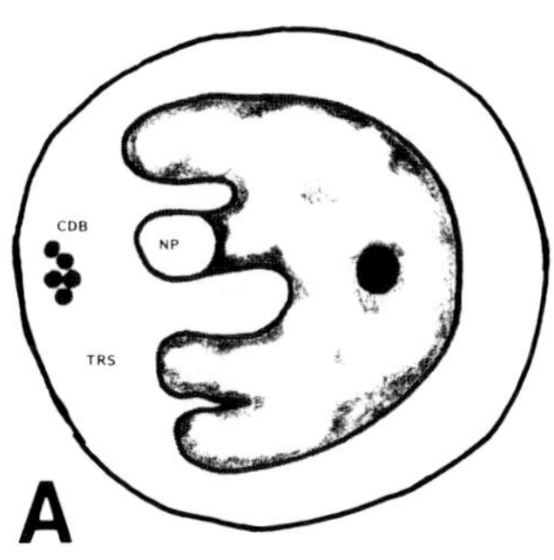

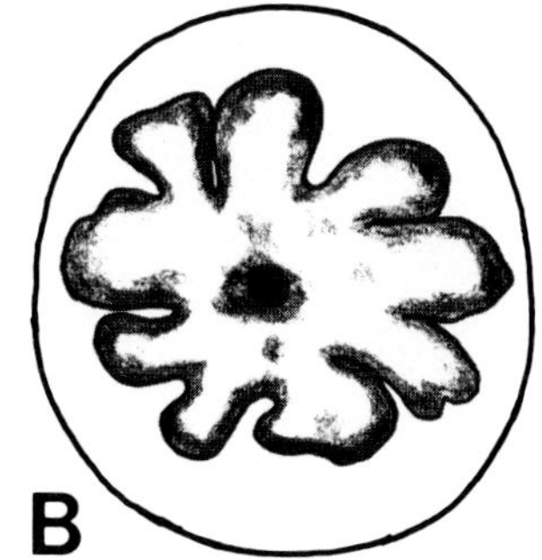

Fig. 16-5. (A) Schematic diagrams illustrating an ATLL cell, and (B) a mycosis fungoides and/or an ATLL cell. CDB: clustered dense body. TRS: tubuloreticular structure. NP: nuclear pocket.

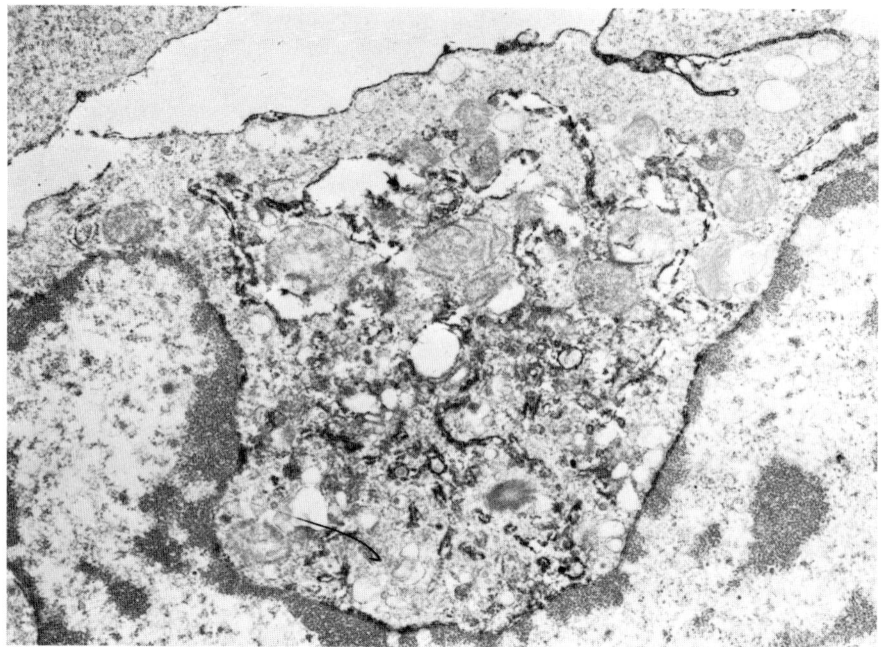

Fig. 16-6. An ATLL case. Not only the plasma membranes, but also the rough endoplasmic reticulum, Golgi apparatus, and nuclear membranes are stained with anti-Tac antibody (× 13,000).

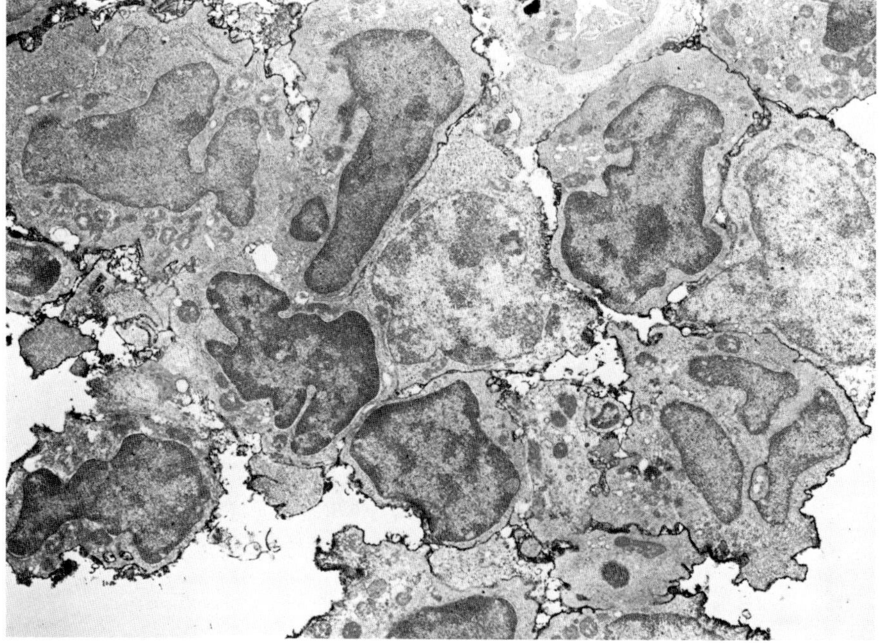

Fig. 16-7. An ATLL case. T4 positive neoplastic cells are seen (× 4,300).

analyses on cell suspension of these tumors revealed that the sum of the percentages of T4 positive and T8 positive cells exceeded 100%. Almost all the neoplastic cells were stained with the T4 antibody (Fig. 16-7), while a slightly smaller number of the cells were stained with the T8 antibody (Fig. 16-8), indicating that many of the cells reacted with both T4 and T8 antibodies, that is, double-marker cells were present. The author likes to call these case T4/T8 type lymphomas.

One case was observed in which most of the neoplastic cells expressed T8 antigen in the early phase of the disease, and gradually T4 positive tumor cells increased with the progress of the disease. Immunoelectron microscopically neoplastic cells at the late stage were positive for both T4 and T8. This case therefore was considered to represent T4/T8 type lymphoma in which biphenotypic expression became apparent with the progression of the disease.

Ultrastructurally, T8 positive cells were again carefully observed in all ATLL cases, in which cell suspension study of the neoplastic cells revealed T4 predominance, but addition of T4 and T8 positive percentage was less than 100%. In one of the ATLL cases, the percentages of T4 and T8 were 44% and 18%, respectively. However, some of the T8 positive cells were large and had irregularly shaped nuclei. There were a few T8 positive cells in metaphase. This case was classified as T4/T8 type lymphoma. It was therefore concluded that 4 cases of the ATLL cases were T4/T8 type lymphomas. In these cases, the appearance of "double-marker" cells, which had both T4 and T8 antigens and/or an admixture of T4 and T8 neoplastic cells, was suggested.

In 6 of the ATLL cases, the localization of FTF 148 antigen was also examined. In cultured cells derived from ATLL patients, KUT-2, Hut 102, and MT-2 cells, FTF 148

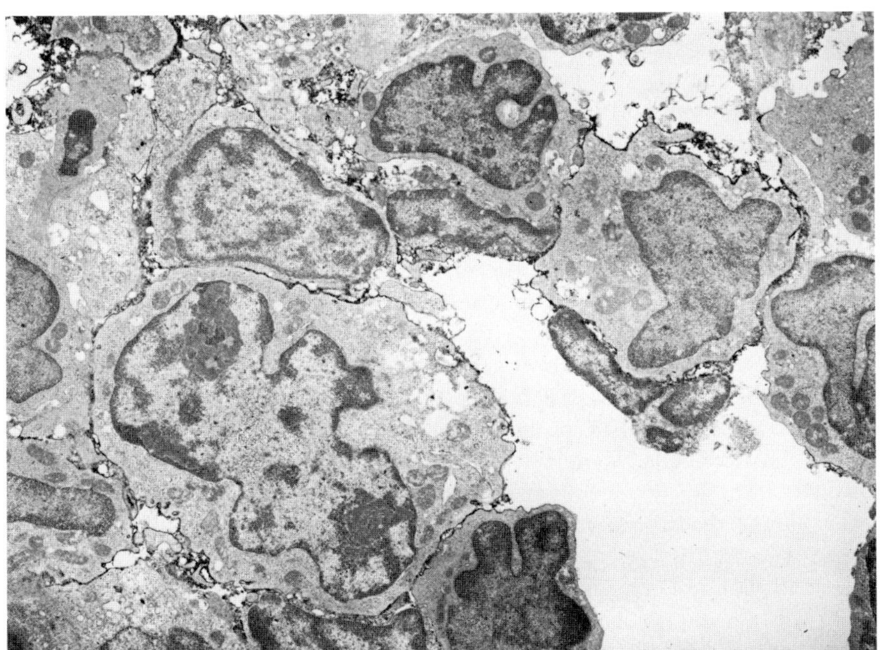

Fig. 16-8. The same case as Figure 16-7. T8 positive cells seem to be also neoplastic (× 4,300).

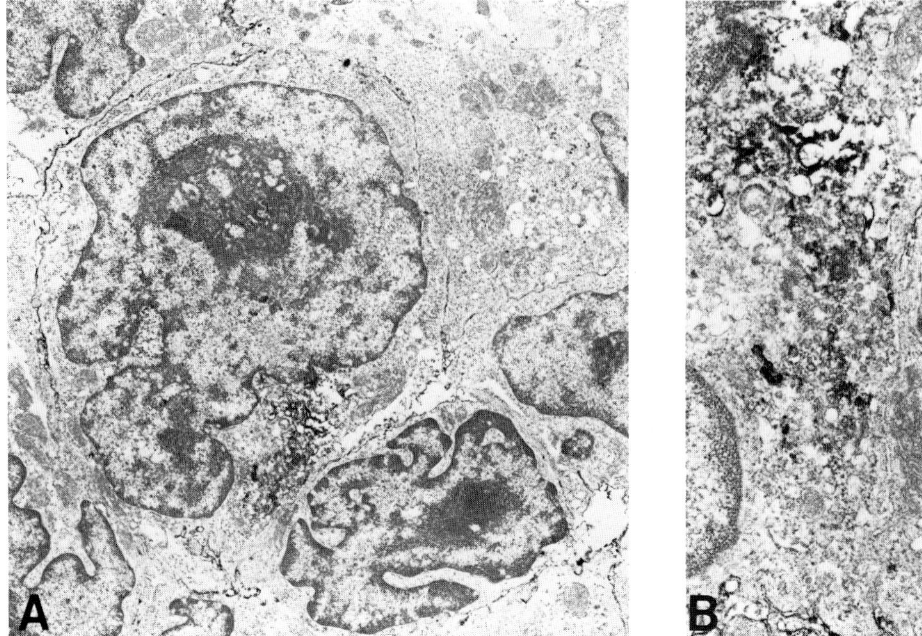

Fig. 16-9. An ATLL case. Both plasma membranes and Golgi apparatrus are positive for FTF 148 antibody (× 4,300). On the right, high magnification of Golgi area of the left photograph (× 13,000).

was mainly expressed on the plasma membranes, and sometimes also on the Golgi apparatus, rough endoplasmic reticulum and nuclear membranes. Virus particles in the cytoplasm and in the cytoplasmic vesicular structures were negative, although the outer membranes of the mature particles of extracellular space were positive. It was therefore speculated that this antigen was not a viral antigen, but a product of certain cellular genes of HTLV-I.[17] Although the number of positive cells amounted to less than 10% of the total, all cases had positive cells. Some cells were only positive on the plasma membranes, but the greater part of the others, especially the rather large blastic cells, were positive on Golgi cisternae, Golgi vesicles and sometimes the rough endoplasmic reticulum near the Golgi complex. In some cells, both the plasma membrances and Golgi complex were stained with FTF 148 antibody (Fig. 16-9).

MYCOSIS FUNGOIDES

The mycosis cells in the skin of the eight cases of mycosis fungoides had the most irregular nuclei of all the T-cell lymphomas. All the cases of mycosis fungoides were T4 type lymphomas (Fig. 16-10). Four cases of mycosis fungoides were stained with FTF 148 antibody. Positive cells in mycosis fungoides cases have not been found so far, although infiltrating neoplastic cells are few in the skin of mycosis fungoides. The expression of FTF 148 antibody may differentiate ATLL cells from mycosis fungoides cells in the skin. Fur-

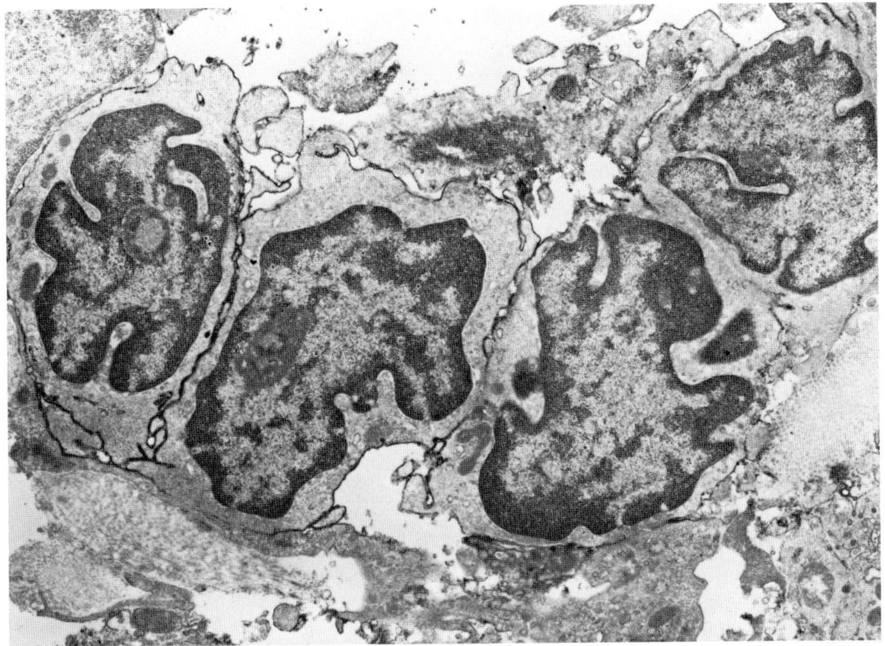

Fig. 16-10. A mycosis fungoides case. The plasma membranes are positively stained with T4 (× 6,500).

ther investigation of mycosis fungoides cases are needed for greater clarification. Mycosis cells were neither T8 positive, nor Tac positive. And needless to say, all cases were positive for T3.[15] The pattern of positive reaction was apparently identical with other T-cell lymphomas. In the lymph node biopsies of 2 cases, typical cells with convoluted nuclei could be observed. They also reacted with both T3 and T4. In the cases of ATLL and mycosis fungoides, Langerhans cells containing Birbeck granules that were positive for OKT-6 could often be found in the lymph nodes and in the dermis, into which the neoplastic cells were infiltrating.[22] It has been speculated that Langerhans cells have a function as antigen-presenting cells to T lymphocytes. This appearance of Langerhans cells in ATLL and mycosis fungoides may indicate the close relationship between Langerhans cells and neoplastic T lymphocytes.

LYMPHOBLASTIC TYPE LYMPHOMA

Ten cases of lymphoblastic type lymphomas were immunohistologically examined. Three cases were T3 positive, and 2 cases were T3, T4, T6, and T8 positive; the rest were single cases, T3, T6, and T8 positive; T3, T4, and T6 positive; T3 and T4 positive; T3 and T8 positive; and T3, T4, and T8 positive. The last 3 cases were available for immunoelectron microscopic studies. T6 positive cells have not been observed by electron microscopy. T4 type, T8 type, and T4/T8 type (Fig. 16-11) lymphomas were ultrastructurally examined. The positive patterns were identical with other T-cell lymphomas. It has been speculated that lymphoid cells at various stages of maturity may develop into malignant lymphomas in lymphoblastic type lymphomas.

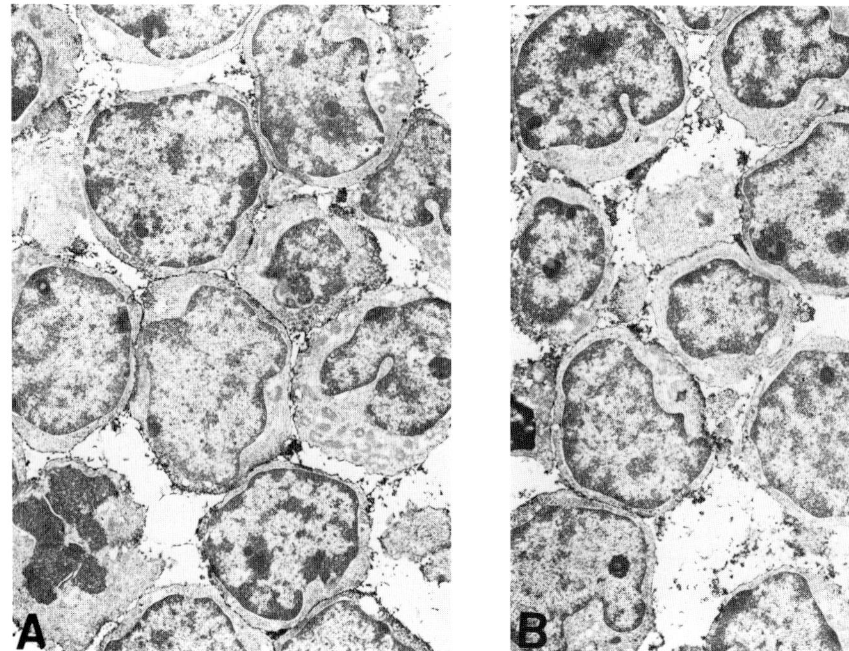

Fig. 16-11A & B. A lymphoblastic type lymphoma case. On the left, the neoplastic cells are positive for T4. On the right, T8 positive neoplastic cells are seen (× 3,400).

REFERENCES

1. Köhler G, Milstein G: Continuous cultures of fused cells secreting antibody of peripheral specificity. Nature 256:495–497, 1975
2. Ledoetter JA, Evans RL, Lipinski M, et al: Evolutionary conservation of surface molecules that distinguish T lymphocyte helper/inducer and cytotoxic/suppressor subpopulations in mouse and man. J Exp Med 153:310–323, 1981
3. Reinzherz EL, Kung PC, Goldstein G, Levey RH: Discrete stages of human intrathymic differentiation: Analysis of normal thymocytes and leukemic lymphoblasts of T-cell lineage. Proc Natl Acad Sci 77:1588–1592, 1980
4. Giorno RC: Immunohistology and Histochemistry of the Lymphoid System. Springfield, Illinois, Charles C Thomas, 1984
5. Sun T, Li CY, Yam LT: Atlas of Cytochemistry and Immunochemistry of Hematologic Neoplasms. Amer Soc Clin Pathol Press, 1985
6. Taylor CR: Immunomicroscopy: A Diagnostic Tool for the Surgical Pathologist. Philadelphia, W.B. Saunders, 1986
7. Nakane PK, Pierce GB, Jr: Enzyme-labeled antibodies-preparation and application for the localization of antigens. J Histochem Cytochem 14:929–931, 1966
8. Leduc EH, Avrameas WS, Bernard W: Ultrastructural localization of SV 40 T antigen with enzyme-labelled antibody. J Gen Virol 4:609–614, 1969
9. Venkatachalam MA, Karnovsky MJ, Cotran RS: Glomerular permeability: Ultrastructural studies in experimental nephrosis using horseradish peroxidase as a tracer. J Exp Med 30:381–399, 1969
10. Avrameas S, Leduc EH: Detection of simultaneous antibody synthesis in plasma cells and specialized lymphocytes in rabbit lymph nodes. J Exp Med 131:1137–1168, 1970
11. Robbins D, Fahimi HD, Cotran RS: Fine structural cytochemical localization of peroxidase activity in rat peritoneal cells: Mononuclear cells, eosinophils and mast cells. J Histochem Cytochem 19:571–575, 1971
12. Steiman RM, Cohn ZA: The interaction of particulate horseradish peroxidase (HRP)-anti HRP immune complexes with mouse peritoneal macrophages in vitro. J Cell Biol 55:616–634, 1972
13. Shamoto M, Suzuki I: An immunoelectron microscopic analysis of Epstein-Barr virus-associated complement-fixing antigen. Cancer 38:2057–2064, 1976
14. Shamoto M, Kito K, Akatsuka H, Suchi T: Immunoelectron microscopic studies on peripheral T-cell lymphomas using monoclonal antibodies. Virchows Arch (Cell Patrol) 47:281–290, 1984

15. Shamoto M, Suchi T: Ultrastructural and immunoelectron-microscopic characteristics of adult T-cell leukemia/lymphoma, Recent Advances RES Res 25:116–123, 1985
16. Shamoto M, Suchi T, Uchiyama T: Immunoelectron-microscopic localization of Tac antigen in adult T-cell leukemia/lymphoma, Amer J Pathol 119:513–516, 1985
17. Tsubai F, Namba Y, Kohno M, et al: A monoclonal antibody detecting a novel antigen expressed in the HTLV-I-infected cells., Blood 69:430–436, 1987
18. Graham RC, Jr, Karnovsky MJ: The early stages of absorption of injected horseradish peroxidase in the proximal tubules of mouse kidney-ultrastructural cytochemistry by a new technique. J Histochem Cytochem 14:291–302, 1966
19. Akatsuka H, Kito K, Shamoto M, Suchi T: Advantages of fixed stored materials for immunoelectron microscopy, with special reference to the study of malignant lymphomas. J Clin Pathol 37:953–955, 1984
20. Watanabe Y, Tamaoki N, Habu S, et al: Fine structural study on huma T- and B-lymphocytes. Acta Haematol Jpn 37:655–666, 1974
21. Shamoto M, Murakami S, Zenke T: Adult T-cell leukemia in Japan: An ultrastructural study. Cancer 47:1804–1811, 1981
22. Shamoto M: Ultrastructure of adult T-cell leukemia in Japan, In Polliack A (ed): Human Leukemias, Boston, Martinus Nijhoff, 1984, 298–307

17

Immunoblastic Lymphadenopathy, Angioimmunoblastic Lymphadenopathy, and IBL-Like T-Cell Lymphoma: A Spectrum of T-Cell Neoplasia

Shaw Watanabe
Hisako Ochi
Kiyoshi Mukai
Kennsei Tobinai
Masanori Shimoyama

Immunoblastic lymphadenopathy (IBL) and angioimmunoblastic lymphadenopathy (AILD) were reported as non-neoplastic lymphoproliferative disorders by Lukes and Tindle[1] and Frizzera et al,[2] respectively. These two disorders have similar histologic findings in many aspects, and the differences between IBL and AIDL are the nature of vascular proliferation and the presence of remnant germinal centers. Both conditions may progress toward malignant lymphoma, so IBL/AILD had been considered to be a premalignant lesion.

Watanabe et al[3–6] have reported that certain examples of peripheral T-cell lymphoma were similar histologically and clinically to IBL and AILD, and that a variety of histologic features could be present at different times in this disease category. Study of further cases suggested that IBL and AILD represented a dysplastic state of T-lymphocytes, initially containing only a small number of neoplastic cells, but that eventually resulted in more overt peripheral T-cell lymphoma in the majority of cases. In the latter condition, the neoplastic character of the proliferating cells was more easily recognized by histology alone.

Several case reports and recent technical developments, such as analyses of immunoglobulin and T-cell receptor gene rearrangements on IBL and AILD support the previous view that the lesion is substantially neoplastic, even though the number of neoplastic cells is too small to reach a definite diagnosis. However, it is still in debate which T-cell subset causes these lesions and what kind of factors modify the various clinical and histologic appearances. This review article, will discuss these points based upon 30 cases in the National Cancer Center series.[6]

NEOPLASTIC NATURE OF IBL AND AILD

Various hypotheses have been considered regarding the nature of IBL and AILD. Lukes

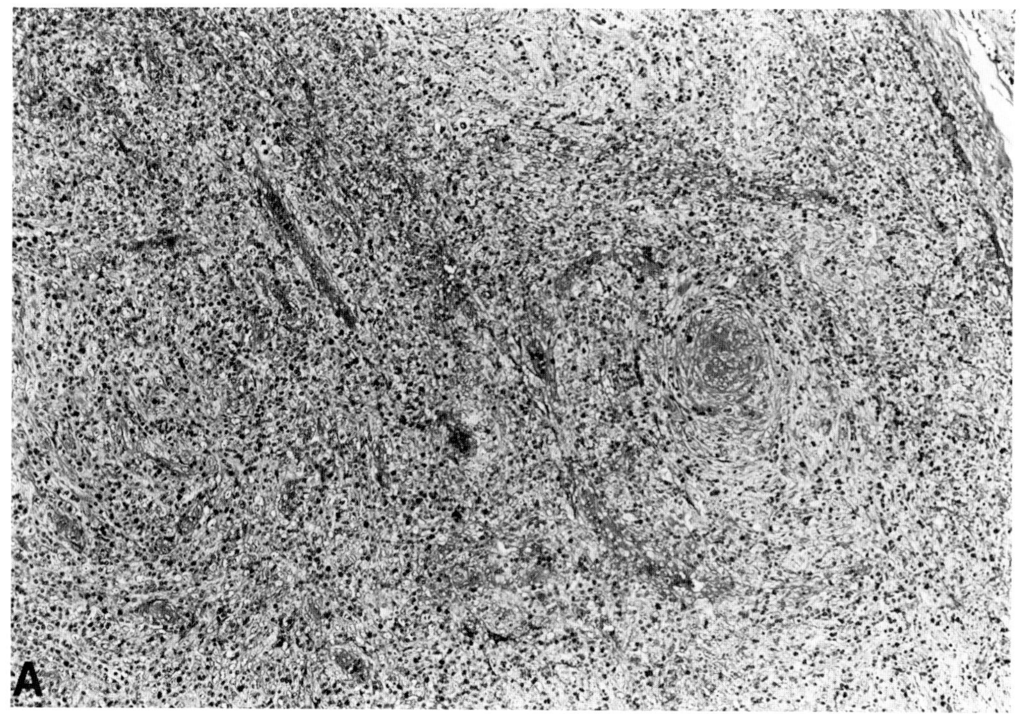

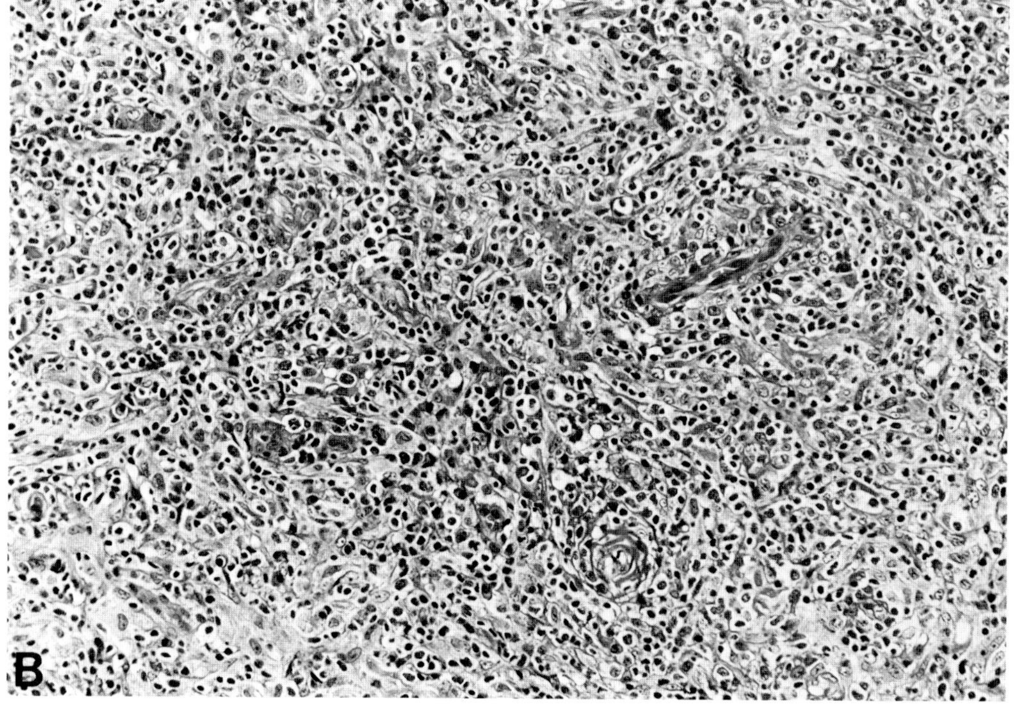

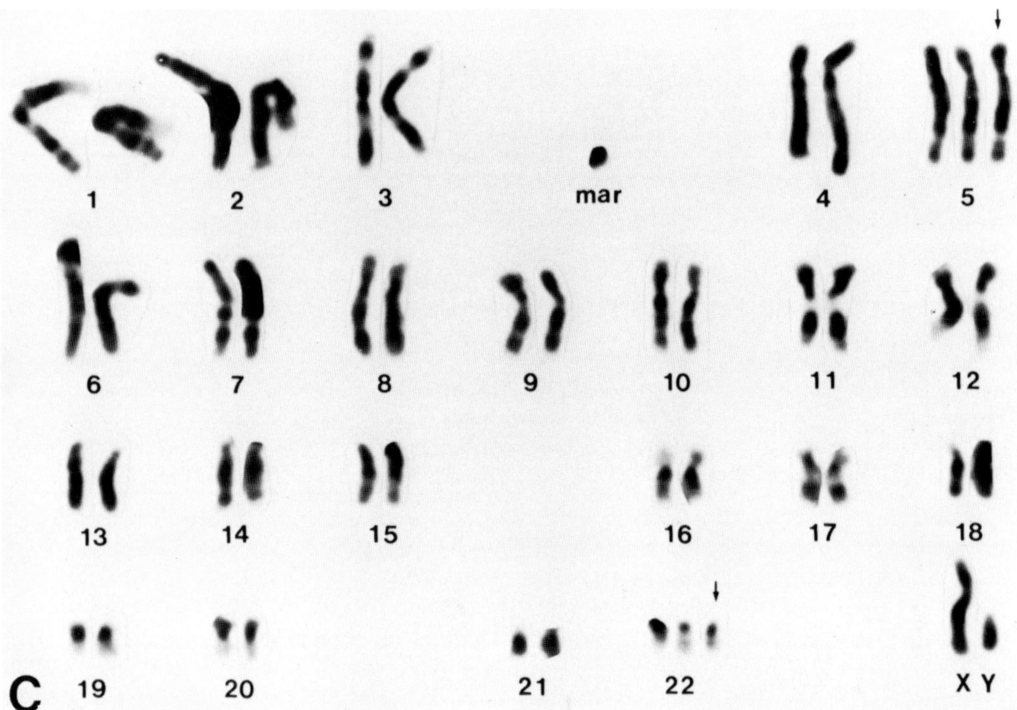

Fig. 17-1. (A) AILD lesion with abnormal karyotype. The burned out germinal center and proliferation of vascular vessels are noted. (B) No atypical cells recognizable to be malignant are present at higher magnifications. (C) Karyotype obtained from the lymph node biopsy, showing 49,XY,+5,+22,+mar.

and Tindle[1,7] considered IBL as to be a preneoplastic stage of B-lymphocytes. There were several reports that immunoblastic sarcoma developed from IBL, but few cases revealed monoclonal growth of B-cells in terms of Ig production.[8–11] Watanabe et al[3–6] reported the presence of peripheral T-cell lymphoma with histologic and clinical similarities with IBL or AILD. Recently, IBL and AILD have been considered as T-cell dysplasia or a prelymphomatous stage of T-cell lymphoma.[6,12]

Confirmation of abnormal clonal growth is one of the strong evidences for malignancy. All 5 cases with initial diagnosis of IBL examined by chromosome analysis in our laboratory showed an abnormal karyotype. One case was histologically diagnosed as AILD, because no definite finding of malignancy could be found (Fig. 17-1a,b). This case was a 72-year-old male with complaints of systemic erythema and lymphadenopathy for 9 months. The biopsied lymph node revealed diffuse involvement with "burned out" germinal centers, proliferation of blood vessels, and mixed composition of cells with predominantly small lymphocytes. Mitotic figures scattered without abnormal ones. However, chromosome analysis revealed an abnormal distribution of chromosome numbers, such as 46 in 48 (61.6%), 47 in 2 (2.9%), 48 in 11 (15.9%), and 49 in 8 (11.6%) metaphases. The karyotypes of these abnormal clones showed clonal evolution from 47,XY,+5 (2 metaphases), 48,XY,+5,+mar (3), 48,XY,+5,−10,+22, +mar (1), to 49,XY,+5,+22,+mar (3) (Fig. 17-1c). Such coexistence of germline and evolved clones suggests that the lesion must develop through a relatively long progression period of at least several years.

Other reported chromosome analyses also showed frequent abnormalities.[13–15] Kaneko et al[13] reported that among the most frequent chromosomal abnormalities in IBL were +3,

TABLE 17-1
Histologic Criteria of IBL, AILD, and IBL-like T-Cell Lymphoma

IBL (Lukes & Tindle)	AILD (Frizzera et al)	IBL-like T-cell lymphoma
Diffuse involvement, no germinal centers	Obliteration of lymph node architecture, burned-out germinal centers	Obliteration of lymph node architecture Diffuse involvement, usually no germinal centers, or burned-out, fibrotic germinal centers
Arborizing blood vessels with PAS positive thick wall	Small vessels with high endothelia	Vascular proliferation
Lymphocyte depletion		
Proliferation of immunoblasts and plasma cells	Polymorphous infiltration with abundant immunoblasts	Cluster or sheet-like proliferation of pale cells Perivascular plasma cells
Deposition of PAS positive material	Eosinophilic amorphous material	

+5, and +19. Apparently, some of their cases seemed to be peripheral T-cell lymphoma by retrospective review, but some IBL showed multiclonal abnormal karyotypes, so the authors considered that the true neoplastic growth seemed to occur from these clones.

Kamada et al[16] collected karyotypes of IBL and AILD in Japan, and reported that simple numerical abnormalities were more frequent than structural ones, and that such changes were compatible with those found in the state of preleukemia. The most frequently involved chromosome was no. 3 (16 out of 26 cases), and then no. 7 (5 out of 26 cases). The sites, 6q21, 14q32, and 14q11 on chromosomes were common sites of breakage or translocation. Trisomy, deletion, or translocation observed in no. 3 chromosomes in IBL/AILD were also frequent in other T-cell lymphomas/leukemias, so that the alteration of chromosome seems to be involved in the early stage of neoplastic change of T-cells.

Clonality of proliferating cells in so-called IBL and AILD lesions were detected in rearrangements of Ig genes and T-cell receptor genes using the Southern blotting method.[17] If a clonal proliferation was present, one or two rearranged bands should be detected. The authors used the restriction enzymes HindIII for J_H probe, and BamHI and EcoRI for T-cell receptor β-chain constant region (CTβ) probe. In all 8 cases examined, no gene rearrangement of J_H was present, while 1 or 2 rearranged bands of CTβ were detected.[18] Ueda et al* reported similar results for IBL/AILD lesions, in which 7 of 10 cases showed rearranged bands.

These findings, in addition to the histologic characteristics and poor prognosis, support the concept that IBL/AILD lesions are malignant.

HISTOLOGIC APPEARANCES

Histologic characteristics of IBL, AILD, and IBL-like T-cell lymphomas are briefly summarized in Table 17-1. The differential diagnosis between these three categories was made by the following points; IBL when there was no germinal center and no pale cell foci; AILD when there was burned-out or fibrotic germinal centers; and IBL-like T-cell lymphoma when the pale cell focus or apparently atypical cell proliferation was recognized in addition to the features of IBL or AILD.[6] Common structural changes were diffuse obliteration of normal lymph node architecture with frequent vascular proliferation and disappearance of germinal centers. Remnants of burned out germinal centers with degener-

* (personal communication)

ated amorphous material or fibrotic germinal centers were sometimes recognized. Capsules and subcapsular lymphatic sinuses were often preserved, even when extracapsular invasion by lymphoid cells was present. Conspicuous blood vessels were not only capillary-venules, but also post-capillary venules and arteriolar-capillary vessels. Perivascular proliferation of plasma cells was recognized in more than one-half of the cases, but it was inconspicuous in almost one-third of them. It was noted that some T-cell lymphomas showed plasmacytoid features. The presence of amorphous eosinophilic material, which was one of the criteria for IBL by Lukes and Tindle, was recognized in less than one-third of the cases. The degree of infiltration of histiocytes and eosinophils was variable, and cases with eosinophilia usually showed moderate to marked eosinophilic infiltration. Decreased T-zone histiocytes in CD8+ cases were in contrast with a marked increase of these histiocytes in CD4+ mycosis fungoides.[19]

The most characteristic finding was the proliferation of lymphoid cells with pale cytoplasm. The nuclei were usually medium-sized, but also they showed nuclear irregularity and variable atypism.[4–6] This was a constant feature of $CD8^+$ cases. Sheet-like proliferation of pale cells in some case formed compartments, but in most cases these pale cells formed irregularly shaped clusters or diffuse small nests (Fig. 17-2). The neoplastic nature was recognized by the increased number of pale cells with nuclear atypsim, occasional mitoses, and sheet-like proliferation. The frequency of large cells with clear cytoplasm and smaller cells with nuclear irregularity varied from case to case. If pathologists recognize clusters of pale cells in addition to the IBL/AILD changes, intensive chemotherapy is recommended. Repeated biopsies and chromosome analyses are necessary, if the T-cell dysplasia is suspected by the mixed composition of cells with scarce pale cells that looked non-neoplastic. Detection of clonal rearrangement of T-cell receptor genes may also help to recognize neoplastic growth.[18]

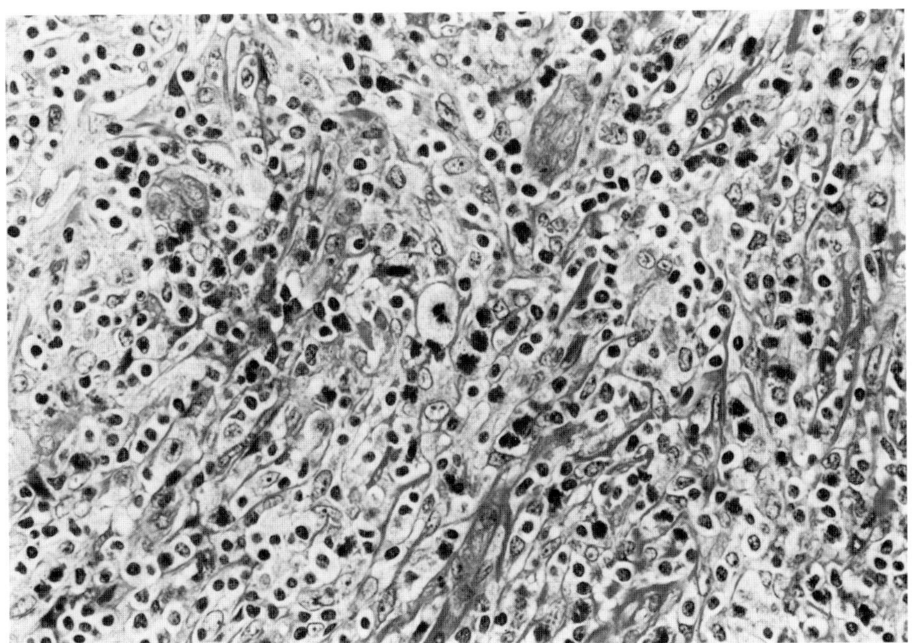

Fig. 17-2. Pale cell focus in the IBL-like T-cell lymphoma. Atypical mitotic figures are present. Irregular nuclei and clear cytoplasmic membrane are noted.

T-CELL SUBSETS PROLIFERATING IN THE PERIPHERAL T-CELL LYMPHOMA WITH IBL/AILD APPEARANCE

Two different proliferative conditions of T-lymphocytes have been distinguished; one is characterized by a predominance of $CD4^+$ (helper/inducer T) cells and another by predominance of $CD8^+$ (suppressor/cytotoxic T) cells. Watanabe et al have reported that the typical IBL-like T-cell lymphoma is mostly a neoplasm of CD8+ T-lymphocytes. However, reports from other institutions described predominance of CD4+ type even in IBL/AILD/IBL-like T-cell lymphoma. Review of almost 100 cases of IBL/IBL-like lymphoma collected in Japan demonstrated that many overt CD4+ peripheral T-cell lymphomas with large watery clear cytoplasm were included. This type, so-called immunoblastic sarcoma of T-cells should be distinguished from IBL-like T-cell lymphoma, because even adult T-cell leukemia/lymphoma, induced by HTLV-I infection, frequently has IBL-like lesions.[20]

Histologic varieties of peripheral T-cell lymphoma are considered to be the result of lymphokine-like materials produced by the neoplastic cells. Functional assays for angiogenic factors, eosinophil chemotactic factor, and histiocyte immobilizing or aggregation factor are necessary in this regard. CD8+ neoplastic cells showed an in vitro helper function for Ig synthesis upon pokeweed mitogen-stimulation of B-lymphocytes and no suppressive effect on normal T-B-cell system for Ig synthesis.[21] This in vitro finding was correlated with clinical hypergammaglobulinemia, although the precise mechanism was not known.

The immunostaining of tissue sections usually revealed patchy distribution of various cells, although $CD8^+$ cell clusters were increased in most cases in accordance with the clusters of pale cells. Watanabe et al experienced one case that showed a dominance of $CD4^+$ cells in the first lymph node biopsy, revealed an increase of $CD8^+$ cells in subsequent biopsies and in cells of the terminal leukemic stage.[6] In some immunohistochemically determined cases, the proliferating cells also stained with Leu7 in addition to CD8 and CD3. Neoplastic cells in one of three such cases contained large azurophilic granules in Giemsa stained imprints. However, clinical and histologic characteristics were not much different from other $CD8^+Leu7^-$ cases. CD8+Leu7+ leukemia was reported by Loughran et al[22] under the term leukemia of

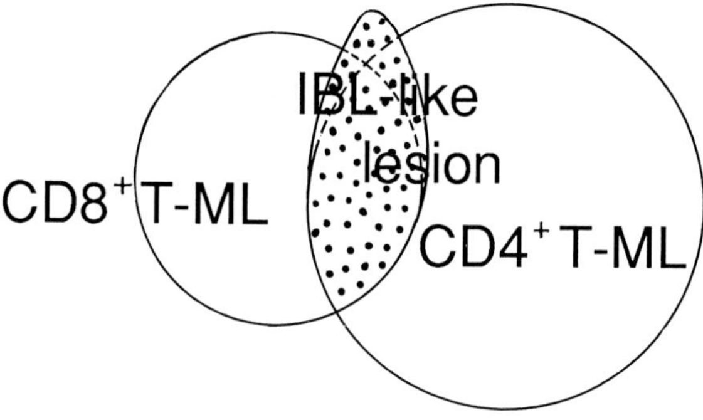

Fig. 17-3. Schema of the disease concept around IBL/AILD and IBL-like T-cell lymphoma.

large granular lymphocytes. All 3 of their cases had a chronic course with autoimmune neutropenia, thrombocytopenia, hemolytic anemia, and polyclonal hypergammaglobulinemia. The relationship between this T-CLL and T8+Leu7+ lymphoma should be examined in the future. The disease category for the differential diagnosis is shown in Figure 17-3.

CONCLUSION

IBL and AILD may be considered as one type of peripheral T-cell lymphoma, although it is not known what substances cause these lesions, and which subpopulation of T-lymphocytes is neoplastic.

Another important problem is the treatment method. Many patients with these disorders have a progressive clinical course with a fatal outcome. The median survival of 18 cases reported by Lukes and Tindle[1] was 18 months, and 47 of 98 cases reviewed by Cullen et al[23] died within 12 months. In our series, the $CD8^+$ cases had a less favorable prognosis than the $CD4^+$ cases, regardless of their age of onset and histologic variations.[6] Almost half of the cases died within one year, and only 5 out of 30 patients survived more than 2 years.

The cause of death of these patients was due to rapidly progressive disease with early recurrence, in spite of intensive combination chemotherapy. More intensive chemotherapy should be considered in this regard to obtain the better quality of life of the patients. Opportunistic infection was the second most common cause of death. Complication with carcinoma of various organs was not rare, so that complete survey at the time of diagnosis was necessary.

By the establishment of criteria for pathologic diagnosis of this entity along with more extensive laboratory and clinical studies we should further clarify the nature of this entity and its correlation with other type of peripheral T-cell lymphomas.

ACKNOWLEDGMENTS

This work was supported in part by the Grant-in-aids for Cancer Research from the Ministry of Health and Welfare (No. 60-S-1)

REFERENCES

1. Lukes RJ, Tindle BJ: Immunoblastic lymphadenopathy: A hyperimmune entity resembling Hodgkin's disease. N Engl J Med 292:1–8, 1975
2. Frizzera G, Moran EM, Rappaport H: Angioimmunoblastic hymphoadenopathy, diagnosis and clinical course. Am J Med 59:803–818, 1975
3. Shimoyama M, Minato K, Watanabe S, et al: Immunoblastic lymphadenoapthy (IBL)-like T-cell lymphoma. Jpn J Clin Oncol 9(Suppl):347–356, 1979
4. Watanabe S, Shimosato Y, Shimoyama M, et al: Adult T-cell lymphoma with hypergammaglobulinemia. Cancer 46:2472–2483, 1980
5. Watanabe S, Shimosato Y, Shimoyama M: Lympohoma and leukemia of T-lymphocytes, in Sommers SC, Rosen P, (eds): Pathology Annual 1981 (Part 2). New York, Appleton-Century-Croft, 1981, 155–206
6. Watanabe S, Sato Y, Shimoyama M, et al: Immunoblastic lymphadenopathy, angioimmunoblastic lymphadenopathy, and IBL-like T-cell lymphoma. Cancer 58:2224–2232, 1986
7. Lukes RJ, Tindle BH: Immunoblastic lymphadenopathy: A prelymphomatous state of immunoblastic sarcoma. Cancer Res 64:241–246, 1978
8. Nathwani BN, Rappaport H, Moran EM, et al: Malignant lymphoma arising in angioimmunoblastic lymphadenopathy. Cancer 41:578–606, 1978
9. Donhuiusen K, Donhuijsen-Ant R, Leder LD: Evolution of angioimmunoblastic lymphadenopathy. N Engl J Med 297:840, 1977
10. Fisher RI, Jaffe ES, Braylan RC, et al: Immunoblastic lymphadenopathy. Evolution into a malignant lymphoma with plasmacytoid features. Am J Med 61:553–559, 1976
11. Toth J, Garam T: Immunoblastic lymphadenopathy proceeding to sarcoma. Lancet 1:102, 1977
12. Nathwani BN, Winberg CD, Berman RM, et al: Angioimmunoblastic lymphadenopathy with dysproteinemia and its progression to malignant lymphoma, in Jaffe ES (ed): Surgical Pathology of the Lymph Nodes and Related Organs. Philadelphia, W.B. Saunders, 1985:57–85
13. Hossefeld DK, Hoeffken K, Schmidt CG, Diedrichs H: Chromosome abnormalities in angioimmunoblastic lymphadenopathy. Lancet 1:198, 1976
14. Volk SLR, Monteleone PL, Knight WAK: Chromosomes in AILD. N Engl J Med 292:975, 1975
15. Kaneko Y, Larson RA, Variakojis D, et al: Nonradom chromosome abnormalities in angioimmunoblastic lymphadenopathy. Blood 60:877–887, 1982

16. Kamada N, Tanaka K, Sakatani K, Hasegawa A. Chromosome aberrations in lymphoid malignancies and transforming gene in adult T-cell leukemia, in Hanaoka, M, et al (eds): Lymphoid Malignancy. Philadelphia, Field & Wood, 1990:57–66
17. Weiss LM, Strickler JG, Dorfman RF, et al: Clonal T-cell proliferation in angioimmunoblastic lymphadenopathy and angioimmunoblastic lymphadenopathy-like lymphoma. Am J Pathol 122:392, 1986
18. Tobinai K, Minato K, Ohtsu T, et al: Immunoblastic lymphadenopathy (IBL)-like T-cell lymphoma: Clinico-pathologic, immunophenotypic and immunogenotypic analyses of 36 cases. Acta Haematol Jpn 50-1668–1676, 1987
19. Igisu K, Watanabe S, Shimosato Y, Kukita A: Langerhans cells and their precursors with S100 protein in mycosis fungoides. Jpn J Clin Oncol 13:693–702, 1983
20. Kikuchi M, Mitsui T, Matsui M, et al: T-cell malignancies in adults: Histopathological studies of lymph nodes in 110 patients. Jpn J Clin Oncol 9 (Suppl):407–422, 1979
21. Oshimi K, Aoyama M, Ohtani T, et al: A case report of T-cell lymphoma with suppressor phenotype and helper function for immunoglobulin synthesis. Cancer 54:2029–2031, 1984
22. Loughran TP, Jr, Kadin ME, Starkebaum G, et al: Leukemia of large granular lymphocytes: Association with clonal chromosomal abnormalities and autoimmune neutropenia, thrombocytopenia and hemolytic anemia. Ann Int Med 102:169–175, 1985
23. Cullen MH, Stansfeld AG, Oliver RTD, et al: Angioimmunoblastic lymphadenopathy: Report of 10 cases and review of literature. Q J Med 48:151–177, 1979

18

T-Zone Dysplasia with Hyperplastic Follicles—An Incipient T-Cell Lymphoma

Taizan Suchi
Ryuzo Ueda
Hirotaka Suzuki
Reiko Namikawa

Abstract

A type of lymphadenopathy termed "T-zone dysplasia with hyperplastic follicles" is described. The lesion is an incipient neoplasia or prelymphomatous state of helper T-cells, and histologically characterized by the presence of markedly hyperplastic germinal centers with only mild atypia of proliferating T-cells in the interfollicular areas, accompanied by many small vessels with swollen endothelial nuclei and variable amounts of epithelioid cell clusters. The results of immunohistochemistry to elucidate the phenotypic character of proliferating cells and of immunoglobulin- and T-cell receptor-gene rearrangement are reported.

T-zone lymphoma was originally defined by Lennert and coworkers[1] as a T-cell lymphoma that grows in the T-zones and consists of cells that normally constitute T-zones of lymph nodes. The follicles are often preserved or even somewhat hyperplastic in its early phase. Suchi previously observed 3 cases of lymphadenopathy in which many markedly hyperplastic germinal centers accompanied by only mild atypia of infiltrating T-cells in rather narrow interfollicular areas had eventually progressed to become overt T-cell lymphomas, and were reported as "atypical hyperplasia of T-zone type" to the International Cancer Congress in 1982.[2]

Since then, the authors accumulated 6 more cases of lymphadenopathy with similar histologic and clinical features, and investigated with immunohistochemistry and immunoglobulin- and T-cell receptor genc rearrangement analysis the clonality of proliferating lymphocytes. In this paper, the results of these studies are reported, with emphasis on the importance of recognition of lymphadenopathy of this type in diagnostic pathology, and the term "T-zone dysplasia with hyperplastic follicles, TZD" for this type of lesion is introduced.

CASE REPORT (CASE 1)

A 54-year-old Japanese male was admitted in November 1979, complaining of rapidly swelling lymph nodes in the right side of neck and swelling of bilateral tonsils. He showed otherwise no significant sign or symptom, nor any remarkable laboratory data.

HISTOPATHOLOGIC APPEARANCE

The biopsied node revealed many markedly hyperplastic germinal centers with variable numbers of tingible-body macrophages throughout the node parenchyma. They were distinctly outlined, round or oval in shape, and endowed with ample mantle zones. The interfollicular areas were rather narrow and contained many vessels with swollen endothelial nuclei and thickened basement membranes. The proliferating cells around them were mostly small to medium-sized, with irregular shaped nuclei in some. They were intermingled with occasional immunoblasts with pale gray cytoplasm. Mitotic figures were frequent. Epithelioid cells were also conspicuous in single cells and in small clusters in the interfollicular areas. (Figs. 18-1 and 18-2) Eosinophiles and plasma cells were rare in this case. The biopsied tonsil showed a few small non-caseating granulomatous foci surrounded by predominantly lymphocytic infiltrates whose nuclei were moderately irregular.

Although malignant character of the lesion could not be definitely established by histologic appearance alone, potential malignancy was suspected. The patient's lymphadenopathy gradually spreaded to the left side of neck, inguinal and axillary regions in the course of disease, during which time the size of the nodes fluctuated with incomplete treatment by radio- and chemotherapy, as well as at

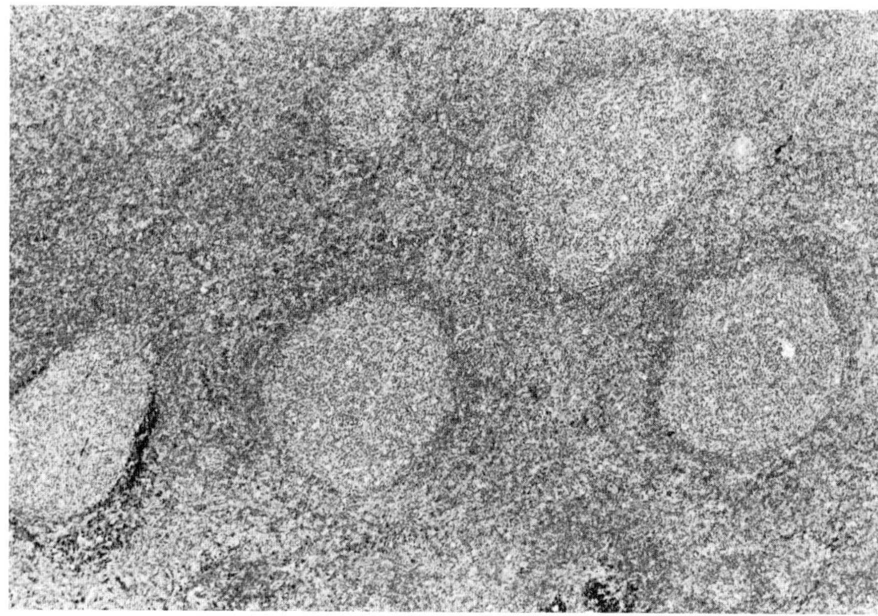

Fig. 18-1. Histologic appearance of the initial biopsy specimen (lymph node) of Case 1. (H&E, $\times$ 40).

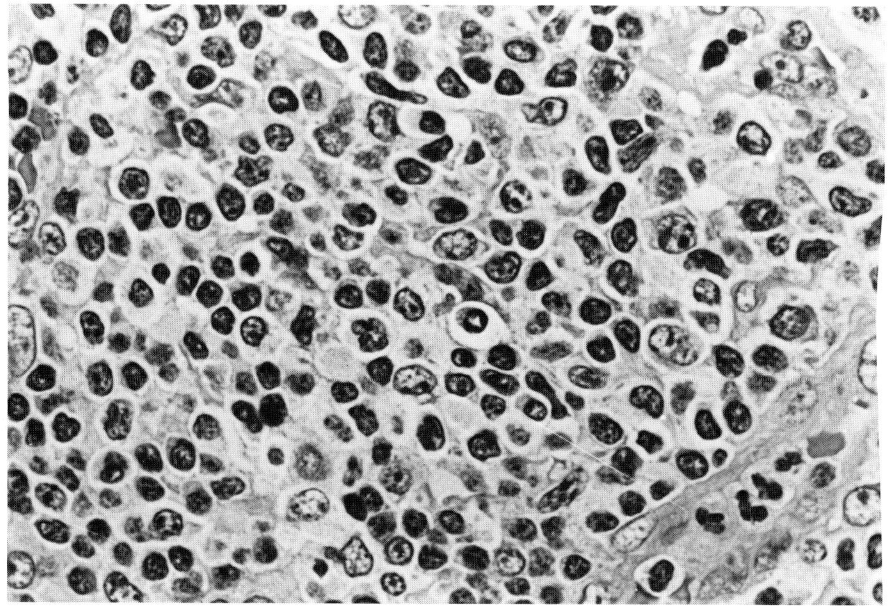

Fig. 18-2. Higher magnification of an interfollicular area of Case 1 (H&E, × 800).

times only with non-steroid anti-inflammatory drugs, or even regressed spontaneously. A lymph node biopsied 2 years later showed similar histologic features with only somewhat smaller germinal centers, broader T-zones, and formation of fibrous bands along portions of the septal structure. The cellular atypism was essentially unchanged.

The biopsy taken in September 1982, however, showed a completely diffuse lymphomatous lesion made up largely of atypical cells with medium-sized nuclei and pale cytoplasm (Fig. 18-3). Abnormal mitoses were seen, and great majority of the composing cells reacted immunohistochemically with the monoclonal antibodies of CD3 and CD4. This was

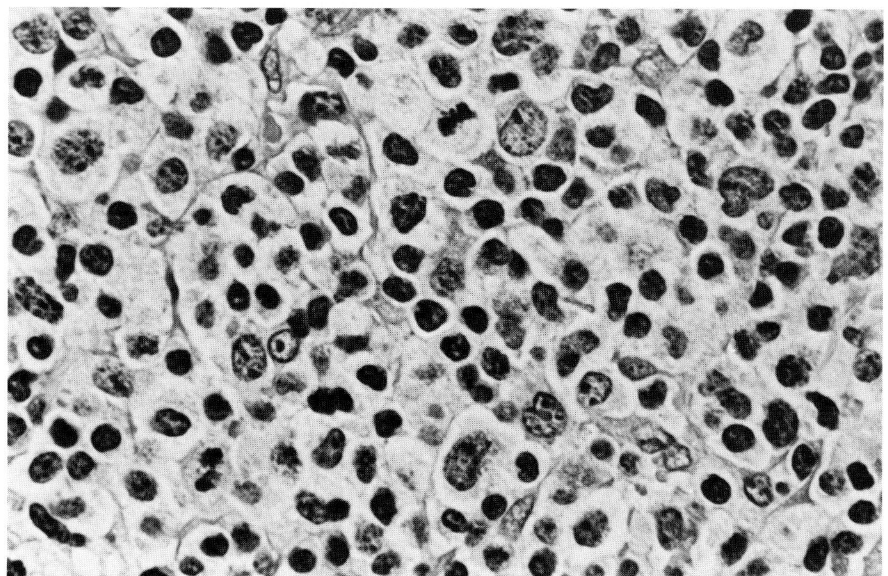

Fig. 18-3. Histologic appearance of the last biopsy specimen (lymph node) of Case 1. Most of the proliferating lymphocytes have medium-sized, round to irregular-shaped nuclei, and pale cytoplasm (H&E, × 800).

thus a peripheral T-cell lymphoma of the helper/inducer phenotype. The patient died of pneumonitis due to *pneumocystis carinii,* while a course of chemotherapy was instituted. It is very likely that the histologic picture of the earlier biopsies of this patient represents an incipient phase of peripheral T-cell lymphoma.

CLINICAL ASPECT OF THE CASES

Altogether nine cases of lymphadenopathy with histologic features similar to the above described have been encountered, and 3 cases including the case reported above (Cases 1–3) were terminated with overt T-cell lymphomas (Group 1). The 6 other cases (Cases 4–9) are in complete remission after courses of chemotherapy at the time of writing of this article (Group 2). The significant clinical findings and laboratory data of these 9 patients as well as the outcome of the patients of Group 1 are summarized in Tables 18-1 and 18-2. All patients except for Case 9 (age 13 years) are in their 6th decade or more, and dominated by female (one male in each group). Lymphadenopathy at the first presentation was localized or semilocalized in 6 cases, and more or less generalized in 3 cases. Symptoms other than lymph node swelling are unremarkable in 2 cases, but there are usually some constitutional symptoms often described as "common-cold like." Among laboratory data, elevation of some serum immunoglobulins are noted fairly frequently, accompanied by accelerated erythrocyte sedimentation rate. Autoimmune phenomena such as Coombs reaction and positive LE and RA factors, as well as anemia, leucopenia, and pancytopenia are observed in some of the cases. In Group I, the length of time from the initial biopsy showing dysplastic lesions to development of overt T-cell lymphomas ranged from 21 to 34 months, and the entire course of disease from 26 to 41 months.

HISTOPATHOLOGY

All these cases showed, in the initially biopsied nodes, similar histopathologic features to those described in the Case Report. They are characterized by the presence of many hyperplastic germinal centers and mild to, at most, moderate atypia of proliferating lymphocytes in the interfollicular areas (T-zones). Cellular atypia can be noticed mainly by irregularity of nuclei and their number, which varied from case to case, and most pronounced

TABLE 18-1
Clinical Findings of Group 1

Case No. Age/Sex	Clinical Findings at Initial Bx: Lymphadenopathy	Symptoms	Lab Data	Length of time to become overt T-L	Histological types of overt T-L	Length of entire course of illness
#1 54M	Neck,bil Tonsils	None	Not Remarkable	2y 7m	Diffuse, Medium-sized T	3y 5m
#2 62F	Neck, lt	Nasal Obstruction Headache Shoulder Stiffness	Not Remarkable	2y 10m	Diffuse, with AILD Feature	2y
#3 61F	Neck,bil Inguinal	Fever, Cough Transient Rash Pitting Edema Weight Loss	WBC: 10500 Anemia M-component in IgM	1y 9m	Diffuse, with AILD Feature	2y 2m

T-L: T-lymphoma

TABLE 18-2
Clinical Findings of Group 2

Case No. Age/Sex	Lymphade- nopathy	Symptoms	Lab. Data
#4 56M	Neck,bil. Axilla,bil. Ing.bil.	Fever	IgG ↑, IgA ↑ CRP(+), ESR ↑
#5 52F	Neck, rt. Supracl.rt.	Headache Cough Hoarseness	ESR ↑, IgM ↑ PPD(−) LE(+), RA(+)
#6 73F	Neck,rt. Supracl.rt. Ing.bil.	Weight Loss	γ-globulin ↑ IgG 2780 ESR ↑, RA(+)
#7 59F	Submax.bil.	Palpebral Swelling Liver Cirrhosis	Pancytopenia γ-globulin ↑
#8 57F	Neck,bil.	Unremarkable	Direct Coombs(+)
#9 13F	Submax.rt. (4x2)	Fever,Rash General Fatigue	Leucopenia

in the Cases 3 and 4. In the interfollicular areas, many small vessels with swollen endothelial nuclei are present. Epitheliod cells, usually in clusters, and eosinophiles are sometimes conspicuously seen, but plasma cells were not numerous. Few to a moderate number of immunoblasts with pale gray cytoplasm and prominent nucleoli were seen.

IMMUNOHISTOCHEMISTRY

In order to characterize the main proliferating cells in the lesions of this type that are of polymorphic composition, the double immunohistochemical staining technique[3] using Ki-67[4] as a marker for proliferating cells and various monoclonal antibodies against lymphocyte differentiation antigens, such as CD3(pan peripheral T), CD4(helper/inducer T), CD8(suppresser/cytotoxic T), and CD22(pan B) were used. It is natural that Ki-67 positive nuclei were most concentrated in the germinal centers in the lesions of this type, and the Ki-67 positive cells there were also CD22 positive. But it is the interfollicular areas (T-zones) that are noteworthy. Table 18-3 summarizes the findings in T-zones in cases of Group B, from which snap-frozen tissues for histochemistry were available. As seen in this table, the interfollicular areas in this type are largely occupied by T-cells (CD3+) and contain only a few to a modest

TABLE 18-3
Characterization of Constituent Cells and of Proliferating Cells in TZD

	Cell Population in T-zone				Estimated % of Ki-67+ cells	
Case	CD3	CD4	CD8	CD22	CD4	CD8
4	+++	++±	±	−	>80	10
5	+++	++±	+	−	90	5
6	+++	++±	+	−	90	<10
7	+++	++±	+	±	85	15
8	++	++±	+	±	>90	< 5
9	++±	++	+	±	>80	< 5

Numbers of cells positive for each MoAb are graded with the scale of: −, ±, +, +±, ++, ++±, +++.

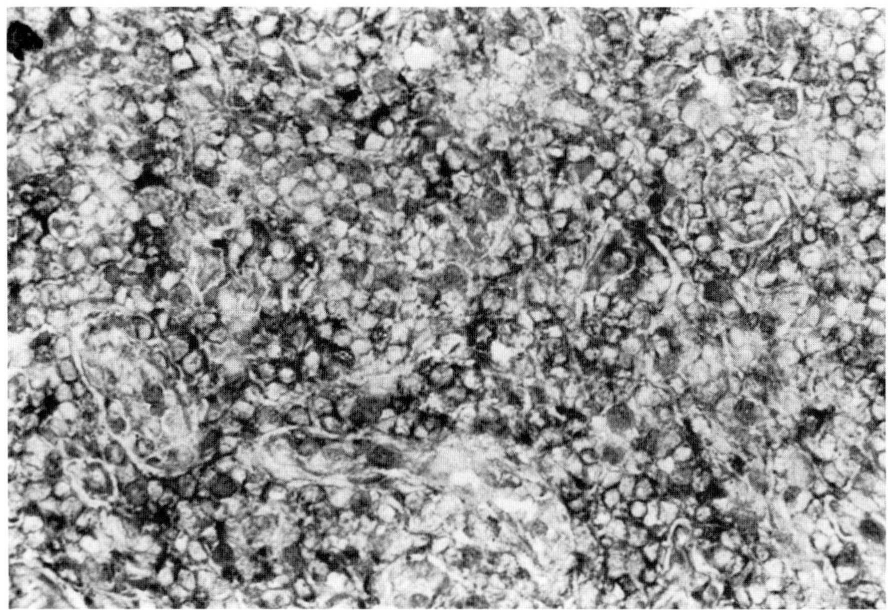

Fig. 18-4. An interfollicular area of Case 4 with double-staining immunohistochemistry using CD4 and Ki-67. Most cells are positive for CD4 on the surface, and some of their nuclei are positive for Ki-67 (× 400).

number of B-cells (CD22+), much fewer than the interfollicular areas in reactive lymph nodes with simple follicular hyperplasia. Among T-cells, most are of the helper/inducer type (CD4+) (Fig. 18-4) and only a small fraction of them are of suppressor/cytotoxic T-cells (CD8+) (Fig. 18-5). Cells labeling with Ki-67 antibody are not numerous among the T-cells in the T-zones. It is apparent from the table that the great majority of proliferating cells in the T-zones are of CD4+ helper T-cells. It should be added that there are naturally many helper T-cells in the hyperplastic germinal centers, but they are usually not proliferating.

GENE REARRANGEMENT STUDY

In order to see if clonal rearrangement of T-cell receptor (TCR) gene[5] or immunoglobulin heavy chain (IgH) gene[6] exists in these cases, Southern blot analyses were done[7] on tissues from all cases. In Case 1, the initial biopsy specimen was not available, but the second node that still showed similar histologic features as described in the Case Report was available for the study. In all other cases, either frozen or fresh tissues of initial biopsy specimens were available for the study. The results are summarized in Table 18-4, which shows that clonal rearrangement of TCR was observed in Cases 3, 4, and 9 only.

Clonal rearrangements are not detected in the dysplastic nodes in Case 1, and 2, even though these patients later developed overt T-cell lymphomas. In Case 9, investigation was done on whole tissue as well as on T-cell rich fraction of suspended cells made from the lymph node and non-T-cell rich fraction, prepared by the E-rosette formation technique. It should be noted that only the T-cell rich fraction showed clonal rearrangement for TCR.[8] In this case the histologic and cytologic atypia were only very mild as shown in Fig. 18-6.

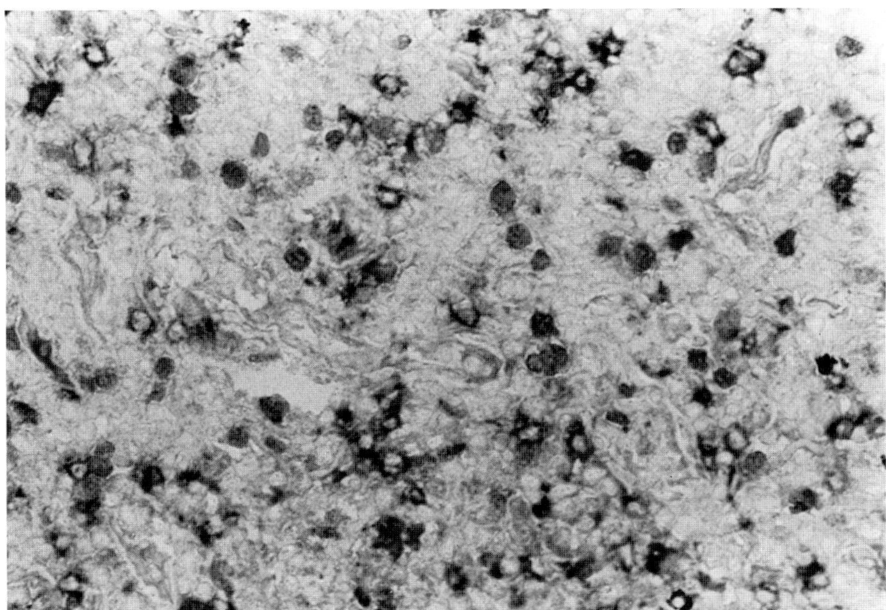

Fig. 18-5. The same area as Fig. 18-4 with double-staining using CD8 and Ki-67. CD8 positive cells are comparatively few, and most of them are Ki-67 negative (× 400).

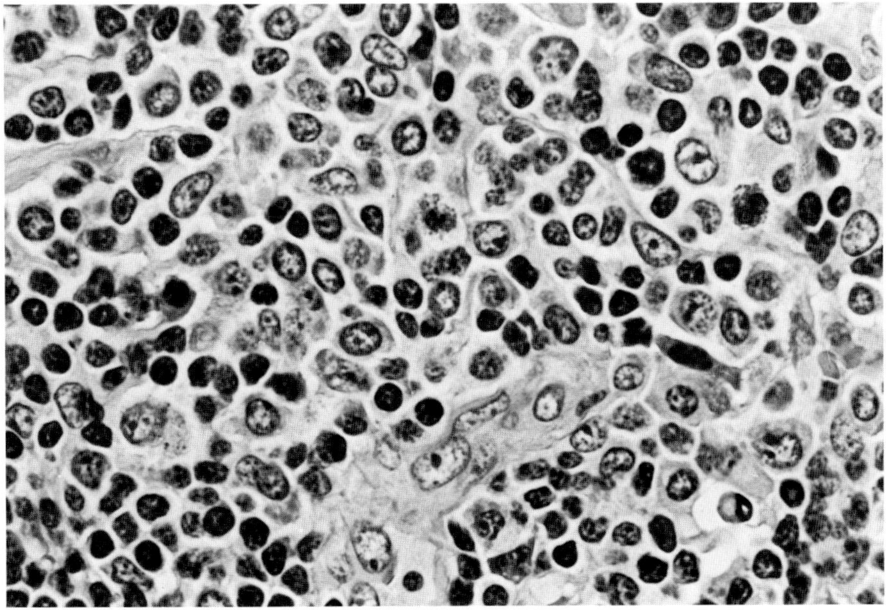

Fig. 18-6. Histologic appearance of an interfollicular area of Case 9. Note very mild atypia of infiltrating cells, in spite of the rearrangement of TCR genes (H&E, × 800).

TABLE 18-4
Clonal Rearrangement of TCR_β Genes in TZD

Case	T_β	J_H
#1	G	G
#2	G	G
#3	R	G
#4a	R	G
b	R	G
#5	G	G
#6	G	G
#7	G	G
#8	G	G
#9a	G	G
b	R	G
c	G	G

4a: first biopsy; 4b: second biopsy; 9a: whole; 9b: T rich; 9c: non-T; G: Germ Line; R: Rearrangement (EcoR1, BamH1, Xba 1)

DISCUSSION

As described above, 3 of the patients with histologic features of T-zone dysplasia with hyperplastic follicles were observed to have progressed into overt T-cell lymphomas, and the lesional tissue from 3 patients showed clonal rearrangements of TCR genes. It is true that 2 (Case 3 and 4) of the 3 cases that showed clonal rearrangement were cases with more noticeable atypism of proliferating cells than in the other cases. But Case 9 with clonal rearrangement detected only in the T-cell rich fraction of the suspended cells showed very moderate atypia in its T-zones. Moreover, the two cases (Cases 1 and 2) that were observed to have progressed to overt T-cell lymphomas within a few years showed no detectable clonal rearrangement band in their earlier biopsies. The possibility, therefore, can not be denied that at least some of the other cases without clonal rearrangement investigated on whole tissues might have been proven to contain some clonal population of T-cells, if the fractionated study was made on them as in Case 9.

Admittedly, the clonal rearrangement alone does not necessarily confirm malignancy, but it is reasonable to assume that those cases with clonal rearrangement contain some population of neoplastic T-cells and thus, in reality, incipient neoplasia. We may extend our inference to suppose that some of the cases without clonal rearrangement may also contain minor populations of clonal T-cells. At any rate, it is apparent that there definitely exists a type of lymphadenopathy of incipient neoplasia or at least prelymphomatous state, which exhibits the histologic features described in this paper. It is a fact that pathologists who deal daily with all kinds of swollen lymph nodes must encounter, though rarely, and therefore should be aware of, the lesions of this type of disease. It is therefore worthwhile to give this type of lesion a definite term, namely "T-zone dysplasia with hyperplastic follicles, TZD."

It should be added that helper/inducer T-cells are the main proliferating cells in the lesions of this type, and thus may well be responsible for the formation of the lesions, that is, activation of germinal centers, through production of a lymphokine. In this respect, it should be remarked that hyperplastic germinal centers are occasionally observed in T-cell lymphomas of high-grade malignancy including the lesion of ATLL.*

One of the most important questions is if we can definitely distinguish lesions of this type by some histologic criteria from those of more innocuous reactive process, and the answer regrettably seems rather negative. It appears that we have to depend largely on the cytologic atypia of proliferating T-cells including T-immunoblasts together with effacement and obliteration of lymph node structures other than germinal centers. Distinction of this type from the lymphadenopathy accompanying autoimmune diseases such as rheumatoid arthritis can be usually made by abundance of plasma cells in the interfollicular areas in the latter. Absence of monocytoid B-cell proliferation may also be

* Kikuchi, personal communication

remarkable in this type (TZD) of lymphadenopathy.

REFERENCES

1. Lennert K: Malignant lymphoma, lymphocytic, T-zone type (T-zone lymphoma), in Malignant Lymphomas, Other Than Hodgkin's Disease, Berlin, Springer-Verlag, 1978, 196–209
2. Suchi T, Tajima K: Histopathology of early lesions of peripheral T-cell lymphomas, in Proceedings of the 13th International Cancer Congress, Seattle, Washington, 1982, p. 350
3. Namikawa R, Ueda R, Suchi T, et al: Double immunoenzymatic detection of surface phenotype of proliferating lymphocytes in situ with monoclonal antibodies against DNA polymerase α and lymphocyte membrane antigens, Am J Clin Path 87:725–731, 1987
4. Gerdes J, Schwab U, Lemke H, Stein H: Production of a mouse monoclonal antibody reactive with a human nuclear antigen associated with cell proliferation, Int J Cancer 31:13–20, 1983
5. Minden MD, Toyonaga B, Ha K, et al: Somatic rearrangement of T-cell antigen receptor gene in human T-cell malignancies, Pro Natl Acad Sci 82:1224–1227, 1985
6. Korsmeyer SJ, Arnold A, Bakhshi A, et al: A. Immunoglobulin gene rearrangement and cell surface antigen expression in acute lymphocytic leukemias of T cell and B cell precursor origins, J Clin Invest 71:301–313, 1983
7. Suzuki H, Ueda R, Obata Y, et al: T cell receptor chain gene rearrangements of leukemias with immature T cell phenotype, Jpn J Cancer Res (Gann) 77:1069–1073, 1986
8. Suzuki H, Namikawa R, Ueda R, et al: Clonal T cell population in angioimmunoblastic lymphadenopathy and related lesions, Jpn J Cancer Res (Gann) 78:712–720, 1987

Part III

Advances in Hodgkin's Disease, Childhood, and B-Cell Lymphomas

19

The Enigma of Hodgkin's Disease: Current Concepts Based on Morphologic, Clinical and Immunologic Observations

Ronald F. Dorfman

Abstract

In contrast to classifications of non-Hodgkin's lymphomas, which have been the subject of debate for decades, the Lukes-Butler classification of Hodgkin's disease (HD) and the Rye modification, have been universally adopted. That pathologists should be conversant with the histopathologic types described by Lukes and Butler, rather than the clinically expedient modification proposed at the Rye conference has repeatedly been emphasized. Recently, the attention of pathologists has been drawn to a number of unusual morphologic forms, (i.e., the syncytial and fibroblastic variants of the nodular sclerosing type (NSHD) and interfollicular HD). Most of these represent morphologic variants with diagnostic implications but with no clinical significance; however, the fibroblastic variant appears to have prognostic implications by virtue of the shorter disease-free survival of patients with this type of NSHD.

Clinical and pathologic staging procedures are of paramount importance in assessing the extent of the disease. Such observations outweigh histologic subclassification in terms of therapeutic decisions. It is nonetheless important for pathologists to subclassify HD since the various subtypes show a correlation with age, sex, and sites of involvement.

Although clinical studies have indicated that HD represents a clinicopathologic entity, with a biological behavior different from that of the non-Hodgkin's lymphomas, immunologic studies provide evidence that the nodular L&H (lymphocyte predominant) subtype represents a distinct and unique entity, affecting B cell domains of the lymph node.

The exact nature of the Sternberg-Reed (SR) cell remains the subject of intense controversy. The most popular current theory holds that SR cells represent activated lymphoid cells of either B or T cell type and that they elaborate lymphokines that activate the tissue reactions, representative of the various histologic subtypes.

The high cure rate of Hodgkin's disease (HD) represents one of the major successes in cancer therapy over the past two decades. Nonetheless the exact nature of this disorder remains the subject of intense controversy, speculation, and investigation! This applies equally to the giant cells that characterize this disorder and have been named Sternberg-Reed (SR) cells.[1,2] These cells are seen amidst reactive cellular elements upon which various classifications have been based. That of Lukes and Butler,[3] proposed in 1966, has received universal recognition by pathologists but was simplified for clinical use and its modified form is known as the Rye classification.[4] HD was first described by Thomas Hodgkin in 1832,[5] but was so named by Sir Samuel Wilkes in 1865.[6]

This paper will review a number of unusual morphologic forms that have recently been reported and will address their clinical and prognostic implications. The importance of clinical and pathologic staging procedures in assessing the extent of the disease will be discussed. New concepts of the nodular L&H (lymphocyte predominant) subtype and its association with so-called "progressively transformed germinal centers" (PTGC) will be reviewed. Finally the impact of immunohistochemical studies on our understanding of HD and of the nature of the SR cell will be critically evaluated.

MORPHOLOGIC OBSERVATIONS

In contrast to classifications of non-Hodgkin's lymphomas, which have been the subject of debate for decades, the Lukes-Butler classification of HD and the Rye modification have been universally adopted. It is essential that pathologists utilize the criteria of Lukes and Butler in their initial evaluation of lymph node biopsies before transposing to the Rye classification of HD.[7] Familiarization with the patterns of the Lukes-Butler classification is essential for accurate diagnosis.

Long continued studies of the influence of histopathologic type on survival have confirmed the validity of the Rye classification; however, in the era of more successful treatment of HD, the prognosis for unfavorable histologies has improved and the differences in prognosis among histologic subtypes have greatly diminished.[8] This has raised the question as to whether we should continue to subclassify HD. The author's answer to this is an emphatic yes! The Rye classification delineates distinct clinicopathologic subgroups correlating with age, sex, and sites of involvement.[9] Examples of such observations are provided by the following clinical histories:

1. A young woman who presents with fever, supraclavicular lymphadenopathy, and a mediastinal mass on X-ray is very likely to have the nodular sclerosing type of HD (NSHD) affecting anterior mediastinal lymph nodes or the thymus.
2. A young patient with biopsy-proven NSHD of the mediastinum, no palpable cervical or supraclavicular lymphadenopathy, normal lymphangiogram and abdominal CT scan is very unlikely to have HD below the diapraghm and can be spared a staging laparotomy.
3. A young patient with lymphocyte predominant HD manifesting in the high right cervical lymph nodes, with normal chest X-ray, normal lymphangiogram and CT scans can similarly be spared a staging laparotomy.

Deliberations of the Committee on Histopathologic Criteria at the Ann Arbor Symposium

This committee (of which the author was a member), under the chairmanship of Henry Rappaport, M.D.[10] made certain recommendations, some of which do not appear to have been recognized by many pathologists. Following are two that warrant repetition:

Minimal Sclerosis Limited to Part of the Section

When only a portion of the biopsy section is typical of nodular sclerosis, while the remaining tissue is devoid of either nodularity or bands, the case should nevertheless be classified as nodular sclerosis. Thus NSHD takes precedence over other histologic types.

Lymphocytic Predominance

The histological criteria include not only an abundance of well differentiated lymphocytes but also a scarcity of SR cells and of mononuclear variants. The paucity of SR cells is as significant for the classification of LPHD as is the abundance of lymphocytes.

Unusual forms of HD: Recent reports by us and others have emphasized the importance of recognizing unusual morphologic patterns that can be encountered within the context of HD, observations which were initially made by Lukes and Butler but have only recently come to the attention of pathologists and clinicians.

The Cellular Phase of Nodular Sclerosing HD

This comprises nodules of varying cellular composition containing lacunar cells and classical SR cells, but there are no surrounding fibrous bands. These features, stressed by Dorfman et al[11,12] have nonetheless become a controversial issue, despite the acknowledgment by Lukes[13] that "lymph node involvement in the cellular phase without collagen bands will be found at times, usually as focal or partial involvement, whereas advanced degrees of sclerosis may become evident subsequently." Moreover, the cellular phase of NSHD was recognized by the histopathology committee at the Ann Arbor symposium. It was stated that, "biopsies in which a nodular pattern and conspicuous lacunar cells are seen but no collagenous bands are evident, should be considered as highly suggestive of nodular sclerosis. Supportive evidence of this subclassification should be sought." The author has favored the retention of this terminology to avoid the inclusion of this pattern in the category of mixed cellularity, which has become somewhat of a wastebasket.

Interfollicular HD

SR cells and variants thereof, in an appropriate cellular background, occupy the expanded interfollicular zones, surrounded by prominant reactive follicles.[14] The degree of reactive follicular hyperplasia may be such as to mask interfollicular involvement by HD. This morphologic variant has received relatively little attention in the literature but was recognized by Lukes[13] as focal involvement of lymph nodes by HD. Interfollicular HD may be confused with nonspecific reactive follicular and paracortical hyperplasia, in addition to benign lymph node disorders in which follicular hyperplasia is a prominent phenomenon,[15] e.g. toxoplasmic lymphadenitis,[16] infectious mononucleosis, rheumatoid arthritis, and giant lymph node hyperplasia (Castleman's disease). Although it has been advocated that interfollicular HD should arbitrarily be included with the mixed cellularity subtype, this is not considered appropriate. Dorfman and coworkers have encountered a number of examples of interfollicular HD in which other nodes removed at the same time showed characteristic nodular sclerosis. Moreover a prominent interfollicular pattern could be seen in lymph nodes which focally showed the features of characteristic NSHD. Recognition of the interfollicular pattern is essential so that unnecessary delays in diagnosis and therapy of a potentially curable disease may be avoided.

The Syncytial Variant of NSHD

Lacunar cells and mononuclear SR variants form cohesive cellular aggregates within nodules.[17] Moreover, these cohesive clusters of "Hodgkin's cells" may be conspicuous around foci of necrosis. The term "syncytial variant" for this unusual morphologic expression of NSHD was first introduced by Butler.[18] Banks[19] designated this pattern as "sarcomatous lacunar Hodgkin's disease" and similarly considered this to be a morphologic variant of the nodular sclerosing type. This lesion may be confused with metastatic neoplasms, especially carcinoma as emphasized by Neiman,[20] in addition to germ cell tumors and melanoma. When the syncytial variant of NSHD occurs in the mediastinum, confusion with thymic carcinoma may be engendered. Pleomorphic large cell lymphoma is also an important consideration in the differential diagnosis.

The Fibroblastic Variant of NSHD

Many, but not all, of the nodules contain proliferating fibroblasts, displacing some of the characteristic cellular elements of NSHD and such nodules characteristically show lymphocyte depletion. Within the context of NSHD, some reported studies have correlated depletion of lymphocytes with a worse prognosis; however, in the report of Colby et al from Stanford,[21] covariate analysis demonstrated that the number of fibroblasts was prognostically more significant than the number of lymphocytes. Morever it was shown that the fibroblastic variant of NSHD was associated with a shorter relapse-free survival.

The author has encountered mediastinal biopsies from patients with this variant, which have been misinterpreted as malignant fibrous histocytoma since the fibroblastic element may show a storiform pattern.

Nodular L&H (Lymphocyte Predominant) HD and Progressive Transformation of Germinal Centers (PTGC)

PTGC was defined by Lennert[22] as "a pathologic variant of germinal centers occurring in chronic nonspecific lymphadenitis." PTGC comprises a phenomenon occurring in reactive follicular hyperplasia whereby the follicles (either in the cortex or central areas of the lymph node) become further enlarged by virtue of an infiltrate of small lymphocytes, which apparently overrun the germinal centers. These become distorted, blurred, or completely masked. Immunophenotyping of the small lymphocytes in these abnormal follicles shows them to represent an admixture of mantle B cells with helper/inducer T cells and there is a relative deficiency of cytotoxic/suppressor T cells.[23]

Poppema, Kaiserling, and Lennert[24,25] have proposed a histogenetic relationship between nodular L&H HD and PTGC. The temporal sequence is that of gradual evolution from PTGC into the nodules of nodular L&H HD (nodular paragranuloma) and a malignant transformation of B immunoblasts (L&H cells). With some reservations, Burns et al have made similar observations.[26] They reviewed 171 cases of nodular L&H HD, and in 18% of these cases, the two processes coexisted in the same lymph node. In some patients PTGC was noted in lymph node biopsies prior to the development of nodular L&H HD, whereas in others with histologically proven HD, subsequent lymph node biopsies post-therapy showed only PTGC. The concept that PTGC may evolve to nodular LPHD is intriguing but remains controversial. Thus, it is imperative that the two lesions be separated for management purposes. For now, PTGC remains a histologic marker of abnormal follicle development that in itself is not neoplastic, but which should alert the pathologist to look for evidence of nodular L&H HD either in the same lymph nodes, or in subsequent lymph node biopsies from these patients.

Necrosis in HD: In the author's experience, necrosis is most often associated with the nodular sclerosing type. SR cells and pleomorphic variants thereof, including so-called "mummified cells" (degenerate SR cells) characteristically aggregate about foci of necrosis. The latter may contain numerous polymorphonuclear leucocytes thus simulating microabscesses of cat-scratch disease.[15]

The section on surgical staging procedures will review the phenomenon of isolated granulomas associated with HD. Eosinophilic granulomas in lymph nodes affected by HD, are composed of a central area of eosinophilic necrosis containing material identical to that described in the Splendore-Hoeppli phenomenon,[27] surrounded by epithelioid histiocytes. Such granulomas give rise to concern for parasitic infestations but repeated studies have failed to identify any organisms. It is of interest to note that the Splendore-Hoeppli phenomenon has been described in the skin lesions of patients with Wells' syndrome (eosinophilic cellulitis)[28] and has been ascribed to the liberation of major basic protein by disintegrating eosinophil leucocytes.[29]

This explanation might well account for this phenomenon in the lesions of HD.

SURGICAL STAGING PROCEDURES

The introduction of laparotomy with splenectomy and biopsy of liver and abdominal lymph nodes in the staging of HD at Stanford University in 1968,[30] disclosed a surprisingly high incidence of clinically unsuspected splenic involvement, an appreciable frequency of microscopic involvement of para-aortic nodes, and a distinctly non-random association between spleen and liver involvement. During the ensuing 10 years, staging laparotomy became a standard diagnostic procedure and the pathologist assumed a vital role in identifying involvement of spleen, liver, lymph nodes, and bone marrow by HD. Hoppe et al[31] at Stanford have made additional observations obligating us to record the number and size of splenic lesions. Those patients with five or more nodules of HD have been shown to have a relatively unfavorable prognosis and thus require more aggressive therapy.

Minimal criteria for identification of HD in staging laparotomy specimens were formulated by the histopathology committee at the Ann Arbor symposium.[10] In essence, the committee recommended that, in patients with an established diagnosis of HD in peripheral lymph node biopsies, the presence of mononuclear SR cells in one of the characteristic cellular environments of HD should be regarded as indicative of involvement of abdominal organs even when serial sections fail to disclose diagnostic SR cells.

In bone marrow biopsies, focal or diffuse fibrosis associated with atypical mononuclear cells should be interpreted as strongly suggestive of marrow involvement by HD. Detection of foci of fibrosis should prompt further sectioning in the search for mononuclear or diagnostic SR cells.

Splenic hilar lymph nodes must be identified by the surgeon and removed with the spleen since these have proven to be the only site of abdominal involvement by HD in a number of patients subjected to staging laparotomy at Stanford.[11]

HD affecting the liver or bone marrow in patients who do not have splenic involvement is yet to be encountered. This provides additional evidence supporting the concept that HD spreads in a predictable fashion, manifesting primarily in peripheral lymph nodes, then involving spleen, abdominal lymph nodes, liver and bone marrow.

Isolated granulomas in HD: Focal sarcoid-like granulomas in tissues involved by HD have long been recognized; however, after the introduction of staging laparotomy in 1968 these granulomas were observed by Kadin et al.[32] in the spleen, abdominal lymph nodes, liver, and bone marrow as an isolated phenomenon unassociated with HD in these organs.[32] It was emphasized that these granulomas did not indicate involvement of these organs by HD[33] and that they should not influence therapeutic decision. Some 5 years later, Sacks et al demonstrated that these isolated granulomas were associated with a more favorable prognosis, and that in all likelihood, they represented the morphologic expression of an immunologic response of the host to HD.[33]

EXTRANODAL HD

We have previously emphasized that the diagnosis of HD in extranodal sites should be made with extreme caution since this is a rare phenomenon, particularly in the skin[34] and in the gastrointestinal tract.[35] As indicated by Smith and Butler,[34] skin lesions occur in patients with advanced disease and invariably involve sites drained by affected regional lymph nodes. In contrast to the frequent involvement of various organs by the non-Hodgkin's lymphomas, only rarely has the author identified HD involving Waldeyer's ring, stomach and intestinal tract, thyroid (by direct extension), skin (advanced disease), dura and brain, and exceptionally, the breast (a recurrent lesion secondary to axillary lymph node involvement).

HD IN HOMOSEXUAL MEN WITH THE AIDS-RELATED COMPLEX

High-grade non-Hodgkin's lymphomas and Kaposi's sarcoma are clearly the most common malignant tumors occurring in immunocompromised patients, whether this be after organ transplantation or in association with the acquired immunodeficiency syndrome. The AIDS-related complex includes the syndrome of persistent, generalized lymphadenopathy. Schoeppel et al have recently observed HD in lymph node biopsies performed on a series of homosexual men with the generalized lymphadenopathy syndrome in the San Francisco bay area.[36] The majority of these patients had advanced stage disease and several patients presented with lesions in unusual sites (e.g., skin). The authors' observations suggest that the natural history of HD in patients at risk for AIDS may be altered to a more aggressive form. Moreover, the effects of treatment modalities used in HD for these patients must be further evaluated.

DIAGNOSTIC AND INVESTIGATIVE TECHNIQUES

Ultrastructural studies, tissue culture, cytogenetic studies, enzyme histochemistry, immunohistochemistry, and immunogenotyping are being applied with increasing frequency in laboratories throughout the world in the diagnosis and investigation of HD.

The Enigma of the SR Cell

Monocytes/histiocytes, interdigitating reticulum cells,[37,38] myeloid cells, and lymphocytes have all been implicated as the cell of origin. Enzyme histochemical studies, performed many years ago,[39] produced results that questioned the origin of SR cells from histiocytes (a popular theory at that time). The electron microscopic studies[40] conducted by Dorfman et al provided some ultrastructural evidence supporting the concept that SR cells may be derived from the transformed lymphocyte. The authors commented on concentrations of lymphocytes around SR cells and the observation of europod formation and adhesion between the cytoplasm of lymphocytes and "Hodgkin's cells," suggesting that interactions between these cell types may be important in the pathogenesis of Hodgkin's disease.

Following the advent of monoclonal antibodies (MoAb) and the development of immunoperoxidase techniques applied to tissue sections, Taylor[41] reported the presence of cytoplasmic immunoglobulins in SR cells, implying their lymphoid origin. On the other hand, Kadin et al[42] and Mason and his associates[43,44] identified both kappa and lambda light chains within these cells suggesting internalization of immunoglobulins and re-introducing the concept of the macrophage origin of SR cells. In 1982 Stein et al[45] reported the identification of Hodgkin and SR cells as a unique cell type derived from a newly detected small cell population that reacted with MoAb directed against the Ki-1 antigen. Subsequently, Stein recognized that the Ki-1 antigen was expressed by reactive and neoplastic lymphoid cells in addition to SR cells and hypothesized that this provided evidence that SR cells were derived from activated lymphoid cells.[46] Subsequent observations by Stein et al[47] that Hodgkin and SR cells contain antigens specific to late cells of granulopoiesis, set in motion a spate of studies utilizing anti-granulocyte antibodies such as Leu M1.[48] Dorfman's studies, in collaboration with Gatter, Pulford, and Mason,[49] indicated that SR cells and variants thereof (including lacunar cells) in NSHD and MCHD expressed the epitope hapten X and reacted with a battery of anti-granulocyte markers. In contrast, these cells did not express leucocyte common antigen, a marker that characterizes the cells of non-Hodgkin's lymphomas. In addition these studies confirmed observations made by Pinkus and Said,[50] who reported a unique staining profile for L&H variants that do express leucocyte common antigen, but are not stained by Leu M1 and other anti-granulocyte markers. Stein et al[51] provided further evidence for the distinctiveness of the nodular lymphocyte predominant type by demonstrating the presence of J chain in the L&H variants. J chain is a polypeptide synthesized exclusively by B cells[52] and is essential for the external transport of secretory immunoglobulins. Cytoplasmic staining indicates endogenous synthesis. Stein et al[51] emphasized that there is a reciprocal relationship between the expression of J chain and hapten X (the epitope identified by anti-granulocyte markers).

Review of reported immunohistochemical studies of nodular lymphocyte predominant HD[25,49–52] indicates that the nodules contain numerous dendritic reticulum cells, in addition to polyclonal B lymphocytes and a lesser number of T lymphocytes, the majority having a helper/inducer phenotype. These findings support the conclusion that nodular LPHD affects the B cell domains of lymph nodes. Further evidence of its distinctive nature is provided by the unique staining profile of the L&H variants when compared with SR cells in other histologic types of HD. L&H variants appear to represent a distinct type of transformed cell, probably of B cell origin and they do not share a common lineage with SR cells in the mixed cellularity, nodular sclerosing, and lymphocyte depleted forms of HD.

The most popular current theory holds that SR cells represent activated lymphoid cells of both B- and T-cell type[53,54] and that they elaborate lymphokines that activate the tissue reactions representative of the various histologic subtypes. According to the concepts of Stein et al[53] and Kadin,[54] SR cells in the nodular sclerosing, mixed cellularity, and lymphocyte depleted forms are derived from activated T cells, while the L&H variants of the nodular lymphocyte predominant subtype derive from activated B cells.

It is clear from various reported studies using MoAb in the investigation of HD, that no marker is specific for SR cells. Leu M1 has been demonstrated to react with a variety of cell types, including normal and malignant epithelial cells.[55] These observations highlight the need always to utilize panels of antibodies for immunohistologic characterization of malignant lymphomas.[56] Distinction of Hodgkin's from non-Hodgkin's lymphomas and from metastatic carcinomas simulating HD, can be facilitated by the additional use of MoAb directed against the leucocyte common antigen T200[57] and keratin, [56] respectively. Tables 19-1 and 19-2 list markers which may be helpful in the study of NSHD, MCHD, and LPHD, respectively.

TABLE 19-1
Immunopathology of NSHD and MCHD

Identification of SR Cells
Antigranulocytic markers (e.g. Leu M1)
Ki-1
Peanut agglutinin
HLA-DR (Ia)
LN-2
Tac (IL2)
Polytypic immunoglobulins
Lack of B, T and macrophage-specific markers.

NSHD = Nodular sclerosing Hodgkin's disease
MCHD = Mixed cellularity Hodgkin's disease

TABLE 19-2
Immunopathology of Nodular LPHD

Identification of "L&H" variants
T200 (leucocyte common antigen)
J chain
Epithelial membrane antigen
Lack of reactivity with Leu M1 and other antigranulocyte markers.

LPHD = Lymphocyte predominant Hodgkin's disease

Genotyping of HD

Conflicting results have been reported in the literature by workers utilizing DNA hybridization techniques for immunoglobulin and T-cell receptor gene rearrangements. Weiss et al[58] from Stanford reported immunoglobulin gene rearrangements in 6 of 7 cases of the nodular sclerosing type selected on the basis of high SR cell content. They reported no rearrangements of T-cell receptor DNA, in accordance with other investigators;[59,60] however, Griesser et al[61] reported occasional clonal T-cell receptor gene rearrangements in Hodgkin's tissues. Weiss et al indicated that, although not conclusive, their observations may support an origin of SR cells from B lymphocytes in NSHD. These findings[58–60] would appear to conflict with the hypotheses proposed by Stein[53] and Kadin,[54] described above.

Weiss et al have also identified Epstein-Barr viral DNA in tissues of Hodgkin's disease.[62] In the light of recent observations that patients with infectious mononucleosis due to Epstein-Barr virus (EBV) have a 2–4 times increased risk of HD,[63,64] the study of Weiss et al[62] may well provide evidence that EBV plays a role in the etiology of HD.

ACKNOWLEDGMENTS

This work was supported in part by Grants CA-34233 and CA-33119 from the National Cancer Institute and National Institutes of Health.

CONCLUSION

The pathologist's role in the management of patients with HD is five-fold; first, to establish a firm and unequivocal diagnosis of HD; second, to utilize the criteria of Lukes and Butler; third, to transpose to the Rye classification; fourth, to identify the extent of disease in staging material, since this influences the clinical course, choice of therapy, and prognosis to a greater extent than does the histologic subtype. Finally, the pathologist is obligated to collect and prepare tissues for the techniques described above, while assuring that adequate material is available for histopathologic evaluation on which patient management decisions are based.

REFERENCES

1. Sternberg C: Über eine eigenartige under dem Bilde der Pseudoleukämie verlaufende Tuberculose des lymphatischen Apparates. Ztschr Heilk 19:21–90, 1898
2. Reed DM: On the pathological changes in Hodgkin's disease with especial reference to its relationship to tuberculosis. Johns Hopkins Hosp Rep 10:133–196, 1902
3. Lukes RJ, Butler JJ, Hicks EB: Natural history of Hodgkin's disease as related to its pathologic picture. Cancer 19:317–344, 1966
4. Lukes RJ, Craver LF, Hall TC, et al: Report of the nomenclature committee. Cancer Res 26(part 1):1311, 1966
5. Hodgkin T: On some morbid appearances of the absorbent glands and spleen. Med Chir Trans 17:68–114, 1832
6. Wilkes Sir S: Cases of enlargement of the lymphatic glands and spleen (or Hodgkin's disease), with remarks. Guy's Hosp Rep 11:56–67, 1865
7. Kaplan HS: Hodgkin's disease (second edition). Cambridge, Massachusetts, Harvard University Press, 1980
8. Torti FM, Dorfman RF, Rosenberg SA, Kaplan HS: The changing significance of histology in Hodgkin's disease. Proc Assoc Cancer Res and ASCO 20:401, 1979 (abstract)
9. Dorfman RF: Relationship of histology to site in Hodgkin's disease. Cancer Res 31:1786–1793, 1971
10. Rappaport H, Berard CW, Butler JJ, et al: Report of the committee on histopathological criteria contributing to staging of Hodgkin's disease. Cancer Res 31:1864–1865, 1971
11. Kadin ME, Glatstein E, Dorfman RF: Clinicopathologic studies of 117 untreated patients subjected to laparotomy for the staging of Hodgkin's disease. Cancer 27:1277–1294, 1974
12. Dorfman RF, Colby TV: The pathologist's role in management of patients with Hodgkin's disease. Cancer Treat Rep 66:675–680, 1982
13. Lukes RJ: Criteria for involvement of lymph node, bone marrow, spleen, and liver in Hodgkin's disease. Cancer Res 31:1755–1767, 1971
14. Doggett RS, Colby TV, Dorfman RF: Interfollicular Hodgkin's disease. Am J Surg Pathol 7:145–149, 1983
15. Dorfman RF, Warnke R: Lymphadenopathy simulating the malignant lymphomas. Hum Pathol 5:519–550, 1974
16. Dorfman RF, Remington J: The value of lymph

node biopsy in the diagnosis of acute acquired toxoplasmosis. N Engl J Med 28:878–881, 1973
17. Strickler JG, Michie SA, Warnke RA, Dorfman RF: The "syncytial variant" of nodular sclerosing Hodgkin's disease. Am J Surg Pathol 10:470–477, 1986
18. Butler JJ: The Lukes-Butler classification of Hodgkin's disease revisited, in Bennett JM (ed): Controversies in the Management of Lymphomas, Boston, Mass. Martinus Nijhoff Publishers, 1983, 1–18
19. Banks PM: Sarcomatous lacunar cell Hodgkin's disease: A morphologic variant of the nodular sclerosing type. Lab Invest 44:3A, 1981 (abstract)
20. Neiman RS: Current problems in the histopathologic diagnosis and classification of Hodgkin's disease. Path Annual 13(2):289–328, 1978
21. Colby TV, Hoppe RT, Warnke R: Hodgkin's disease: A clinicopathologic study of 659 cases. Cancer 49:1848–1858, 1982
22. Lennert K, Stein H, Mohri N, et al: Malignant lymphomas other than Hodgkin's disease. Berlin, Springer-Verlag, Heidelberg, (a p. 38), (b p. 46), 1978
23. Stein H, Gerdes J, Mason DY: The normal and malignant germinal center. Clin Haematol 11:531–559, 1982
24. Poppema S, Kaiserling E, Lennert K: Hodgkin's disease with lymphocytic predominance, nodular type (nodular paragranuloma) and progressively transformed germinal centers—a cytohistological study. Histopathol 3:295–308, 1979
25. Poppema S, Kaiserling E, Lennert K: Nodular paragranuloma and progressively transformed germinal centers. Ultrastructural and immunohistologic findings. Virchows Archiv B Cell Pathol 31:211–225, 179
26. Burns BF, Colby TV, Dorfman RF; Differential diagnostic features of nodular L&H Hodgkin's disease, including progressive transformation of germinal centers. Am J Surg Pathol 8:253–261, 1984
27. Symmers W. St: Systemic pathology (second edition), Vol 2, Churchill Livingstone, Edinburgh, London, New York, 1979, 679, 750
28. Wells GC, Smith NP: Eosinophilic cellulitis. Brit J Dermatol 100:101–109, 1979
29. Peters MG, Schroeter AL, Gleich GJ: Immunofluorescence identification of eosinophil granule major basic protein in the flame figures of Wells' syndrome. Brit J Dermatol 109:141–148, 1983
30. Kaplan HS, Dorfman RF, Nelsen TS, Rosenberg SA: Staging laparotomy and splenectomy in Hodgkin's disease. Analysis of indications and patterns of involvement in 285 consecutive, unselected patients. International Symposium on Hodgkin's Disease. Nat Cancer Instit Monogr 36:291–302, 1973
31. Hoppe RT, Rosenberg SA, Kaplan HS, Cox RS: Prognostic factors in pathologic stage IIIA Hodgkin's disease. Cancer 46:1240–1246, 1980
32. Kadin ME, Donaldson SE, Dorfman RF: Isolated granulomas in Hodgkin's disease. N Engl J Med 283:859–861, 1970
33. Sacks EL, Donaldson SS, Gordon J, Dorfman RF: Epithelioid granulomas associated with Hodgkin's disease. Cancer 41:562–567, 1978
34. Smith JL, Jr, Butler JJ: Skin involvement in Hodgkin's disease. Cancer 45:354–361, 1980
35. Lewin KJ, Ranchod M, Dorfman RF: Lymphomas of the gastrointestinal tract. A study of 117 cases presenting with gastrointestinal disease. Cancer 42:693–707, 1978
36. Schoeppel SA, Hoppe RT, Dorfman RF, et al: Hodgkin's disease in homosexual men with generalized lymphadenopathy. Ann Int Med 102:68–70, 1985
37. Kadin ME: Possible origin of the Reed-Sternberg cells from an interdigitating reticulum cell. Cancer Treat Rep 66:601–608, 1982
38. Hsu SM, Yang K, Jaffe ES: Phenotypic expression of Hodgkin's and Reed-Sternberg cells in Hodgkin's disease. Am J Pathol 118:209–217, 1985
39. Dorfman RF; Enzyme histochemistry of the cells in Hodgkin's disease and allied disorders. Nature 190:925–926, 1961
40. Dorfman RF, Rice DF, Mitchell AD, et al: Ultrastructural studies of Hodgkin's disease. Natl Cancer Instit Monogr 36:221–238, 1973
41. Taylor CR: An immunohistological study of follicular lymphoma, reticulum cell sarcoma and Hodgkin's disease. Eur J Cancer Clin Oncol 12:61–75, 1976
42. Kadin ME, Steites DP, Levy R, Warnke RA: Exogenous immunoglobulin and the macrophage origin of Reed-Sternberg cells in Hodgkin's disease. N Engl J Med 299:1208–1214, 1978
43. Mason DY, Bell JI, Christensson B, Biberfeld P: An immunohistological study of human lymphoma. Clin Exp Immunol 40:235–248, 1980
44. Abdulaziz Z, Mason DY, Stein H, et al: An immunohistological study of the cellular constitutents of Hodgkin's disease using a monoclonal antibody panel. Histopathol 8:1–25, 1984
45. Stein H, Gerdes J, Schwab V, et al: Identification of Hodgkin and Sternberg-Reed cells as a unique cell type derived from a newly detected small cell population. Int J Cancer 30:445–459, 1982
46. Stein H, Mason DY, Gerdes J, et al: The expression of Hodgkin's disease-associated antigen Ki-1 in reactive and neoplastic lymphoid tissue. Evidence that Reed-Sternberg cells and histiocytic malignancies are derived from activated lymphoid cells. Blood 66:848–858, 1985
47. Stein H, Uchanska-Ziegler B, Gerdes J, et al: Hodgkin and Sternberg-Reed cells contain antigens specific to late cells of granulopoiesis. Int J Cancer 29:283–298, 1982
48. Hsu S, Jaffe ES: Leu M1 and peanut agglutinin stain the neoplastic cells of Hodgkin's disease. Am J Clin Pathol 82:29–32, 1984
49. Dorfman RF, Gatter KC, Pulford KAF, Mason DY: An evaluation of the utility of anti-granulocyte and anti-leucocyte monoclonal antibodies in the diagnosis of Hodgkin's disease. Am J Pathol 123:508–519, 1986
50. Pinkus GS, Said JW: Hodgkin's disease, lymphocyte predominant type, nodular—a distinct entity? Unique staining profile for L&H variants of Reed-Sternberg cells defined by monoclonal antibodies to leucocyte common antigen, granulocyte specific antigen and B cell specific antigen. Am J Pathol 118:1–6, 1985
51. Stein H, Hansmann ML, Lennert K, et al: Reed-Sternberg cells and Hodgkin's cells in lymphocyte

predominant Hodgkin's disease of nodular subtype contain J chain. Am J Clin Pathol 86:292–297, 1986
52. Isaacson P: Immunohistochemical demonstration of J chain: A marker of B cell malignancy. J Clin Pathol 32:802–807, 1979
53. Stein H, Gerdes J, Lemke H, Mason DY: Evidence of Sternberg-Reed cells being derived from activated lymphocytes. Haematol Blood Transf 29:441–444, 1985
54. Kadin ME: Activated helper-T-cell origin for lymphomatoid papulosis, mycosis fungoides and some types of Hodgkin's disease. Lancet 2:864–865, 1985
55. Sheibani K, Battifora H, Burke JS, Rappaport H: Leu-M1 antigen in human neoplasms. An immunohistologic study of 400 cases. Am S Surg Pathol 4:227–236, 1986
56. Gatter KC, Heryot A, Alcock C, Mason DY: Clinical importance of analyzing malignant tumors of uncertain origin with immunohistochemical techniques. Lancet 1:1302–1305, 1985
57. Warnke RA, Gatter KC, Falini B, et al: Diagnosis of human lymphoma with monoclonal anti-leucocyte antibodies. N Engl J Med 309:1275–1281, 1983
58. Weiss LM, Strickler JG, Hu E, et al: Immunoglobulin gene rearrangments in Hodgkin's disease. Hum Pathol 17:1009–1014, 1986
59. Sundeen J, Lipford E, Uppenkamp M, et al: Rearranged antigen receptor genes in Hodgkin's disease. Blood 70:96–103, 1987
60. Brinker MGL, Poppema S, Buys CHCM, et al: Clonal immunoglobulin gene rearrangments in tissues involved by Hodgkin's disease. Blood 70:186–191, 1987
61. Weiss LM, Strickler JG, Warnke RA, et al: Epstein-Barr viral DNA in tissues of Hodgkin's disease. Am J Pathol 129:86–91, 1987
62. Griesser H, Feller A, Lennert K, et al: Rearrangement of the Beta chain of the T cell antigen receptor and immunoglobulin genes in lymphoproliferative disorders. J Clin Invest 78:1179–1184, 1986
63. Gutensohn NM, Cole P: Childhood social environment and Hodgkin's disease. N Engl J Med 304:135–150, 1981
64. Munoz N, Davidson RJL, Whitthoff B, et al: Infectious mononucleosis and Hodgkin's disease. Int J Cancer 22:10–13, 1978

20

Comparative Pathology of Giant Cells in Lymphoid Malignancies: Evidences That They Are Proliferating Stem Cells

Koji Nanba
Naomi Sasaki

Abstract

Malignant-appearing giant cells are found in various forms of malignant lymphoma (ML), but their nature is only poorly understood. Nanba and Saski studied 76 cases of ML containing such giant cells with the aid of a recently developed high resolution immunohistochemical technique.

Giant cells in HD were always positive for FTF148, K-1, Ki-67, transferrin receptor (TFR), and mostly for Leu M1, and IL2-R-positivity was observed in one-half of the cases. A pan B marker, L26, was simultaneously expressed in their cytoplasm in some cases, however, T-cell and histiocytic markers were consistently negative.

Giant cells of peripheral T-cell lymphoma were also positive for Ki-67, TFR, IL2-R, Leu 1, and FTF148, and occasionally for Ki-1, but not for other markers. Giant cells of IBL, plasmacytoid were positive for L26, Ki-67, and TFR, and in some cases for FTF148 and Ki-1, but not for Leu M1 and IL2-R. In addition, there were other cases in which histologic distinction between HD and NHL was not possible (ML, unclassified). Giant cells in these cases were positive for Ki-1, IL2-R, TFR, FTF148, Leu M1, and MT-1, and were partially positive for L 26, Leu 4, and 5.

These results indicated that neoplastic giant cells were actively proliferating cells and at the same time, some kind of stem cells in particular forms of lymphoma.

Since the first description in 1932,[1] Hodgkin's disease (HD) has been an enigmatic disease. Characteristic neoplastic giant cells delineated by Sternberg[2] and Reed[3] have been the subject of big controversies on their origin and nature with many cells proposed as their normal counterparts.[4]

Recent developments in immunohistochemistry using monoclonal antibodies and in the rearrangement study of genes for immunoglobulin (Ig) and T-cell receptor (TCR) in malignant lymphoma (ML) have brought some newer findings.

Reed-Sternberg (RS) and mononuclear giant (H) cells were demonstrated to be positive for Ki-1,[5] and Leu M1-positivity was also reported.[6] Although Ki-1-positive cells are only rarely encountered in normal lymphoid tissues, the peripheral blood lymphocytes became positive after stimulation.[7] Based on these, the activated lymphocyte theory has been proposed[7] and is currently popular.

RS and H cells are characterized by their giant nuclei and prominent eosinophilic single nucleoli and abundant, clear to amphophilic cytoplasm,[4] (Fig. 20-1). Variants of these, (i.e., lacunar cells in nodular sclerosing type[8] and the other in the mixed lymphocytic and histiocytic [L&H], nodular type), have also been recognized.[9]

Giant cells with these features are, however, not pathognomonic for HD. These have been described in various neoplastic and nonneoplastic lymphoid tissues as well as in nonhematopoietic conditions.[4] Among hematopoietic malignancies, certain types of non-Hodgkin's lymphoma (NHL) are well known for the appearance of RS-like cells, (e.g., polymorphous immunoblastic lymhoma [IBL] and plasmacytoid IBL). Actually the polymorphous IBL that is a form of peripheral T-cell lymphomas has long been erroneously diagnosed as HD in Japan, because of the frequent presence of such cells[4] (Fig. 20-2).

A recently developed new monoclonal antibody, FTF148,[10] was incidentally found to react, not only with giant cells of peripheral T-cell lymphoma, but also with those in HD.[11] Therefore, a further characterization of giant cells in lymphoid malignancies was undertaken. The authors' study demonstrated that neoplastic giant cells not only shared many common features, regardless of the histologic type, but also represented the proliferating

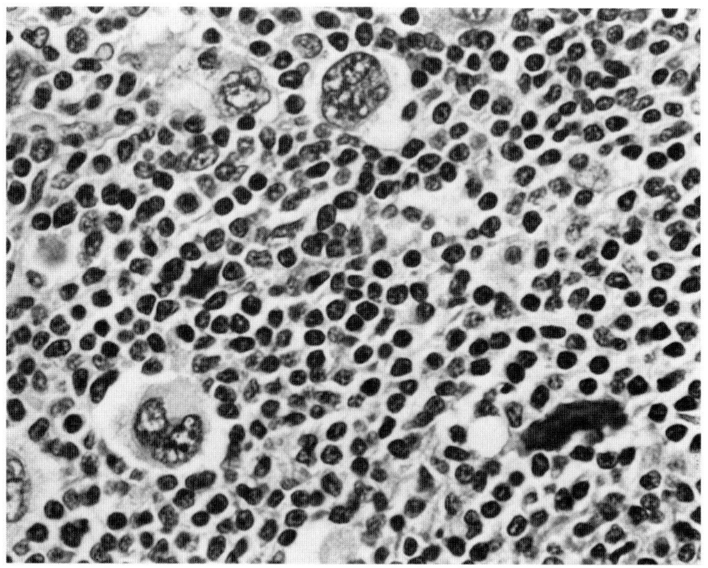

Fig. 20-1. Giant cells observed in Hodgkin's disease, Mixed Cellularity (MC). An elongated dark cell at the lower right was the "mummified" cell (paraffin section, H&E stain, × 600).

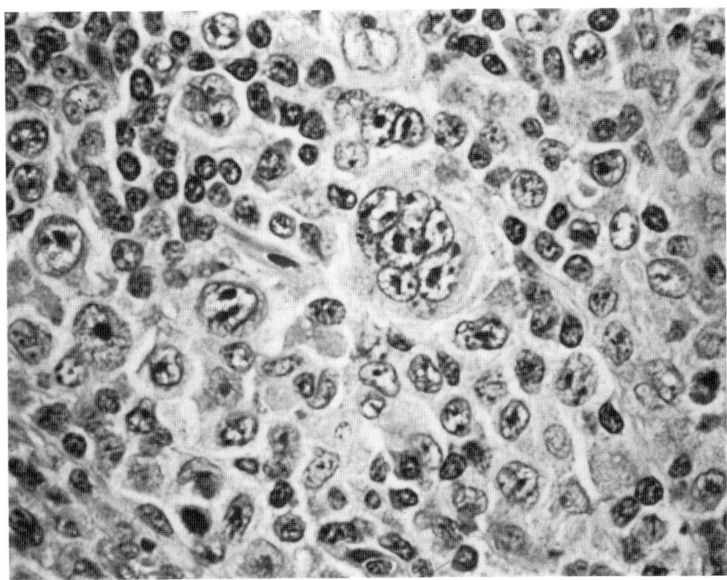

Fig. 20-2. A multinucleated giant cell observed in a HTLV-1-positive immunoblastic lymphoma, polymorphous (Paraffin section, H&E stain, × 800).

cells. Furthermore, an origin from the common stem-cell for lymphocytes and monocytes/histiocytes was suggested.

THE CASES AND METHOD

A total of 76 cases was studied. The tissue was all obtained by the excisional biopsy and was mostly the lymph node. HD was classified according to the Rye classification,[12] and NHL was with the International Working Formulation (IWF).[13] A breakdown of the cases was listed in the Table 20-1. Formalin-fixed paraffin blocks and snap-frozen tissues with liquid nitrogen were used.

A panel of monoclonal antibodies including Leu M1, CD30(Ki-1), FTF148,[11] Ki-67, CD25(IL2-R), L27,[14] (close to CD20) and anti-transferrin receptors (TFR) have been utilized as well as more common antibodies defining T- and B-cell subsets. All antibodies except FTF148 and L27 were commercially obtained.

A new method of alkaline phosphatase (ALP) labeled avidin-biotin technique[15] was used to visualize the antigen-antibody reaction on the tissue section. Since the reaction product was bright red and insoluble in alcohol and xylene, the permanent slides with hematoxylin counterstain were prepared.

TABLE 20-1
Studied Cases in Which Giant Cells are Frequently Observed

Histology	Paraffin	Frozen
Hodgkin's	13	8
IBL,polymorphous	7	7
IBL,plasmacytoid	6	6
ML,unclassified	10	3
Others*	14	2
Total	50	26

* include D-mix., IBL, clear, mycosis fungoides and lymphomatoid papullosis

CHARACTERISTICS OF LYMPHOMATOUS GIANT CELLS

Evidences That Giant Cells Are Proliferating Cells

Ki-67 and TFR were expressed in more than 10% of giant cells in all the cases studied irrespective of the histologic type (Table 20-2).

In HD, TFR was mostly found in RS and H cells as well as in reactive histiocytes, and is rarely found in other cells. The Golgi area of RS cells also showed strong reactivity. (Fig. 20-3A)

Ki-67 was found in the nuclei of giant cells in both HD and NHL. In HD, Ki-67-positivity with the range of 16 to 78% among the giant cells was mainly localized in the nucleolar area of RS and H cells, but diffuse nuclear staining was also observed among the neighboring medium-sized lymphocytes. The reactivity tended to be more diffuse in the nuclei of NHL cells, although there were some cells with clear nucleolar localization indistinguishable from those of RS cells (Fig. 20-3B).

Ki-67 is expressed within the nuclei of cells except G_0 phase and is considered a marker of the cell in proliferative phase.[16] TFR is the receptor for transferrin, which transports iron required by the cell in proliferation.[17] The presence of these two important markers in all the giant cells strongly indicate that these cells are acutally in proliferation in spite of a widely held understanding that these are the result of tumor anaplasia and represent a non-proliferative and degenerative fraction.

Giant Cells Share Common Features

Results of FTF148, Ki-1, Leu M1, and IL2-R staining were summarized in the Table 20-2. It is obvious that these antigens were found at high frequencies in the giant cells of various types of lymphomas. IL2-R reactivity was always membranous (Fig 20-4A), and that of FTF148 was mostly localized at the Golgi area. The reactivity of Ki-1 and Leu M1 was membranous or Golgi-associated. T-IBL and B-IBL were, however, different from the rest by the weak or low expression of FTF148 and Ki-1.

Giant cells also variably expressed membrane antigens like EMA, L26, and MT1, irrespective of the markers observed in the majority of normal-sized cell population in the same tissue. A redundancy of surface membrane in the giant cell was often observed on paraffin sections (Fig. 20-4B). The exuberant membrane corresponded to the villous projections observed with the tranmission electron microscopy.

TABLE 20-2
Expression of Various Antigens in Giant Cells According to Histologic Types of Lymphoma

Histology	TFR (%)	Ki-67 (%)	FTF148(%)	Ki-1(%)	Leu M1(%)	IL2-R (%)
HD(LP)	1/1 (100)	1/1 (100)	1/1 (100)	1/1 (100)	0/1 (0)	1/1 (100)
HD(MC)	3/3 (100)	3/3 (100)	3/3 (100)	3/3 (100)	2/3 (66)	2/3 (66)
HD(LD)	2/2 (100)	2/2 (100)	2/2 (100)	2/2 (100)	1/2 (50)	2/2 (100)
HD(NS)	2/2 (100)	2/2 (100)	2/2 (100)	2/2 (100)	2/2 (100)	2/2 (100)
B-IBL	6/6 (100)	6/6 (100)	1/6 (17)	1/4 (25)	0/4 (0)	2/5 (40)
T-IBL	5/5 (100)	5/5 (100)	6/7 (86)	2/7 (29)	0/7 (0)	5/5 (100)
ML,UC	3/3 (100)	3/3 (100)	3/3 (100)	1/3 (33)	2/3 (66)	2/3 (66)

Positive in more than 10% giant cells. TFR; transferrin receptor
See text for other abbreviations.

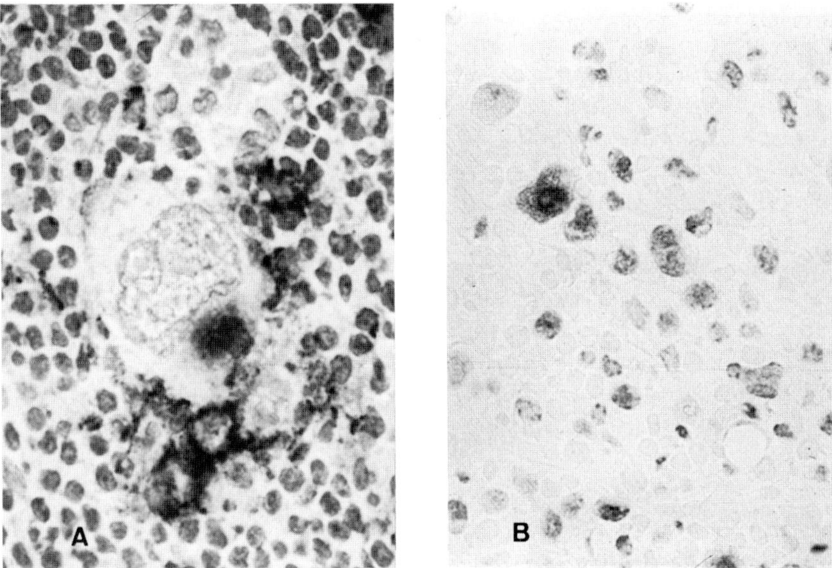

Fig. 20-3. (A) Transferrin receptor was positive on the surface membrane and in the Golgi area of RS cell in a Hodgkin's disease (MC). Two strongly positive cells in the lower center were normal macrophages (frozen section, ALP-labeled immunostain, hematoxylin counterstain, × 800). (B) Ki-67 (Dako-PC) reactivity of immunoblastic lymphoma, polymorphous. Nuclei of giant cells were strongly positive (frozen secion, ALP-labeled immunostain, methylgreen counterstain, × 600).

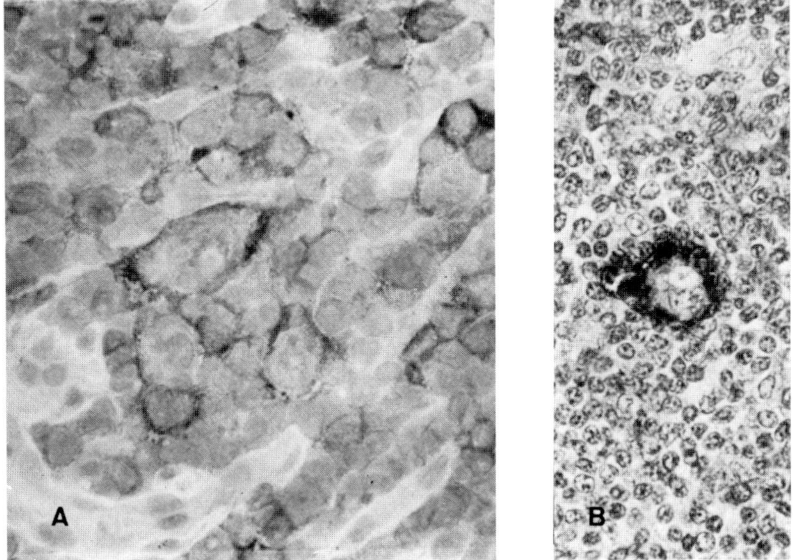

Fig. 20-4. (A) Interleukin 2 receptor (IL2-R) was strongly expressed on the surface membrane of a giant cell (center) in a immunoblastic lymphoma, polymorphous. Notice a huge nucleolus (frozen section, ALP-labeled immunostain, hematoxylin counterstain, × 800). (B) A pan-B antigen (L26) strongly expressed on the surface membrane (which is undulating) of a giant cell in a Hodgkin's disease (MC). Small lymphocytes were completely negative (paraffin section, ALP-labeled immunostain, hematoxylin counterstain, × 600).

On the formalin-fixed paraffin sections, the giant cells were polyclonally stained for cytoplasmic IgG and occasionally for IgA. This phenomenon was not observed if the frozen sections immediately fixed with formol-ethanol were treated in the same manner. Poppema et al[18] initially reported this on HD, but it turned out to be a common feature of giant cells. Although interpreted as the fixation artefact in routinely processed tissue, (i.e., penetration of low molecular proteins into the cell from outside), it suggested a peculiar membranous fragility shared by the neoplastic giant cells.

Giant Cells Express Diverse Differentiation Antigens

Only in a single case among NHLs, were giant cells found to have similar differentiation antigens expressed on the neoplastic lymphocytes in their vicinity. In HD, however, a dissociation between the giant cells and the surrounding lymphocytes was observed as to their antigen expressions: H and RS cells consistently lacked T-cell antigens, but small lymphocytes surrounding them usually carried Th/i markers. The expression of T- and B-cell antigens were generally weak for lymphocytes in HD compared to normal controls.

Furthermore, in a series of the cases classified as ML, unclassified (UC) because of the simultaneous occurrence of RS cells and morphological atypism in the nuclei of lymphocytes (Fig. 20-5A), the following interesting findings were observed.

First, the expression of differentiation antigens in giant cells was variable, even in the single case depicted in the Table 20-3. They had both T and B antigens, and at the same time, expressed histiocytic markers, (e.g., alpha-1-antichymotrypsin [AACT], lysozyme [LYZ], S100-protein, etc.) (Fig. 20-5B). Second, atypical lymphocytes were found to be composed of both T and B cells that were

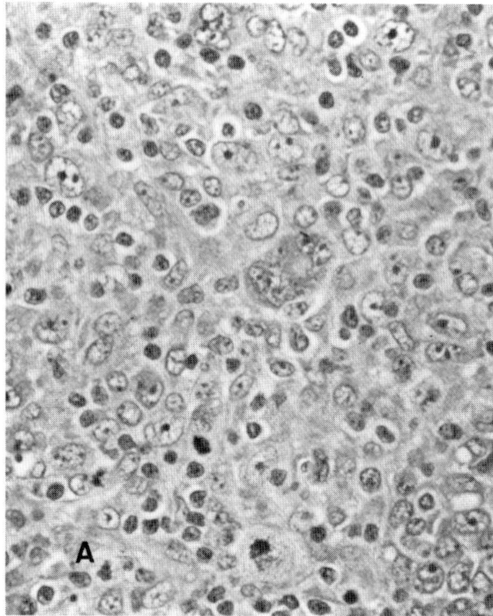

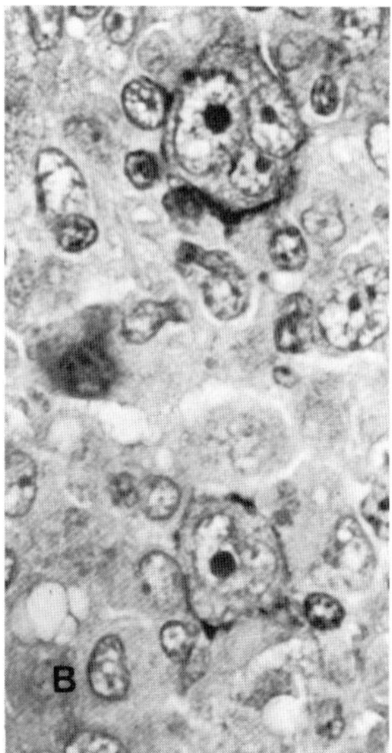

Fig. 20-5. (A) A histology of malignant lymphoma, unclassified (corresponding to Case 5 in Table 20-3). Numerous mononulear and multinucleated giant cells were intermingled with atypical lymphocytes. Both types of cells were in mitosis (parrafin section, H&E stain, × 400). (B) Reactivity to L26 of the same case as in Fig. 5A. Some of giant cells revealed positivity on the surface but admixed lymphocytes were negative (paraffin section, ALP-labeled immunostain, hematoxylin counterstain, × 800).

TABLE 20-3
Giant Cells in ML, Unclassified Express Amazingly Various Antigens

Case #	Age, Sex	Leu M1	L26	MT1	UCHL-1	κ & λ	Leu1	Leu4	S100	Lyz	Phenotype
1 (861620)	46M	+	+	+	+	+	+	+			H,T,B
2 (C-792)	68M	+	+	+	+	+					H,T,B
3 (871693)	72M	+	+	+	+						H,T,B
4 (C-960)	42M	−	+	+	+	+					T,B
5 (872744)	53M	+	+	−	−	+	−	−	+	+	H,B
6 (C-795)	32M	+	−	+	+	+					H,T
7 (C-825)	38M		+	−		λ					B
8 (C-938)	60M		+	−	−						B
9 (C-756)	59M	−	+	−	−						B
10 (863823)	66M	+	−	−	−	+		−			G

Positive in more than 10% giant cells. LYZ; lysozyme, H; histiocyte, T; T cell, B; B cell, G; granulocyte

forming irregular foci segregated within a single lymph node.

NATURE OF GIANT CELLS INCLUDING RS AND H CELLS

H and RS cells were reported to be positive for HLA-DR,[19–20] Leu M1,[6] IL2-R,[20] and Ki-1.[5] The Nanba and Sasaki study not only confirmed these reports, but also clearly demonstrated that giant cells morphologically resembling RS and H cells likewise possessed similar antigens expressed in RS and H cells in HD and, furthermore, shared other features in common. Since the morphology is an integration of numerous kinds of molecules, these findings were not surprising.

Giant cells including RS and H cells are actively proliferating cells as indicated by the positivity for Ki-67 and TFR. The proliferating nature of H and RS cells have also recently been demonstrated by the simultaneous staining of Ki-1 and Ki-67 on the tissue sections of HD.[21] Since Ki-67 also reacts with the nucleus in G_1 phase, a high positivity for this antibody does not automatically mean that the cells are rapidly proliferating. On the contrary, considering rare mitotic figures among these cells on the tissue section and a rather indolent clinical course, it is highly probable that these cells have an exceedingly long G_1 phase.

Giant cells are also known as hyperdiploid cells. Karyotypic studies[22] as well as microphotometric measurements of DNA[23] demonstrated that giant cells in HD were triploid (3N) or mostly tetraploid (4N), and rarely octaploid (8N). It is not an uncommon experience for hematopathologists to observe tetraploid cells in mitosis, with four poles, on the tissue section of HD. In the normal bone marrow, megakaryocytes with the nuclei of up to 16N were reported to be able to undergo cell division.[24]

Based on these evidences, it would not be unreasonable to postulate that giant cells in 4N range of ploidy can duplicate their DNA, hence chromosomes, and give rise to similar giant cells. (Fig. 20-6)

By means of a similar mechanism with the megakaryocte, 4N giant cells might be able to produce daughter 4N cells by mitosis and 8N giant cells by endomitosis[25] (i.e., nuclear fission without cell division). The latter cell may further increase the ploidy by endomitosis or may be destined to degenerate and become "mummified cells" often observed in the tissue slide (Fig. 20-1), since mitosis of 8N cells have not been observed at least by the authors.

Small lymphocytes in the vicinity of giant

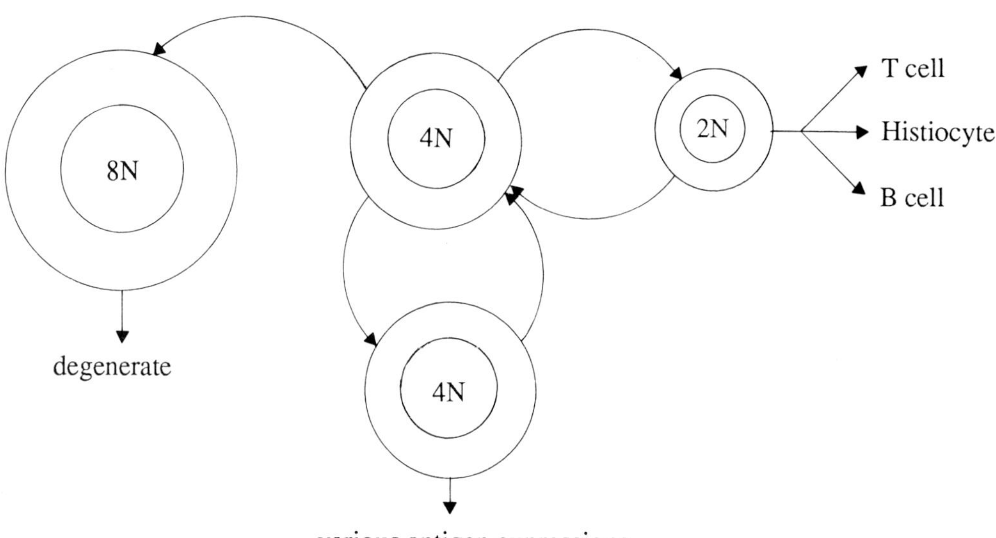

Fig. 20-6. A schematic representation of the relationship of the ploidy of neoplastic lymphoid cells and their differentiation. In this scheme, a 4N giant cell in the upper center is considered as the stem cell for a neoplastic clone. The 8N giant cells are postulated to degenerate and to change into the mummified cells, which are found in Hodgkin's disease and in IBL, polymorphous and ML, unclassified. The 2N cells derived from a 4N cell are considered to have a capability for further differentiation into T, B cells, and histiocytes.

cells are, of course, diploid cells and generally considered as non-neoplastic components. However, Nanba and Saski marker study in HD and ML, UC demonstrated various antigen defects on their surface. This may be due to intrinsic defects in the host cells. The other interpretation is that these cells also derive from neoplastic 4N giant cells and represent end-stage cells incapable of further division. This hypothesis includes the existence of cell division from 4N to 2N, which is only known in the case of germ cells as the meiosis (in this case from 2N to N), and is hard to accept for the somatic cells. However, if we presume the existence of such a mechanism, many of paradoxical behaviors and peculiar features of HD and other ML with giant cells would be more easily explained.

Most of the past study on the nature of RS and HD cells had taken it for granted that the fully differentiated cell should be the physiologic counterpart. Therefore, T and B cells, monocytes, interdigitating reticulum cells (IDC) among others, have been proposed as the normal counterparts of these giant cells. However, any theory presuming a differentiated cell or a cell committed to a single lineage for the origin of RS and H cells cannot explain successfully the discrepancies between the heterogeneity of markers expressed on these cells and a remarkable homogeneity of clinical behavior in the disease, a situation so different in the case of NHL.

Recently, the proposed activated lymphocyte theory[5] could explain the presence of unusual markers like Ki-1 and Leu M1 on these cells but again failed to explain the diversity of other markers found in them unless subdividing HD into T, B, and null cell types. Weiss et al[26] studied 8 cases of lacunar cell-rich nodular sclerosing HD with immunohistochemical and immunogenetic methods. Although the phenotype of neoplastic giant cells were typical of HD, none disclosed rearranged TCR genes in spite of Leu 4(CD3) and 5(CD2) expression in two cases. On the contrary, the rearranged joining region gene of heavy chain was observed in four cases, although the monoclonal band was faint, after digestion with only 1 of 3 restriction enzymes, a very strange phenomenon as discussed by others.[27]

Likewise, IDC theory[20] is hard to accept, not only because of the apparent absence of ATPase activity (a well known characteristic of IDC) in RS cells, but because of the clinical features completely different from a proven IDC proliferation, (e.g., histiocytosis X).

The other explanation, which is schematized in the Figure 20-6, is to assume that: (1) non-committed stem cells for T, B, and histiocytes exist even after birth throughout life in the lymph node, at least in humans. An exceptionally long G_1 phase, presence of HLA-DR, leucocyte common antigen (LCA, CD45), and TFR are consistent with the feature of such stem cells; (2) malignant lymphoma with RS-like giant cells derives from these uncommitted stem cells, but they are capable of differentiation even after the neoplastic transformation; (3) the neoplastic stem-cells are tetraploid and are able to proliferate. However, since they are the tumor of non-committed stem cells with tetraploidy and prolonged G_1 phase, they can not recirculate be-

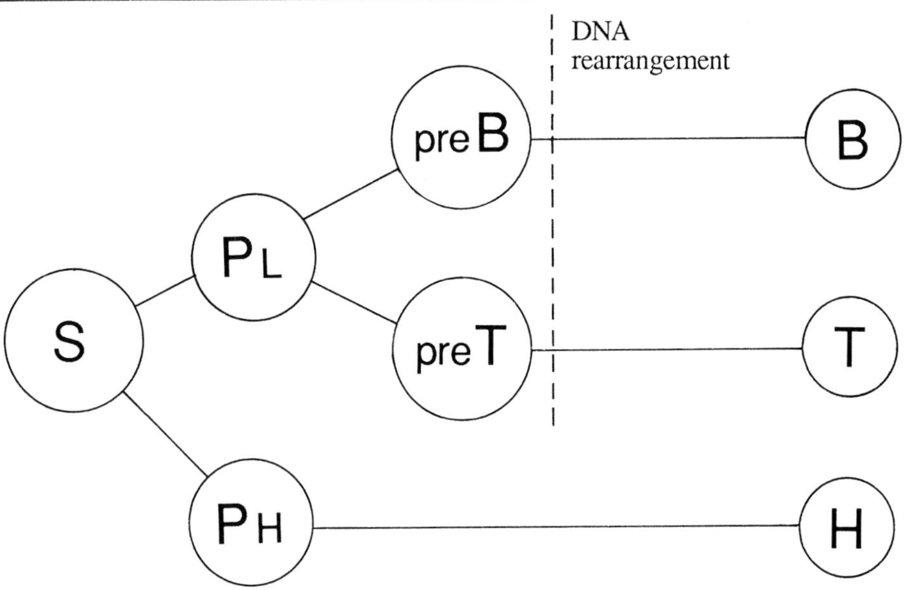

Fig. 20-7. A schematic representation of the relationship between the cell lineage and the corresponding malignant lymphomas. A stem cell (S) for lymphocytes and histiocytes is postulated, and this gives rise to prolymphocyte (P_L) and prohistiocyte (P_H). The prolymphocytes, then, can produce pre-B cells (preB) and pre-T cells (preT), but at this stage the immunogenes are still in germline; DNA rearrangement of these takes place beyond this (broken line). Since most non-Hodgkin's lymphomas including true histiocytic lymphoma occur from the cell that crossed the broken line, their phenotype and genotype are in good agreement. Hodgkin's disease and ML, unclassified, in contrast, arise from the cells at the stage before the broken line. As a result, their expression of differentiation antigens is not necessarily compatible with the genotype.

tween blood vessels and lymphatics in contrast to the committed 2N cells in G_0 phase.[28] This theory is not only able to very well explain a contradiction between a remarkable clinicopathologic homogeneity and the diversity of markers observed in giant cells, but it is also compatible with the available cytogenetic, immunogenetic, and cytokinetic data. The contiguous spread of the neoplastic cells, a peculiar feature observed in HD, is similarly well explainable.

In this connection, so-called Ki-1 positive lymphoma,[5] which demonstrated bimodal incidence peaks in the young and old like HD, could also be explained as having originated from these uncommitted stem cells. The immunophenotype of Ki-1-positive lymphoma was heterogenous,[5] with no correlation between the phenotype and the genotype.[29]

In another word, as is shown in the Figure 20-7, malignant lymphomas could be divided in two major groups; one that derives from the stem cell for lymphocytes and histiocytes, and the other that arises from the committed cell either for T, B cells or histiocytes; the latter is designated as NHL.

Through the study of angioimmunoblastic lymphadenopathy[30] and IBL-like T-cell lymphoma,[31] which had been frequently confused with HD in the past, the authors have presented evidences that both T and B cells are abnormally proliferating in these conditions and that so-called immunoblasts, which sometimes morphologically mimick H and RS cells are devoid of differentiation antigens of T or B cells. Based on these and other immunogenetic as well as clinical data, they proposed a concept of lymphodysplastic syndrome (LDS).[32] LDS may also be related with abnormal and non-neoplastic proliferation of such uncommitted stem cells.

ACKNOWLEDGMENTS

The authors thank Mrs. J. Aoki, Y. Koura, Y. Maeda, and Ms. K. Orisaki for technical assistance; Drs. F. Tsubai and M. Hanaoka, Kyoto University, for providing FTF148; and Drs. T. Takami and K. Kikuchi, Sapporo Medical College, for supplying L26.

Supported in part by the Grant-in-Aid for General Scientific Research (#62570146) of the Ministry of Education, Science and Culture of Japan.

REFERENCES

1. Hodgkin T: On some morbid appearance of the absorbent glands and spleen. Med Chir Soc Tr 17:68–114, 1832
2. Sternberg C: Über eine eigenartige unter dem Bilde der Pseudoleukämie verlaufende Tuberculose des lymphatischen Appartes. Ztschr f Heilk 19:21–90, 1989
3. Reed DM: On the pathological changes in Hodgkin's disease, with special reference to its relation to tuberculosis. Johns Hopkins Hosp Rep 10:133–196, 1902
4. Nanba K, Sasaki N: Histopathologic classification of Hodgkin's disease. Jpn J Clin Radiol 30:1153–1165, 1985 (Japanese)
5. Stein H, Gerdes J, Schwab U, et al: Identification of Hodgkin and Sternberg-Reed cells as a unique cell type derived from a newly-detected small-cell population. Int J Cancer 30:445–459, 1982
6. Hsu S-M, Jaffe ES: Leu M1 and peanut agglutinin stain in the neoplastic cells of Hodgkin's disease. Am J Clin Pathol 82:29–32, 1984
7. Stein H, Mason DY, Gerdes J, et al: The expression of the Hodgkin's disease associated antigen Ki-1 in reactive and neoplastic lymphoid tissue: Evidence that Reed-Sternberg cells and histiocytic malignancies are derived from activated lymphoid cells. Blood 66:848–858, 1985
8. Lukes J, Butler JJ: The pathology and nomenclature of Hodgkin's disease. Cancer Res 26:1063–1081, 1966
9. Poppema S, Kaiserling E, Lennert K: Hodgkin's disease with lymphocytic predominance, nodular type (nodular paragranuloma) and progressively transformed germinal centers—a cytohistologic study. Histopathol 3:295–308, 1979
10. Tsubai F, Namba Y, Kohno M, et al: A monoclonal antibody detecting a novel antigens expressed in the HTLV-I-infected cells. Blood 69:430–436, 1987
11. Sasaki N, Nanba K, Tsubai F, et al: The FTF 148 monoclonal antibody recognizes not only THLV-1 infected cell lines but also neoplastic giant cells in non-Hodgkin's lymphoma and Hodgkin's disease. J Jap Soc Res 27:110, 1987 (Japanese)
12. Lukes RM, Craver LF, Hall TC, et al: Report of the nomenclature committee. Cancer Res 26:1311, 1966
13. The Non-Hodgkin's Lymphoma Pathologic Classification Project: National Cancer Institute sponsored study of classification of non-Hodgkin's lymphomas: Summary and description of a Working Formulation for Clinical Usage. Cancer 49:2112–2135, 1982
14. Ishii Y, Takami T, Yuasa H, et al: Two distinct

antigen systems in human B lymphocytes; identification of cell surface and intracellular antigens using monoclonal antibodies. Clin Exp Immunol 58:183–192, 1984

15. Nanba K, Aoki J, Sasaki N: A new enzyme immunohistochemical technique using alkaline phosphatase-labeled avidin and new fuchsin. Pathol Clin Med 5:333–339, 1987 (Japanese)
16. Gerdes J, Lemke H, Baish H, et al: Cell cycle analysis of a cell proliferation-associated human nuclear antigen defined by the monoclonal antibody Ki-67. J Immunol 133:1710–1715, 1984
17. Trowbridge IS, Omary MB: Human cell surface glycoprotein related to cell proliferation is the receptor for transferrin. Proc Natl Acad Sci (USA) 78:3039–3043, 1981
18. Poppema S, Elema JD, Halie M: The significance of intracytoplasmic proteins in Sternberg-Reed cells. Cancer 42:1793–1801, 1978
19. Poppema S, Bhan AK, Reinherz EL, et al: In situ immunologic characterization of cellular constitutents in lymph nodes and spleens involved by Hodgkin's disease. Blood 59:266–232, 1982
20. Hsu SM, Yang K, Jaffe ES: Phenotypic expression of Hodgkin's and Reed-Sternberg cells in Hodgkin's disease. Am J Pathol 118:209–217, 1985
21. Gerdes J, Van Baarlen J, Pileri S, et al: Tumor cell growth fraction in Hodgkin's disease. Am J Pathol 129:390–393, 1987
22. Rowley JD: Chromosomes in Hodgkin's disease. Cancer Treat Rep 66:639–643, 1982
23. Anastasi J, Bauer KD, Variakojis D: DNA aneuploidy in Hodgkin's disease; a multiparameter flowcytometric analysis with cytologic correlation. Am J Pathol 128:573–582, 1987
24. Pennington DG: The cellular biology of megakaryocytes. Blood Cells. 5:5–10, 1979
25. Therman E, Sarto GE, Stubblefield PA: Endomitosis: A reappraisal. Hum Genet 63:13–18, 1983
26. Weiss LK, Stricker JG, Hu E, et al: Immunoglobulin gene rearrangements in Hodgkin's disease. Hum Pathol 17:1009–1014, 1986
27. O'Connor N: J_H rearrangement in Hodgkin's disease. Hum Pathol 18:871, 1987
28. Nanba K, Hanaoka H: Malignant lymphoma and lymphatic leukemia; their interrelationship. GANN Monogr Cancer Res 28:91–105, 1982
29. O'Connor NTJ, Stein H, Gatter KC, et al: Genotypic analysis of large cell lymphomas which express the Ki-1 antigen. Histopathol 11:733–740, 1987
30. Frizzera G, Moran EM, Rappaport H: Angio-immunoblastic lymphadenopathy with dysproteinemia. Lancet I:1070–1073, 1974
31. Shimoyama M, Minato K, Saito H, et al: Immunoblastic lymphadenopathy (IBL)-like T-cell lymphoma. Jpn J Clin Oncol 9 (Suppl.);347–356, 1979
32. Nanba K, Sasaki N: Pathology of diffuse lesion of the lymph node with cellular atypism—A proposal for diffuse lymphoid dysplasia or lymphodysplastic syndrome. Acta Haematol Jpn 50:1635–1643, 1987

21

Lymphomatoid Papulosis and Ki-1+ Large Cell Lymphomas of the Skin: Pathology, Immunology, Natural History, and Relevance to Hodgkin's Disease

Marshall E. Kadin

Abstract

The author studied and compared the large atypical cells in lymphomatoid papulosis (LyP), Ki-1+ lymphomas, and Hodgkin's disease. The atypical cells in each disorder are characterized by nuclear pleomorphism with prominent nucleoli, aneuploidy, and expression of cellular activation antigens Ia(DR), Tac(CD25), T9, and Ki-1(CD30). An aberrant helper T-cell phenotype is also detected in lymphomatoid papulosis (80%), Ki-1 lymphoma (70%), and Hodgkin's disease (30%). Skin lesions are nonepidermotropic and lymph node involvement, absent in LyP, is often focal within sinuses (Ki-1 lymphoma) and paracortex (Ki-1 lymphoma and Hodgkin's disease). Possible mechanisms to explain the spontaneous regression of skin tumors observed in lymphomatoid papulosis and Ki-1 lymphoma, and waxing and waning of lymph nodes in Hodgkin's disease are also discussed.

INTRODUCTION

This paper summarizes the author's experience with cutaneous tumors of activated T-cells including lymphomatoid papulosis, Ki-1+ large cell lymphomas, and unusual examples of primary cutaneous Hodgkin's disease. From this experience, a hypothesis was made that Reed-Sternberg cells in some types of Hodgkin's disease are derived from activated T-cells. This concept is supported by studies done directly on tissues from patients with Hodgkin's disease, using an improved histochemical technique. Additionally, a working hypothesis for the multistep progression of lymphomatoid papulosis to T-cell lymphoma or Hodgkin's disease is presented. This hypothesis includes possible mechanisms to explain the spontaneous regression of skin lesions typical of lymphomatoid papulosis, which are sometimes observed in skin, and the occasional waxing and waning of lymph nodes affected by Ki-1+ lymphomas and Hodgkin's disease.

Lymphomatoid Papulosis

Histology

Lymphomatoid Papulosis (LyP) was best characterized and described as a clinicopathologic entity in 1968 by Warran Macaulay, a dermatologist practicing in Fargo, North Dakota.[1] LyP is a recurrent, continuous cutaneous eruption that is clinically benign, but histologically malignant. The clinical appearance is that of generalized self-healing papules and nodules that resemble the earliest clinical manifestations of Adult T-cell Leukemia-Lymphoma (ATL);[2] however, unlike ATL, no atypical cells are detected in the blood in LyP. The classical histologic appearance of LyP is that of a wedge-shaped lesion comprising atypical lymphoid cells within the dermis and focally infiltrating the epidermis. In early stages, the lymphoid cells may be confined largely to perivascular regions, whereas in late stage lesions, there is usually an admixture of inflammatory neutrophils and eosinophils with focal ulceration of the epidermis. Plasma cells are rare, although there is frequently cuffing of dermal vessels by small lymphocytes. This feature plus swelling and hypertrophy of endothelial cells closely resembles the appearance of a delayed hypersensitivity reaction.[3]

Willemze[4] classified lymphomatoid papulosis into two principal histologic types: type A, in which large atypical cells with characteristics of Reed-Sternberg (RS) cells are prominent; and the less common type B, in which atypical cerebriform cells, similar to mycosis fungoides cells, predominate. A transition between the two cell types is often found.

Immunophenotype

The large atypical cells are activated T-cells which express Hodgkin's disease associated antigens Ki-1, la, Tac, and T9[5] As shown in Table 21-1, these large atypical cells have an aberrant T-cell phenotype that is characteristic of peripheral T-cell lymphoma.[6] There is frequently absence of pan-T-cell antigens CD2, CD5, CD3, and especially, CD7. CD7 is frequently absent in cutaneous T-cell lymphomas, such as mycosis fungoides and the Sezary syndrome.[7] As shown in these representative cases, a helper T-cell phenotype, CD4+, is found in 70% of LyP cases; a CD8 phenotype, characteristic of cytotoxic suppressor T-cells, is found in a smaller percentage (10%) of cases. No T-cell specific antigens can be detected in approximately 20% of LyP cases. In these cases, the phenotype of large atypical cells in LyP is similar to that of Reed-Sternberg cells in most cases of Hodgkin's disease (HD).[8]

TABLE 21-1
Phenotype of Atypical Cells in Lymphomatoid Papulosis

All cases positive for activation antigens Ia(DR), Tac, T9, Ki-1(CD30)
All cases have aberrant T-cell phenotype lacking one or more pan-T-cell antigens, especially 3A1(CD7)
Helper T-cell phenotype T4(CD4) in 70% of cases
Cytotoxic suppressor phenotype T8(CD8) in 10% of cases
Hodgkin's/Reed-Sternberg cell phenotype Ki-1(CD30) lacking all T-cell specific antigens in 20% of cases

Ploidy

Aneuploidy, often with hypertetraploid cells, is another malignant feature shared by RS cells in Hodgkin's disease and RS-like cells in LyP.[4,9] Figure 21-1 shows a DNA histogram with bi-modal peaks of diploid and hypertetraploid cells made from a skin biopsy of a patient with lymphomatoid papulosis type A. An abnormal hypertetraploid karyotype was confirmed in dividing cells from a skin lesion of LyP studied by Espinosa et al.[10]

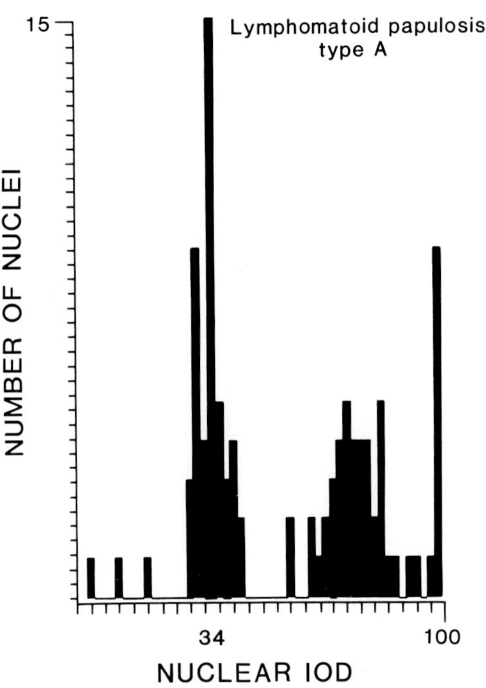

Fig. 21-1. Abnormal DNA histogram in lymphomatoid papulosis, type A, showing normal diploid peak with mode at integrated optical density (IOD) of 34 and many nuclei in tetraploid, hypotetraploid, and hypertetraploid range.

Clonality

Most LyP skin lesions are comprised of clonal T-cells as shown by T-cell antigen receptor beta chain gene rearrangement studies.[11,12] The absence of a 10.8 Kb band and no rearranged band in Eco RI, Hind-III, or Bam HI digests, indicates a likely T-cell hyperplasia in a minority of skin lesions from patients with lymphomatoid papulosis.[12] Multiple separate skin lesions have been analyzed from too few patients to determine whether one or multiple T-cell clones are usually involved. In separate skin lesions obtained 11 months apart from one of our patients, the same gene rearrangement pattern was found.[12] This result is different from that of Weiss et al who found varying patterns of gene rearrangement in each of three separate specimens from one of their patients.[11] However, these authors indicate a likely non-lymphoid source for the 9 Kb DNA band, which provided evidence for a different gene rearrangement pattern in biopsy A, the first of the three skin lesions. If this 9 Kb band were removed, the pattern of rearranged bands in biopsies A and B would be identical, indicating that both lesions may have been derived from the same T-cell clone. Subsequently, Weiss et al reported identical T-cell antigen receptor gene rearrangements in two separate lesions biopsied from each of two patients with pityariasis lichenoides et variola formis acuta (PLEVA) which they considered to be closely related to, if not the same entity as lymphomatoid papulosis.[13]

Secondary Lymphomas

The malignant potential of lymphomatoid papulosis is further indicated by its progression to systemic lymphoma in an estimated 20% of patients.[14,16] Mycosis fungoides, Hodgkin's disease, and large cell lymphoma, usually of the large cell immunoblastic type, are the most common secondary lymphomas occurring in LyP patients.[14–16] We have postulated that these lymphomas arise from clonal expansions of lymphoid subpopulations in the primary skin lesions of LyP patients, accounting for the similar morphology and immunologic phenotype of cells in the skin lesions and secondary lymphomas.[17] Direct molecular genetic or cytogentic evidence demonstrating the clonal derivation of the secondary lymphoma from the primary skin lesions is presently lacking. The development of systemic lymphoma is a slow process, usually longer than 10 years, and is consistent with a multistep process of lymphomagenesis.

Regression of Skin Lesions

The mechanism of usual regression of skin lesions in the pre-malignant stage of LyP is unclear. The presence of small lymphocytes surrounding blood vessels and other histologic features of a delayed hypersensitivity reaction are supportive of the view that a host immune response may contribute to the spontaneous resolution of skin lesions. An alternative hypothesis is shown in Figure 21-2. Upon activation, possibly by a retrovirus, the lymphoid cells secrete interleukin 2 (IL-2) and express receptors for IL-2. This autocrine mechanism promotes their rapid short-term growth. However, as is characteristic of normal activated T-cells, the clonal expansion of these cells is subsequently inhibited by their elaboration of transforming growth factor beta (TGF-beta), which is known to suppress IL-2-dependent T-cell proliferation, apparently by down regulating the IL-2 receptor.[18] This hypothesis is supported by our studies of a clonal T-cell line derived from circulating malignant cells of a patient with cutaneous T-cell lymphoma. This patient had clinically regressing skin lesions. The malignant T-cells produced biological activity of TGF-β, as shown by support of anchorage independent growth of normal rat kidney and AKR-84B fibroblasts in soft agar. In vitro growth of the malignant T-cell clone was 20–40% inhibited by exogenous TGF-β added in nanogram quantities. No growth inhibition was shown when similar quantities of TGF-β were added to the Hodgkin's disease cell line L428, which has no receptors for TGF-β or IL-2.[19]

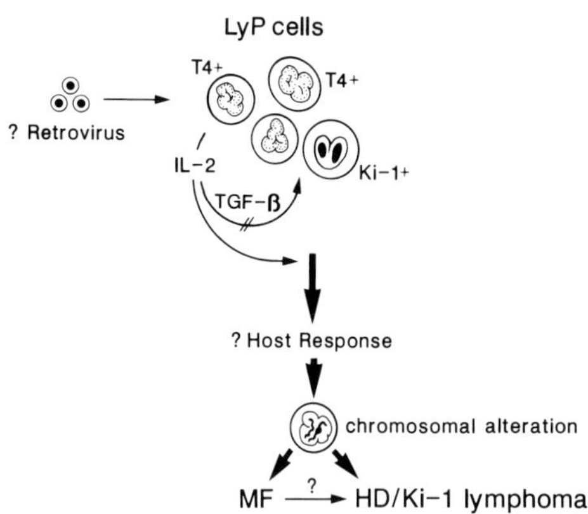

Fig. 21-2. A retrovirus related to HTLV activates T4+ cells, changing their appearance to T4+ Sezary-like cells or Ki-1+ Reed-Sternberg-like cells. The activated T-cells secrete IL-2 and express receptors for IL-2 sustaining their growth. Clonal expansion is limited by the secretion of TGF-β, which suppresses the mitogenic effect of IL-2. A host immune response of the delayed hypersensitivity type can also suppress the growth of individual skin lesions. Repeated crops of skin lesions eventually lead to a mutation or chromosomal alteration. The resulting subclone no longer responds to normal growth regulation signals nor control by the host immune response. The outcome is a systemic lymphoma, usually mycosis fungoides, Hodgkin's disease, or a large cell Ki-1+ immunoblastic lymphoma. The coexistence of mycosis fungoides and Hodgkin's disease, which may result from progressive transformation of T4+ cerebriform cells to Ki-1+ Reed-Sternberge-like cells[17] is also shown.

Etiology

The etiology of LyP is uncertain, although a retrovirus related to HTLV-I can be suspected because of the usual adult onset of the disease, skin lesions, the transformed appearance of the cells, and the usual activated helper T-cell phenotype, resembling the malignant cells of ATL.

Ki-1+ LARGE CELL LYMPHOMA

A large cell Ki-1 lymphoma, which appears morphologically and immunologically similar to LyP, yet clinically resembles regressing atypical histiocytosis (RAH) has recently been described.[20] In contrast to LyP, the skin lesions of Ki-1 lymphoma typically are larger than 2 cm, few in number, and regress only temporarily. Histologically they are deeper, extend into the subcutis, lack epidermotropism, and have fewer small lymphocytes sur-

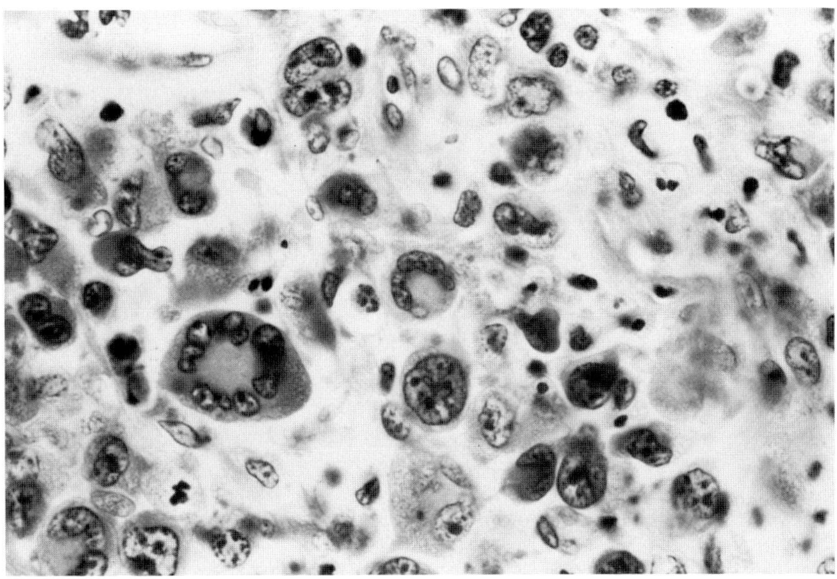

Fig. 21-3. Abnormal histiocyte-like cells in skin lesion of patient with Ki-1+ lymphoma.

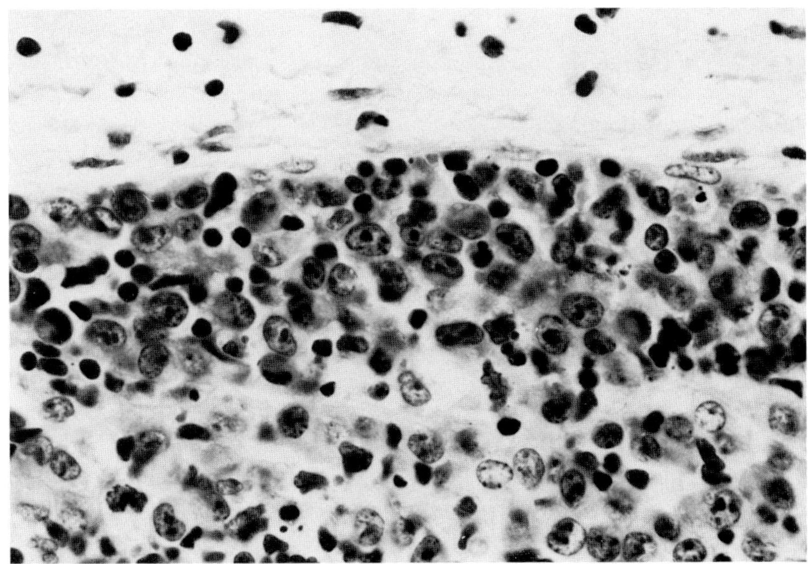

Fig. 21-4. Lymphoma cells with appearance of immunoblasts in subcapsular sinus of lymph node from patient with Ki-1+ lymphoma.

rounding the margin of the lesion and blood vessels than the lesions of LyP. The tumor cells are uniformly large, have fewer convolutions, more cytoplasm, and more often resemble histiocytes than LyP cells (Fig. 21-3).

Lymph nodes are often involved, with characteristic intrasinusoidal and paracortical infiltration of tumor cells (Fig. 21-4). Occasionally, the lymph nodes resemble Hodgkin's disease. However, the atypical cells in Ki-1 lymphoma can be distinguished from Reed-Sternberg cells by their lack of expression of Leu M1(CD15) and expression of LCA(CD45). The immunophenotype is similar to that of LyP cells, but usually with fewer T-cell specific antigens (CD2, CD4, CD3).

A TCR β-chain rearrangement has been detected in the absence of T-cell specific surface markers in Ki-1+ lymphoma.[20] In one patient, separate lesions from the arm and leg were studied, and the same T-cell receptor gene rearrangement pattern was found, indicating a monoclonal origin for the separate lesions.

The initial group of Ki-1+ lymphoma patients presenting with skin lesions were children and adolescents, and there was an unexpectedly high frequency of Black and Oriental patients. A second group of adult patients, 40–70 years of age, have now been identified. The clinical presentation is often deceptive, with a frequent history of insect bite, inflammation, and initial tumor regression, leading to a false impression of benign disease. However, the tumors eventually recur with progressive skin lesions and lymphadenopathy. Radiation may be inadequate for control. Many patients can achieve durable remissions with multi-agent chemotherapy.[20]

PRIMARY CUTANEOUS HODGKIN'S DISEASE

The diagnosis of primary cutaneous Hodgkin's disease has been made for a few patients who have large cutaneous or subcutaneous lesions indistinguishable from Hodgkin's disease, and without associated lymphadenopathy. Three such elderly patients were previously reported by Szur et al.[21] The tumor cell phenotype is similar to that of Reed-Sternberg cells, but with more frequent expression of T-cell antigens. The clinical course may be remarkably benign. Some investigators regard primary cutaneous Hodgkin's disease to be a variant of lymphomatoid papulosis.

RELEVANCE TO HODGKIN'S DISEASE

From these observations, we made the hypothesis that RS cells are derived from activated T-cells in some types of HD. To test this hypothesis, we examined RS-cells in lymph nodes and spleen of patients with HD for expression of T-cell antigens using a method that allowed the distinction of surface antigen staining of RS-cells from surrounding lymphocytes, and confirmation of results by immunoelectronmicroscopy.[22] We found expression of T-cell antigens by RS cells in 8 of 30 or 27% cases of HD. CD2, CD4, and CD3 were the only T-cell specific antigens detected. RS cells were negative for leukocyte common antigen (CD45), in contrast to CD45+ RS-like cells in T-cell lymphomas. The percentage of RS cells expressing T-cell antigens was less than 20% (2 cases), 20–50% (3 cases), more than 50% (3 cases). The percentage of positive cells and the specific T-cell antigens expressed, varied in tissues from different sites in each of two cases suggesting a variable density of surface antigen expression on RS-cells. Expression of T-cell antigens by RS cells was found in nodular sclerosis (6 of 20 cases), and mixed cellularity (2 of 5 cases) types of HD. One case of nodular sclerosing Hodgkin's disease (NSHD) occurred in a patient with a 7-year history of mycosis fungoides. This patient had Ki-1+, T4+, tumor cells in skin and lymph nodes. Two other T-antigen positive cases were associated with the syncytial variant of NSHD, previously reported to be associated with mycosis fungoides.[22] This is consistent with our hypothesis of a common activated helper T-cell origin for lymphomatoid papulosis, mycosis fungoides, and some types of Hodgkin's disease.[17]

CONCLUSION

In summary, this study of lymphomatoid papulosis and other cutaneous lymphomas has improved our understanding of Hodgkin's disease, which appears in some cases to be a proliferation of activated T-lymphocytes. Further analysis of lymphomatoid papulosis may led to clarification of the mechanisms of spontaneous tumor regression in this disorder, and new methods for treatment of Hodgkin's disease.

ACKNOWLEDGMENTS

Supported by Grant 254A from the American Cancer Society.

REFERENCES

1. Macaulay WL: Lymphomatoid papulosis. A continuing self-healing eruption, clinically benign—histologically malignant. Arch Dermatol 97:23–30, 1968
2. Yamaguchi K, Mishimura H, Kawano F, et al: A proposal for smoldering adult T-cell leukemia—diversity in clinical pictures of adult T-cell leukemia. Jpn J Clin Oncol 13 (Suppl 2):189–200, 1983
3. Dvorak HF, Galli, SJ, Dvorak AM: Cellular and vascular manifestations of cell-mediated immunity. Human Pathol 17:122–137, 1986
4. Willemze R, Scheffer E, Ruiter DJ, et al: The clinical and histological spectrum of lymphomatoid papulosis. Brit J Dermatol 107:131–144, 1982
5. Kadin ME, Nasu K, Sako D, et al: Lymphomatoid papulosis: A cutaneous proliferation of activated helper T-cells expressing Hodgkin's disease associated antigens. Am J Pathol 119:315–325, 1985
6. Weiss LM, Crabtree GS, Rouse RV, et al: Morphologic and immunologic characterization of 50 peripheral T-cell lymphomas. Am J Pathol 118:316–324, 1986
7. Haynes BF, Metzgar RS, Minna JD: Phenotypic characterization of cutaneous T-cell lymphoma. Use of monoclonal antibodies to compare with other malignant T-cells. N Engl J Med 304:1319–1323, 1981
8. Hsu SM, Yang K, Jaffe ES: Phenotypic expression of Hodgkin's and Reed-Sternberg cells in Hodgkin's disease. Am J Pathol 118:209–217, 1985
9. Seif GSF, Spriggs Al: Chromosome changes in Hodgkin's disease. J Natl Cancer Inst 39:557–570, 1967
10. Espinosa CG, Erkman-Balis B, Fenske NA: Lymphomatoid papulosis: A premalignant T cell disorder. J Am Acad Dermatol 13:736–743, 1985
11. Weiss LM, Wood GS, Trela M, et al: Clonal T-cell populations in lymphomatoid papulosis: Evidence of a lymphoproliferative origin for a clinically benign disease. N Engl J Med 315:475–479, 1986
12. Kadin ME, Vonderheid ED, Sako D, et al: Clonal composition of T-cells in lymphomatoid papulosis. Am J Pathol 126:13–17, 1987
13. Weiss LM, Wood GS, Ellisen LW, et al: Clonal T-cell populations in *pityariasis lichenoides et varioliformis acuta* (Mucha-Habermann Disease). Am J Pathol 126:417–421, 1987
14. Sanchez NP, Pittelkow MR, Muller SA, et al: The clinicopathologic spectrum of lymphomatoid papulosis—study of 31 cases. J Am Acad Dermatol 8:81–94, 1983
15. Tucker WFG, Leonard JN, Smith N, et al: Lymphomatoid papulosis progressing to immunoblastic lymphoma. Clin Exp Dermatol 9:109–115, 1984
16. Madison JF, O'Keefe TE, Meier FA, Clendenning WE: Lymphomatoid papulosis terminating as cutaneous T-cell lymphoma (mycosis fungoides). J Am Acad Dermatol 9:743–747, 1983
17. Kadin ME: Common activated helper T-cell origin for lymphomatoid papulosis, mycosis fungoides, and some types of Hodgkin's disease. Lancet 2:864–869, 1985
18. Kehrl JH, Wakefield LM, Roberts AM, et al: Production of transforming growth factor-beta by human T lymphocytes and its potential role in regulation of T cell growth. J Exp Med 163:1037–1050, 1986
19. Newcom SE, Kadin, ME, Ansari AE: Production of transforming growth factor-beta activity by Ki-1 positive lymphoma cells and analysis of its role in the regulation of Ki-1 positive lymphoma growth. Am J Pathol 131:569–579, 1988
20. Kadin ME, Sako D, Berliner N, et al: Childhod Ki-1 lymphoma presenting with skin lesions and peripheral lymphadenopathy. Blood 68:1041–1049, 1986
21. Szur L, Harrision CY, Levene GM, Samman PD: Primary cutaneous Hodgkin's disease. Lancet 1:1016–20, 1970
22. Kadin ME, Muramoto L, Said J: Expression of T-cell antigens on Reed-Sternberg cells in subset of patients with nodular sclerosing and mixed cellularity Hodgkin's disease. Am J Pathol 130:345–353, 1988

22

Childhood Lymphoma in Japan, Immunohistologic and Clinicopathologic Review

Atsuo Mikata
Tenjun Mizukami
Hiroshi Horie

Abstract

The authors reviewed childhood lymphomas occurring in the past 15 years in a suburban area of Tokyo, and compared the results with other reports. They also compared children's lymphomas occurring in southwestern Japan, namely Fukuoka and those in the Tokyo area. No meaningful differences were observed, though the number of cases were small. The study showed that childhood non-Hodgkin's lymphomas did not differ significantly from those of western countries. Comparison of childhood and adult lymphomas revealed characteristic differences and some similarities. These facts may give a clue to elucidate the etiology of these lymphomas.

The incidence of lymphomas, especially of Hodgkin's disease is much lower in Japan than in western countries.[1,2] This appears also to be true of childhood lymphomas.[3,4] Large scale clinicopathologic studies have been hampered because of the rarity of childhood lymphomas in any single institute in Japan,[4] although a national survey ranks lymphoma as the fourth most common malignancy in children.[5] The situation seems to be the same even in Europe and the U.S.A.[6–8]

T-cell lymphomas comprise one-third of the cases in middle and eastern Japan, while two-thirds of lymphomas are of T-cell origin, including adult T cell leukemia/lymphoma (ATLL), in south-western Japan.[9] Such predominance of T-cell lymphomas characterize Japanese cases in contrast to those of western countries.[1,9] It is, therefore, most interesting to see if such geographic or racial differences exist in the childhood lymphomas of Japan. The authors reviewed cases collected in Tokyo and Fukuoka areas to clarify these points.

HISTOLOGICAL CLASSIFICATION AND INCIDENCE

Non-Hodgkin's lymphomas in children are different from adult cases, due to the frequency of histologic subtypes,[8] and also the clinical features.[4]

Currently, there are at least four different classification schemes in widespread use in the United States and Europe,[10–13] and one used in Japan.[14] The modified Rappaport classification retains its proven clinical usefulness both in adults and children.[15] Since childhood non-Hodgkin's lymphomas in the U.S. are virtually limited to three major histologic types, Dorfman[16] adopted Rappaport's scheme for the classification of childhood lymphomas. He classifies lymphoblastic, large lymphoid, Burkitt, undifferentiated, and histiocytic types.

The authors used the Japanese Lymphoma Study Group (LSG) classification[14] for the review of the present material, since this scheme has been developed from the Rappaport classification to meet the situation rich in varieties of T-cell lymphomas. LSG scheme can easily be translated into Rappaport or W.F. classification (Table 22-1).

There are only a few well documented series of the childhood lymphomas reported in Japan. Fujimoto[4] reported on 349 cases registered to the nationwide survey program. Pathologic diagnosis made by institutional or local pathologists was entered as such without an authorized review system. In his series, 28% of the cases were lymphoblastic lymphomas. Wakasa[17] reviewed cases from the National Cancer Center, Tokyo University Hospital, and from Fukushima University Hospital. Of 119 cases 70 were the lymphoblastic

TABLE 22-1
Correlation of Japanese LSG Classification to Rappaport and WF Schemas

Rappaport	L.S.G.	W.F.
Nodular	Follicular	Low grade malignancy
poorly differentiated lymphocytic	medium-sized cell(B)	Diffuse small lymphocytic
		Follicular, small cleaved
mixed lymphocytic & histiocytic	mixed cell(B)	Follicular, mixed
histiocytic	large cell(B)	Intermediate malignancy
		Follicular, large cell
Diffuse	Diffuse	
well differentiated lymphocytic	small cell(B,T)	Diffuse small cleaved*[1]
		Diffuse mixed
poorly differentiated lymphocytic	medium-sized cell(B,T)	
		Diffuse large cell
mixed lymphocytic & histiocytic	mixed cell(B,T)	High grade malignancy
histiocytic	large cell (B,T)	Immunoblastic*[2]
	large cell, immunoblastic(B)	polymorphous
Undifferentiated	Burkitt(B)	Diffuse small non-cleaved
Burkitt	Pleomorphic(T)	Burkitt
non-Burkitt	Lymphoblastic(T)	Lymphoblastic

W.F. = Working formulation for clinical usage. --- indicates partial correlation. (*[1] medium-sized T cell lymphoma is not inclued,*[2] immunoblastic includes both T and B cell tumors)—indicates more complete correlation.

TABLE 22-2
Childhood Non-Hodgkin's Lymphomas, Frequency of Histologic Types

	Fujimoto[4]	Wakasa[17]	Present Series
	%	%	%
Follicular	11 (3.2)	1 (0.8)	0
Diffuse	338 (96.8)	118 (99.2)	49 (100.0)
Lymphoblastic	99 (28.4)	70 (58.8)	26 (53.0)
Large cell	68 (19.5)	16 (13.4)	10 (20.2)
Medium-sized cell	65 (18.6)	2 (1.7)	4 (8.2)
Burkitt	51 (14.6)	30 (25.2)	9 (18.4)
Others	55 (15.8)		

type (58.8%), 30 cases, Burkitt lymphomas (25.2%); followed by large cell lymphoma (Table 22-2). Fourty-nine cases were reviewed at Tokyo Metropolitan Children's Hospital, Chiba University Hospital, Matsuo Municipal Hospital, and at Keio University Hospital.[18] The frequency distribution was similar to Wakasa's report.

Since Fukuoka in Kyushu Island is in the endemic HTLV-1 infected area, it was interesting to analyze the children's cases in such a special environment. With courtesy of Professor Kikuchi, the authors personally reviewed 40 cases collected at Fukuoka University during the same period as the cases in Tokyo area were collected (Table 22-3). Though medium-sized cell lymphomas were somewhat more frequent, no pleomorphic lymphomas, as seen in adult cases, were encountered. No special forms of peripheral T-cell lymphoma were found in the children examined of southwestern Japan. The possibility, however, should be explored in a survey of a much larger population.

Although no follicular lymphomas were ob served, Wakasa reported one in his series, and Fujimoto's registration series contained 11 cases of 3.2% (Table 22-2). Burkitt lymphomas made up 18.4% in the Mikata et al series,[19] while they were 25.2% in Wakasa's report. In the U.S.A., Burkitt type was reported to be 86 out of 407 cases (21%) analyzed by Kjeldsberg,[8] and only 4 of 193 cases (2%) of the total by Wieslaw.[20] Lennert reported 8 in his series of 107 cases.[21] Wide variation in the frequency of Burkitt lymphoma in non-endemic countries may reflect the difference in the diagnosis of this entity. In the LSG classification, the undifferentiated non-Burkitt type is included either in the large-cell type, mixed cell type or in immunoblastic type.

In general, the present review did not disclose much difference in the incidence of each subtype of Japanese children's lymphomas from those reported in the western countries.

LYMPHOBLASTIC LYMPHOMAS

Lymphoblastic lymphomas can be divided into pre-B cell, non-T non-B cell, and the T-cell type.[22] With the use of monoclonal

TABLE 22-3
Childhood non-Hodgkin's Lymphomas—Tokyo Area vs Kyushu

	Tokyo	Kyushu
Lymphoblastic	26 (53.0%)	13 (32.5%)
Burkitt	9 (18.4%)	10 (25.0%)
Diffuse large cell	5 (10.2%)	9 (22.5%)
Immunoblastic	5 (10.2%)	
Diffuse medium/mixed	4 (8.2%)	8 (20.0%)
Total	49	40
T : B	26 : 14	
Male : Female	35 : 12	32 : 8

antibodies, most of the lymphoblastic lymphomas are found to be of the cortical thymocyte stage, whereas tumor cells of acute lymphoblastic leukemia are of earlier T cells.[22] Detailed immunologic studies on this lymphoma have not yet been reported in Japan.

Monoclonal MT_1 and MB_1 antibodies were used to determine phenotypes in the paraffine-embedded tissues.[23,24] Of 26 lymphoblastic lymphomas, 21 cases were MT_1 positive and MB_1 negative, while in 2 cases, tumor cells did not react with either of the antibodies (Table 22-4). Two other cases showed no reactivity at all, possibly because of poor fixation. Terminal deoxynucleotidyl transferase (TdT) was positive on the nuclei in 16 of 18 cases examined; with one case TdT positive from both MT_1 and MB_1 reactivity. Since MT_1 can react with immature B cell tumors and TdT is positive in pre-B tumors, bitypic expression may reflect such B-cell tumors, or alternately may well be artefact. Isaacson and Norton[25] recommend the use of a combined panel of LN_1, MB_1, MB_2, MT_1 and UCHL-1 for the phenotypic determination on paraffin sections. Of these 26 lymphoblastic cases, LCA was positive only in 13 cases, cyte common antigen positive (LCA). It appears that immunohistologically, immature T cells did not react with LCA in paraffine sections. One-half or more of patients with lymphoblastic lymphoma presented with a mediastinal mass. Most patients also had peripheral lymphadenopathy and no splenomegaly. Extranodal manifestations in skin, breast, or tonsils were common.[8] Of 26 lymphoblastic lymphomas, 15 patients had a mediastinal mass at diagnosis and, of these, 12 patients also had peripheral lymphadenopathy. Seven patients presented with lymphadenopathy but without mediastinal mass, and 3 patients had cutaneous manifestations at presentation. Non-B non-T lymphoblastic lymphoma showed a possible predilection to develop cutaneous tumors.[26] Only four of the cases developed leukemia.

BURKITT LYMPHOMAS

The first Burkitt lymphoma in Japan was reported by Oboshi et al.[27] in 1969, and more than 50 cases have since been reported. Miyoshi reviewed 14 Japanese cases, including 7 cases of his own series, in which information concerning surface markers, EBV-determined nuclear antigen (EBNA) and chromosomal analysis were available.[28] Age of the patients ranged from 4 to 51 years. Six patients presented with an abdominal mass and 5 with jaw tumors. Most of the patients had a rapid clinical course in spite of combination che-

TABLE 22-4
T : B Classification by Immunostaining

Histology	T	B	NTNB	TB	NR	ND
Lymphoblastic	21	0	2	1	2	0
Diffuse large	3	0	1	0	1	0
Immunoblastic	0	5	0	0	0	0
Burkitt	0	5	0	0	0	4
Diffuse medium/mix	1	0	0	1	0	2
Total	25	10	3	2	3	6*
Final	26	14				

T: Tumor cells positive with MT-1 negative with MB-1 CIg
B: Tumor cells positive with MB-1 and/or CIg, negative MT-1
TB: Tumor cells positive with both MT-1 and MB-1
NTNB: Tumor cells negative with both MT-1 or MB-1, non-tumorous lymphocytes positive
NR: No staining reaction (poor specimen)
* 5 cases were determined immunocytologically as one T- and four B-lymphomas.

motherapy. Only 2 of 14 patients were EBNA-positive. The surface immunoglobulin was Mκ in 7, Mλ in 4, M only in 2 and Gλ in one. Nine patients had the t(8;14) (q24;q32) translocation; and 3 had t(2;8) (p12;q24) or t(8;22) (q24;q13).

In the authors' series 9 Burkitt type lymphomas were found (Table 22-2). Three of them presented with abdominal tumors, 3 with epidural tumors, and 2 others with lymph node enlargement. One of the last had an abdominal tumor also. Except for one patient who underwent intestinal resection, all other patients died within one year. Immunohistologically, Burkitt tumors were MT_1 negative, TdT negative, and MB_1 positive (Table 22-4). In three cases cytoplasmic immunoglobulin was stained as IgMκ, IgM and λ. These findings were entirely consistent with those of non-African or non-endemic Burkitt lymphoma.

Mikata et al encountered three primary spinal epidural Burkitt lymphomas during the review of the present series.[29] This primary site has not been recorded in the literature. Surprisingly, 2 of these 3 cases came from a small rural city in northern Kanto area. Time-space clustering, however, could not be proven.

LARGE CELL LYMPHOMAS AND OTHER TYPES

The Mikata et al series[19] contained 10 large cell lymphomas. Of these, 5 cases were of the immunoblastic type with large central nucleoli and plasmacytoid features. All immunoblastic cases were of B-cell type judged from MB_1 and cytoplasmic immunoglobulin staining. Two of them had ileocecal tumors and the histology might be compatible with undifferentiated non-Burkitt lymphoma. Five other cases showed larger and more irregularly shaped nuclei. Three cases showed infiltration in the T-zone of biopsied lymph nodes. MT_1 was positive and histiocytic markers were negative.

The large-cell lymphoma appears heterogenous in childhood as in adult. Immunologic studies report tumors of both T and B lymphocytes and of null cells.[29,30] Fifty to 60 percent are of B-cell origin[31] in the U.S.A. In eastern Japan, approximately 80% of diffuse large cell lymphoma in adults are B-cell tumors.[32] Data on a significant number of children's cases have not yet been reported in Japan.

Mikata et al classified 3 cases into medium-sized cell type and one case into the mixed cell type. One patient of the former group had anterior mediastinal mass with lymphadenopathy and later developed central nervous system involvement. Since nuclear chromatin and other findings were not of lymphoblastic type, this case was excluded from the lymphoblastic type. Two other cases had lymphadenopathy and MT-1 was positive. The mixed cell type was a case with a frontal skin lesion. Recently, fresh tissues of this case were located, and immunostaining of frozen sections showed OKT-3 and OKT-8 positivity of the tumor cells.

Although Wilson et al.[15] have shown excellent reproducibility of results among hematopathologists separating lymphoblastic from other types, in some instances when tissues are not satisfactory, differentiation of lymphoblastic lymphoma from other medium-sized cell lymphomas is difficult. Immunostaining on a paraffin section of TdT (ABC method) is very useful in such situation.[33] Apparently, further investigation and collection of cases are needed to clarify non-lymphoblastic medium-sized cell lymphomas of children.

CHILDREN'S VERSUS ADULT LYMPHOMAS

Mikata et al compared findings of children's lymphomas with 164 adult cases. There were 80 diffuse large cell cases that accounted 48.7% of the total. Diffuse medium-sized cell type was the second most common subtype, followed by follicular lymphomas (19 or 11.5%), while lymphoblastic lymphoma was 6 or 3.7% of the total. There were 7 pleomorphic T-cell cases. All together, 102 or 66.7% were of B-cell origin and 47 (30.7%) were T-cell tumors, while in children 60% of all

TABLE 22-5
Frequency of S-100 Positive Cells in Lymphomatous Tissue

Histology	Case	−	+	++	+++
Lymphoblastic	24	19	3	1	1
Diffuse large cell	4	0	1	1	2
Immunoblastic	5	5	0	0	0
Burkitt	5	4	1	0	0
Diffuse medium/mix	3	2	1	0	0

+: Average 1–5 positive cells in one field (200×)
++: Average 5–10 positive cells in one field (200×)
+++: Over 20 positive cells in one filed (200×)

cases were T-cell tumors. No Burkitt lymphoma occurred in this period in adults and no small lymphocytic lymphomas or follicular lymphomas were encountered in children.

As for the primary presenting lesions, 63.2%, or 61B and 29T lymphomas, had lymphadenopathy; and mediastinal tumor occurred only in 1.8% in adults. In children, 32.7% showed mediastinal mass at presentation and lymphadenopathy in 30.6%. Most of these differences were due to the predominance of lymphoblastic lymphoma in the children.

Since S-100 protein-positive reticular cells are usually found in the T-cell area of the lymph nodes and are frequently associated with tissues of peripheral T cell lymphoma,[34] the presence of S-100 positive cells in childhood cases was investigated (Table 22-5). Most of the B-cell tumors, such as Burkitt or immunoblastic lymphomas, did not contain S-100 positive cells. Most of the lymphoblastic lymphomas did not show presence of S-100 positive cells. Prominent infiltration was found, however, in diffuse large cell lymphomas, and at least one of these cases was MT_1 positive. Therefore, the authors' experience

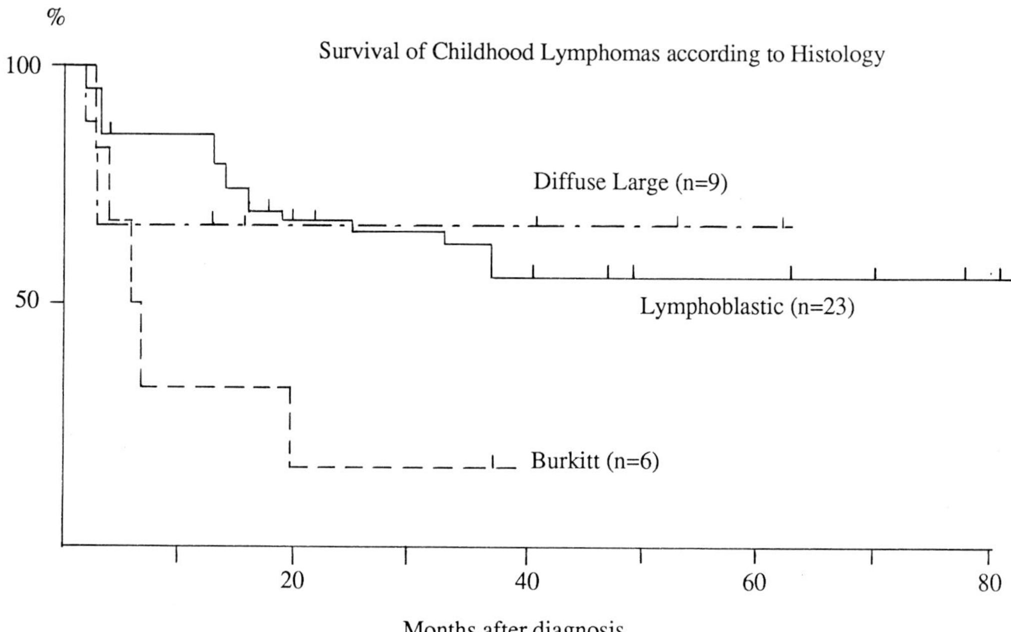

Fig. 22-1. Histologic data outlining survival of childhood lymphomas.

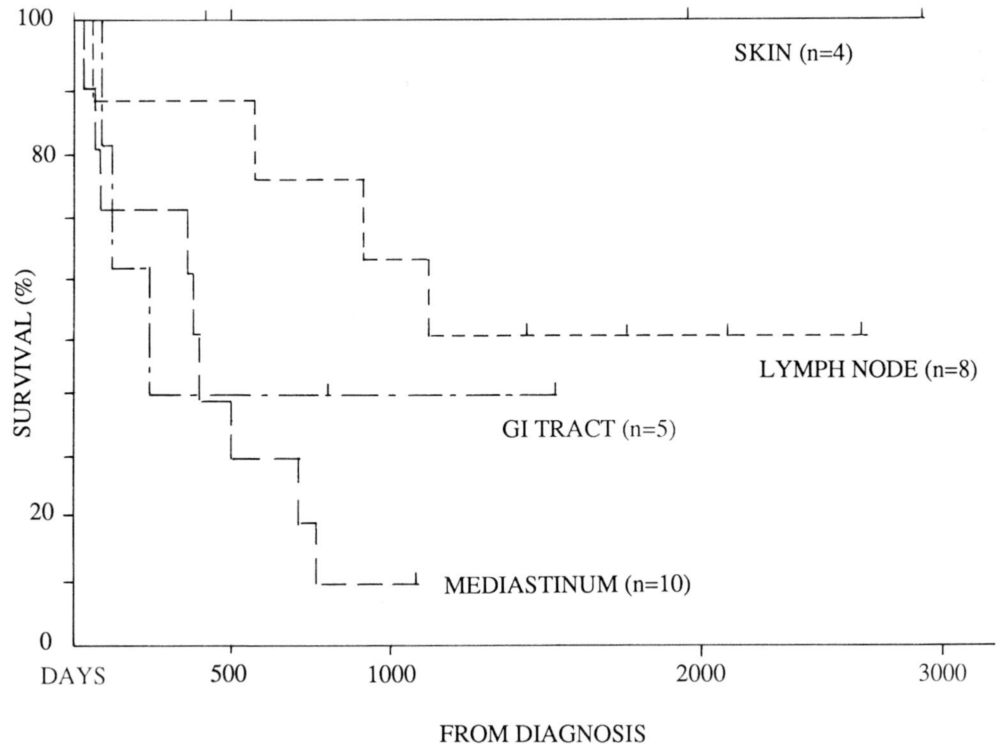

Fig. 22-2. Failure-free survival according to primary sites in childhood NHLs.

is quite compatible with the fact that S-100 protein-positive reticular cells are associated with peripheral T-cell lymphomas. This is also the rule in children.

It is interesting, to note as far as prognosis is concerned, that lymphoblastic lymphoma is not the worst group in children, while the same histologic subtype is usually regarded as one of the most malignant lymphomas in adults[12] (Figure 22-1).

In the present study, no significant difference in survival was demonstrated between B-cell and T-cell groups.[18] The survival curves in relation to the primary sites differ among the skin, peripheral lymph nodes, gastrointestinal tract, mediastinum, and the spinal epidura (Figure 22-2). The authors agree that the prognostic influence of histology and immunophyenotype in childhood lymphoma is of less importance than the site or stage of the disease.[35,36]

ACKNOWLEDGMENTS

We appreciate the cooperation given by Drs. H. Hajikano, Metropolitan Children's Hospital; K. Asanuma, Matsuo Municipal Hospital; H. Sato, Department of Pediatrics, Chiba University Hospital; and M. Aoki, Metropolitan Bokuto Hospital.

REFERENCES

1. Kadin ME, Berard CW, Nanba K, Wakasa H: Lymphoproliferative diseases in Japan and western countries. Human Pathol 14:745–772, 1983
2. Kageyama K, Mikata A, Watanabe S: Hodgkin's disease in Japan, in Akazaki K, Rappaport H, Berard CW, Bennett E, Ishikawa E (eds): Malignant disease of the hematopoietic system. Tokyo, University Tokyo Press, 1973, 239–252
3. Ise T: Malignant lymphoma in children. Jpn J Clin Radiol 30:1415–1425, 1985 (in Japanese)
4. Fujimoto T: Malignant lymphoma of childhood; clinical and biological specificity and its treatment.

Annual Report of the Cancer Research. Ministry of Health and Welfare. 1986 60–16, 191–195 (in Japanese)
5. Sasaki K, Kawai S, Fujimoto T, et al: Treatment of childhood non-Hodgkin's lymphoma with multidrug combination protocol including high dose methotrexate and citrovorum factor rescue; a report from Japanese Children's Cancer and Leukemia Study Group. Jpn J Clin Hematol 26:721–730, 1985 (in Japanese)
6. Growicz TS, Ackerman M: A clinicopathological study of non-Hodgkin's lymphomata in childhood. Brit J Cancer 31 (Suppl. II) 332–336, 1975
7. Weinstein HJ, Link MP: Non-Hodgkin's lymphoma in childhood. Clin Haematol 8:699–716, 1979
8. Kjeldsberg CR, Wilson JF, Berard CW: Non-Hodgkin's lymphoma in children. Hum Pathol 14:612–627, 1983
9. Tajima K, Shimoyama M et al: The T- and B-cell Malignancy Study Group: Statistical analysis of clinicopathological, virological and epidemiological data on lymphoid malignancies with special reference to adult T-cell/leukemia lymphoma: A report of the second nationwide study of Japan. Jpn. J. Clin. Oncol. 15:517–535, 1985.
10. Rappaport H: Tumors of the hematopoetic system. Atlas of Tumor Pathology. Section 3, Fascicle 8, A.F.I.P., 1966, 91
11. Lukes RJ, Collins RD: The Lukes-Collins classification and its significance. Cancer Treatment Rep 61:971–979, 1977
12. National Cancer Institute Sponsored Study of Classification of non-Hodgkin's lymphoma; Summary and description of a working formulation for clinical usage. Cancer 49:2112–2135, 1982
13. Lennert K, Stein H, Kaiserburg E: Cytological and functional criteria for the classification of malignant lymphoma. Brit J Cancer 31: 29–33, 1975
14. Suchi T, Tajima K, Nanba K, et al: Some problems on the histopathological diagnosis of non-Hodgkin's malignant lymphoma—a proposal of a new type. Acta Pathol Jpn 29:7551nd776, 1979
15. Wilson JF, Jenkin RDT, Anderson JR, et al: Studies on the pathology of non-Hodgkin's lymphoma of childhood. I. The role of routine histopathology as a prognostic factor; a report from the Children's Cancer Study Group. Cancer 53:1695–1704, 1984.
16. Dorfman RF: The non-Hodgkin's lymphomas, in Rebuck JW, Berard CW and Abell R. (eds): International Academy of Pathology Monograph. Baltimore, Williams and Wilkins, 1975 262–281
17. Wakasa H, Segami H, Ono N, et al: Pathological characteristics of the childhood lymphoma, in Fujimoto T (ed): Hematological Malignancies in Children. Tokyo, Cancer and Chemotherapy Publishing Co., 1987, 90–103 (in Japanese)
18. Mizugami T, Mikata A, Hajikano A, et al: Primary spinal epidural Burkitt's lymphoma. Surg Neurol 28:158–162, 1987
19. Mizugami T, Mikata A, Hajikano H, Asanuma K: Childhood Lymphoma, a clinicopathological and immunohistological study of 58 cases. Acta Pathol. Jpn. 38, 1149–1166, 1988
20. Wieslaw TD, Molgorzata J, Gladkowska-Dura MJ, Johnson WW: Non-Hodgkin's lymphoma in the first two decades. Virchow's Arch (Pathol Anat) 390:23–62, 1981
21. Lennert K: Malignant lymphomas other than Hodgkin's disease, Histology, Cytology, Ultrastructure and Immunology. New York, Springer-Verlag, 1978
22. Cossman J, Berard CW: Histopathology of childhood non-Hodgkin's lymphoma, in Graham-Pole J (ed); non-Hodgkin's lymphoma in children (Masson Monograph in Pediatric Hematology/Oncology) New York, Masson Publishing Company, 1980, 13–36
23. Tsutsumi Y, Kawai K: Immunohistochemical demonstration of lymphocyte surface markers in formalin-fixed and paraffin embedded specimens. Jpn J Clin Immunol 19:163–175, 1987 (in Japanese)
24. Poppema S, Hollema H, Visser L, Vos H: Monoclonal antibodies (MT_1, MT_2, MB_1, MB_2, MB_3) reactive with lymphocyte subsets in paraffine-embedded tissue sections. Amer J Pathol 127:418–429, 1987
25. Norton AJ, Isaacson PG: The diagnosis of malignant lymphoma using monoclonal antibodies reactive in routinely fixed wax embedded tissue. J Pathol 151:183–184, 1987
26. Bernard A, Murphy SB, Melvin S, et al: Non-T non-B lymphomas are rare in childhood and associated with cutaneous tumor. Blood 59:549–554, 1982
27. Oboshi S, Ise T, Hanawa Y: A childhood lymphoma of jaw resembling Burkitt tumor; the first case in Japan. Gann 60:347–350, 1969
28. Miyoshi I: Japanese Burkitt lymphoma, clinciopathological review of 14 cases. Jpn J Clin Oncol 13:489–496, 1983
29. Koh S, Vargas GS, Cases JN, et al: Malignant histiocytic lymphoma in childhood. Amer J Clin Pathol 74:391–425, 1980
30. Strauchen JA, Young RC, DeVitta VR Jr, et al: Clinical relevance of the histopathological subclassification of diffuse histiocytic lymphoma. New Engl J Med 299:1382–1387, 1978
31. Berard CW, Jaffe ES, Bryalan RC, et al: Immunologic aspects and pathology of the malignant lymphomas. Cancer 42:911–921, 1978
32. Shimoyama M, Minato K, Saito H, Tobinai K: Non-T cell lymphoma and chronic lymphocytic lymphoma, immunologic and clinicopathologic study. Jpn J Clin Oncol 10:241–254, 1980
33. Sawada U, Uchida T, Sakabe T, Amaki I: Detection of terminal deoxynucleotidyl transferase in paraffine sections of malignant lymphoma. Igaku no Ayumi 135:1083–1084, 1985 (in Japanese)
34. Watanabe S, Nakajima T, Shimosato Y: T-zone histiocytes with S 100 protein. Development and distribution in human fetus. Acta Pathol Jpn 33:15–22, 1983
35. Murphy SB: Classification, staging and end results of treatment of childhood non-Hodgkin's lymphomas; dissimilarities from lymphomas in adult. Semin Oncol 7:332–339, 1980
36. Wollner N, Exelby PR, Lieberman PH: Non-Hodgkin's lymphoma in children, a progress report on the original patients treated with the LSA2-L2 protocol. Cancer 44:1990–1999, 1979

23

Non-Hodgkin's Lymphomas in Childhood

Junichiro Fujimoto
Jun-ichi Hata

Abstract

Fifty cases of childhood non-Hodgkin's lymphoma (NHL)s in Japan were analyzed histologically as well as immunohistochemically. Major histologic types were lymphoblastic (LB) (40%), Burkitt's (BU) (34%), and large types (LA) (22%). In each subtype, considerable heterogeneity existed, which first became evident by immunohistochemical approach. Thus, the majority of LB were T cells, most of which corresponded to thymocyte differentiation stage I, while a significant number of B-cell LB having phenotypes of common acute lymphoblastic leukemia (ALL) was also identified. Stage I, T-cell LB had many characteristics comparable to T-cell ALL. Fresh sporadic BUs were found to be heterogenous regarding antigenic phenotypes, all of which were derived from common ALL antigen positive early activated B cells. Finally, childhood LA type was also heterogenous. About half of the LAs were B cell type and three cases of Ki-1 lymphomas were identified. Immunohistochemical and electron microscopic analysis of Ki-1 lymphomas indicated that they might arise from non-lymphoid cell lineage and that epithelial membrane antigen could be used as another marker to characterize this tumor. The results indicate that childhood NHLs are histogenetically heterogenous and that they provide a unique opportunity to study the cellular differentiation mechanism.

With the advent of hybridoma and DNA technology, precise analysis, especially in the determination of cell lineages of non-Hodgkin lymphoma (NHL) has been achieved.[1] This has also been true in childhood NHLs,[2,3] but a precise analysis on the histogenesis of them is not well characterized. Furthermore, the detailed histologic and immunohistochemical study of childhood NHLs in Japan has not been well documented. In this paper the authors describe the histologic and immunohistochemical features of NHLs in childhood emphasizing, the histogenesis of these tumors. The data described in this study confirm that NHLs in childhood are considerably heterogenous, although they are relatively simple in histology as compared with that of NHLs in adults. Such a heterogeneity may include am important clue to understand the cellular differentiation mechanism which can not otherwise be obtained.

Histological Classification of NHL in Childhood

Fifty cases of non-Hodgkin's lymphoma (NHL)s were studied. All cases were diffuse of the types. Histological classification was done by the working formulation (Table 23-1) and it was found that major types were lymphoblastic (LB), Burkitt's (BU), and large cell (LA) types. The incidence for each type was 40%, 34%, and 22%, respectively. A small number (4%) of the small, cleaved-cell type derived from mature T cells was also identified. Consistent with previous observations, LBs arose from mediastinum and lymph nodes, while BUs tended to arise from extranodal sites.

The overall results of the immunophenotypes studied are summarized in Table 23-1. Determiantion of cell lineage was effectively done on paraffin sections by using two monoclonal antibodies: MT1[4] and L26[5] for labeling T cells and B cells, respectively (Fig. 23-1). The reliability of these two antibodies was confirmed by monitoring the same tumors with a panel of monoclonal antibodies used on frozen sections (Tables 23-2 and 23-3). With these two antibodies, most NHL of childhood can be classified. Namely, most of the LB cases were T cells (Figs. 23-1A&B), although a small number of LB was B cells. These B cell LBs had phenoytypes corresponding to common ALL (Table 23-3). All the BUs were positive for B-cell antigen L26 (Fig. 23-1C&D). The details of this type will be discussed later. In the LA type, one half of the cases were diagnosed as B cells (Figs. 23-1E and 23-1F). The remaining cases could not be diagnosed regarding their cell lineage, although three of them were found to be Ki-1 lymphomas[6,7] (Fig. 23-2) which will also be described later.

TABLE 23-1
Histological Classification and the Clinical Manifestation of Childhood Non-Hodgkin's Lymphomas

Histology*	No.		M:F	Mean Age	Primary Site† MED	LN	TON	GIT	RP	Other
LB	T‡	17	11:6	8.3yo	6	9	0	1	0	1(Spine)
	B	3	0:3	5.3yo	0	1	0	0	0	2(Bone, Spine)
BU	B	17	13:4	8.3yo	0	8	2	4	2	1(Oral submucosa)
LA	R	6	3:3	7.8yo	0	2	1	2	0	1(Testis)
	U	5	3:2	8.6yo	0	2	0	0	0	3(Skin, Testis, Bone)
SC	T	2	2:0	12.0yo	0	0	0	1	0	1(Skin)
		50	32:18	8.2yo	6	22	3	8	2	9

* Histological classification was done according to working formulation. LB;Lymphoblastic, BU;Burkitt's, LA; Large, SC;Small cleaved.
† Primary site:MED;Mediastinum, LN;Lymph node, TON;Tonsil, GIT:Gastrointestinal tract, RP;Retroperitoneum.
‡ Cell lineage was determined by MT1 and L26 reactivities. T;T cell type, B;B cell type, U;Undefined.

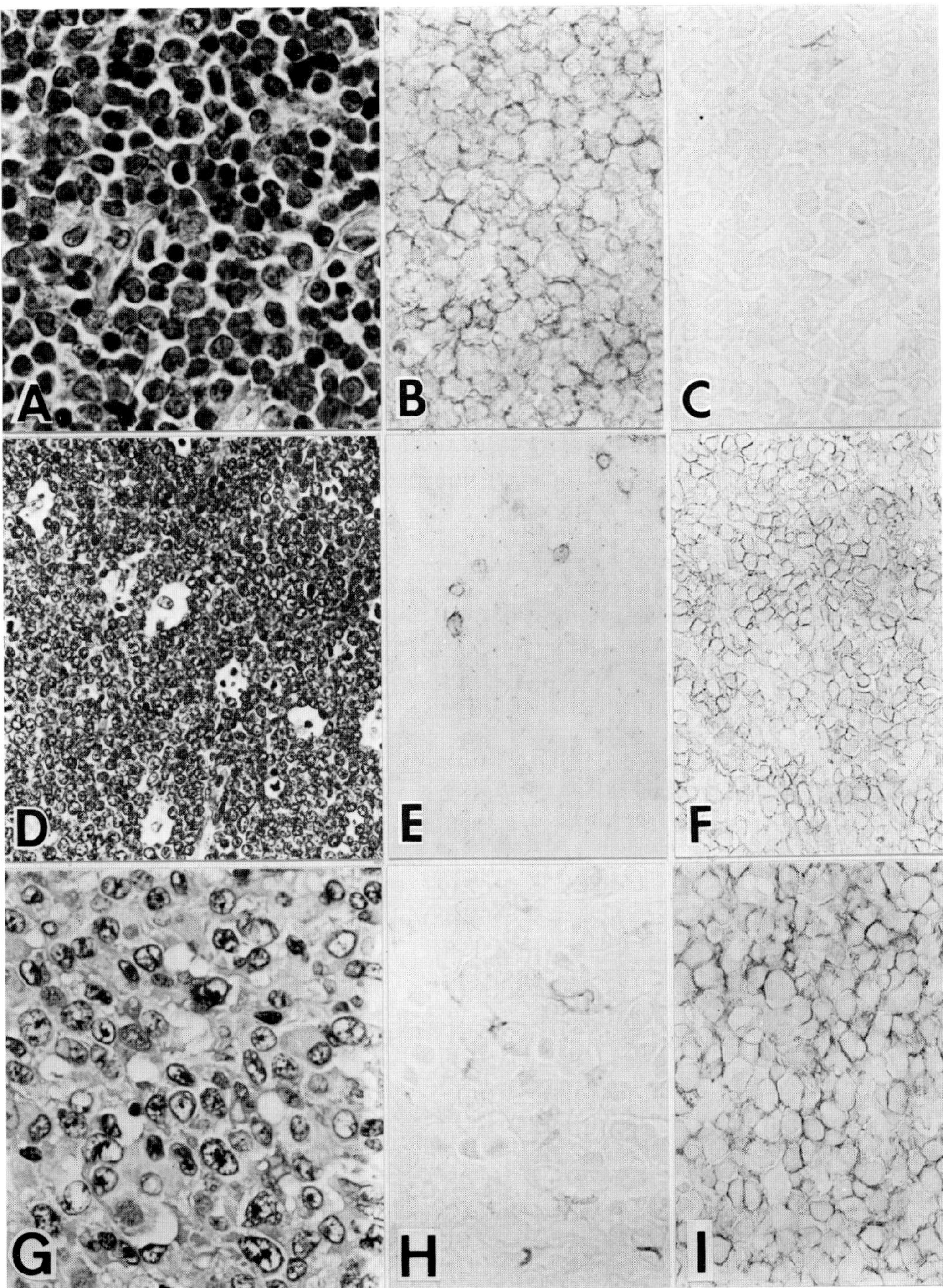

Fig. 23-1. Histologic and immunohistochemical features of non-Hodgkin's lymphomas in childhood. (A) Lymphoblastic type (B) MT-1 immunoperoxidase staining, (C) L26 immunoperoxidase staining, (D) Burkitt's type, (E) MT-1, (F) L26, (G) Large cell type, (H) MT-1, (I) L26. Immunostaining was done on paraffin sections.

TABLE 23-2
Immunophenotypical Classification of Lymphoblastic Lymphomas in Childhood

	CD Classification*																	
	1	2	3	4	5	7	8	10	19	20	T9	T10	MT1	DR	Ig	L26	TdT	Stage†
T Cell Type																		
Case 1 4Y,M	−‡	−	−	−	−	+	−	−	−	−	+	−	+	±	−	−	+	I
Case 2 12Y,M	−	−	−	−	+	+	−	+	−	−	+	+	+	−	−	−	+	I
Case 3 8Y,M	−	+	−	−	+	+	−	−	−	−	+	+	+	−	−	−	+	I
Case 4 10Y,M	−	+	−	−	+	+	−	−	−	−	+	+	+	−	N	N	+	I
Case 5 18Y,F	−	+	−	−	+	+	−	−	−	−	N	N	+	+	−	−	+	I
Case 6 14Y,M	−	−	+	−	+	+	−	−	−	−	±	N	+	−	−	−	+	I
Case 7 9Y,M	−	−	−	+	−	+	−	±	−	−	−	−	+	+	−	−	±	I
Case 8 10Y,M	+	+	+	+	+	+	+	+	−	−	+	+	+	−	−	−	+	II
Case 9 14Y,M	+	N	+	+	+	+	+	N	−	−	N	N	+	−	−	−	N	II
Case 10 15Y,M	+	+	+	+	+	+	+	−	−	−	+	+	+	−	−	−	+	II
B cell Type																		
Case 11 2Y,F	N	N	N	N	N	−	N	±	+	N	N	N	−	+	N	+	+	
Case 12 5Y,F	−	−	−	−	−	−	−	+	+	+	+	±	−	+	−	+	+	
Case 13 9Y,F	−	−	−	−	−	−	−	+	+	−	+	−	−	+	−	+	+	

* Cluster designation of human leukocyte differentiation antigen.
† Stage of thymocyte differentiation.
‡ Reactivity was judged as negative(−), weakly positive(±), or positive(+). N;not tested.

Heterogeneity of Lymphoblastic Lymphomas

The phenotypical results of 13 LBs are summarized in Table 23-2.

Ten were T cells with variable positivity to T cell antibodies. Among the T cell antigens, CD7 and MT1 were most reliable to make the diagnosis. When these cases were judged regarding T cell maturation proposed by Reinherz et al,[8] most cases (Cases 1–7) were stage I (early thymocyte), while only 3 cases (Cases 8–10) were stage II (common thymocyte). In contrast to the observations in western countries,[9] the proportion of stage I T-LB was significantly higher. This may be due to the limited number of cases tested, but the clinical manifestations were typical. Thus stage I T-LB frequently (3 cases out of 7) showed bone marrow involvement at their initial manifestations and they tended to lack a mediastinal mass. From these observations it may be likely that stage I T-LB has characteristics comparable to those of T-cell acute lymphoblastic leukemias.

LBs having phenotypes corresponding to common ALL were also identified (Cases 11–13). These cases tended to arise from extranodal sites (bone and spine). Identification of three immature B cell lymphomas in 50 childhood cases (6%) was quite a high incidence indicating that immature B-cell lymphoma is not rare in childhood NHLs.

Heterogeneity of Sporadic Burkitt's Lymphomas

Eight fresh cases of sporadic BU lymphomas (Table 23-3) were studied using various monoclonal antibodies. All the cases were positive for Ig M, pan B cell antigens such as B4, B1, and L26. In addition, CALLA was positive in all cases. When the resting B cell antigen, L30, and the activation-related antigen, L29, were examined on these cases, heterogenous phenotypes were isolated. The majority of cases (Cases 1–5) were L30+L29−, while L30+L29+ cases (Case

TABLE 23-3
Immunophenotypical Heterogeneity of Sporadic Burkitt's Lymphomas in Childhood

	CALLA	L30	L29	L26	B4	B1	OKB2	sIg	TdT	MT1
Case 1	+	+	−	+	+	+	+	IgMk	−	−
Case 2	+	+	−	+	+	+	+	IgMk	−	−
Case 3	+	+	−	+	+	+	+	IgMk	−	−
Case 4	+	+	−	+	+	+	+	IgMk	−	−
Case 5	+	+	−	+	+	+	+	IgMk	−	−
Case 6	+	+	+	+	+	+	+	IgMk	−	−
Case 7	+	+	+	+	+	+	+	IgMk	−	−
Case 8	+	−	+	+	+	+	−	IgMk	−	−

6 and 7) and a L30−L29+ case (Case 8) were also identified.

In normal tonsillar tissue, L30 was expressed mainly on mantle zone lymphocytes, while L29 was present in germinal center B cells. CALLA positive B cells were located in the germinal center. Judging from these normal tissue distributions of L30, L29, and CALLA, it is likely that sporadic BUs arise from the activated B cells normally present in the germinal center. In endemic fresh BUs, such heterogeneity has not be observed, although it can easily be established from in vitro cultivation.[10] These observations are important because a recent study in DNA analysis, especially on breakpoint position involved in the translocation of chromosome, indicates different mechanisms in endemic and sporadic BUs.[11] In endemic BUs breakpoint regions are in VDJ region in Ig heavy chain gene, whereas in sporadic BUs, translocation occurs at the isotype switching level. It is yet unknown how the different translocation mechanisms result in an almost identical histologic appearance. The phenotypical differences in endemic and sporadic BUs may reflect different events at the DNA level.

Heterogeneity of Large Cell Type Lymphomas

Recent studies by Stein et al[6] and Kadin et al[7] clearly indicate the existence of a certain type of malignant tumor, called Ki-1 lymphoma, showing typical histologic and immunohistochemical characteristics. The authors studied three childhood malignant tumors with characteristics that were compatible to those of Ki-1 lymphomas.[12] Histologically, three cases were the large cell type with highly atypical nulcei and abundant cytoplasm (Figs. 23-2A&B). Lymph node involvement was characterized by subcapsular sinus and perifollicular involvement. The typical proliferation pattern is shown in Fig. 23-2C where Ki-1 positive tumor cells were present in subcapsular marginal sinus, and also in parafollicular area. These cases were postivie for Ki-1, HLA-DR, Interleukin 2 receptor, and OKT9, but negative for Leu M1. All T or B cell antigens were negative except for CD4 in two cases. Electron microscopically, tumor cells had atypical nuclei with peripheral chromatin condensation and contained abundant cytoplasmic organells (Fig. 23-2E). Marked interdigitation of the cell membrane was clearly shown by Ki-1 immunoelectron microscopy (Fig. 23-2F). Interestingly all cases were positive for epithelial membrane antigen (EMA) on cell membrane as well as in cytopasm (Fig. 23-2D). When additional ten LA lymphomas (8 B cell types and 2 unclassified) and two malignant histiocytosis in childhood were studied, two were positive, one case in each type, for EMA. All the B-cell LA types were negative for EMA. One EMA+ LA lymphoma showed a typical sinus

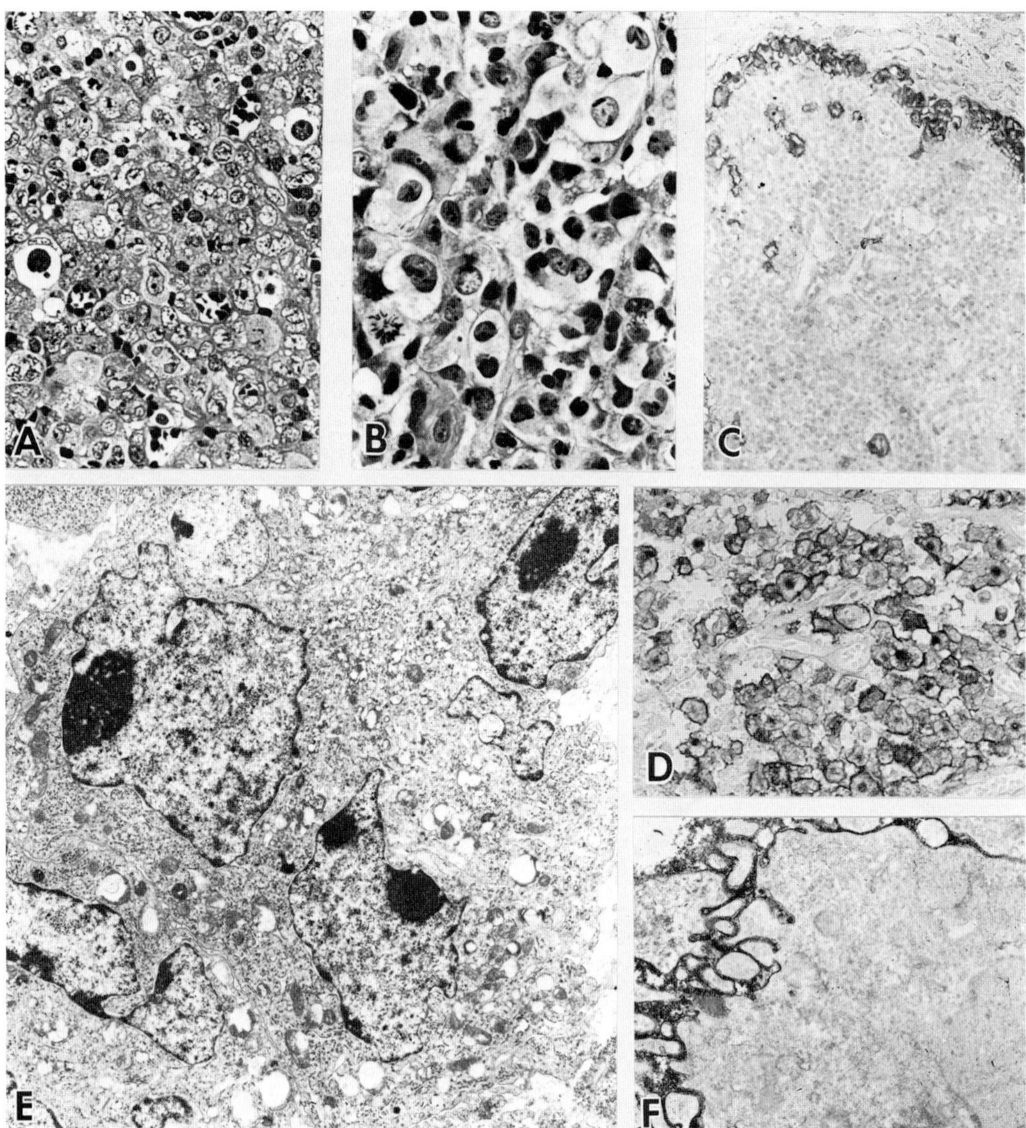

Fig. 23-2. Histologic and immunohistochemical features of Ki-1 lymphomas. (A) Case 1 (8 y.o. male) lymph node; (B) Case 2 (3 y.o. male) testis; (C) Ki-1 immunostaining of Case 1 on frozen section: note the infiltration of Ki-1 positive tumor cells in the marginal sinus; (D) EMA immunostaining of Case 2 on paraffin-section, cell membrane as well as cytoplasm were positive; (E) Electron microscopy of Case 1 (× 8,000); (F) Immunoelectron microscopy of Case 1 stained with Ki-1: marked interdigitation of cell membrane is clearly shown.

infiltration pattern, thus consistent with Ki-1 lymphoma. The results strongly suggest that Ki-1 lymphoma accounts for a significant part of LA type lymphomas in childhood and that EMA can be used as an another marker for Ki-1 lymphomas. Although these cases can be classified as Ki-1 lymphomas, immunohistochemical and electron microscopic studies suggest that possibility that they are derived from non-lymphoid cell lineage. Consistently, Stein et al described Ki-1 lymphomas whose cell lineage were not well characterized.

Therefore, it is likely that lymphoma seems to include tumors of various cell lineages. However, phenotypical as well as histologic similarities clearly show the existence of tumors of the activated cell stage. Of note to add, marked granulocytosis was observed in two our Ki-1 cases, suggesting strongly that they were functional tumors.

CONCLUSION

Consistent with other reports,[2,3] most of NHLs in childhood in Japan fell into three major histologic types: LB, SNC, and LA. But, as described in this paper, there was considerable heterogeneity in each of the histologic subtypes. For example, T-cell LB, Stage I was the most common in Japan, in contrast to the observation in western countries.[9] Sporadic BU was also found to be heterogenous, being derived from CALLA-positive early activated B cells. Last, in LA type, Ki-1 lymphomas in childhood exhibited unique characteristics regarding their proliferation pattern and antigen phenotypes. Finding three fresh Ki-1 lymphomas in 50 childhood non-Hodgkin's lymphomas during a 2-year survey was a relatively high incidence, thus making it possible to accumulate cases to establish their histogenesis. In summary, childhood NHLs in this study in most instances were derived from immature lymphocytes, in contrast to the observations in NHLs in adults where many were derived from the termination stage of differentiation. Childhood lymphomas, therefore, provide important opportunities to study cellular differentiation mechanisms, which could not otherwise be achieved.

ACKNOWLEDGMENT

This work was supported by a Grant-in-Aid for Cancer Research (62–16, 62–19) from the Ministry of Health and Welfare and from the Ministry of Education in Japan. This work was also supported by funds provided by the Entrustment of Research Program of the Foundation for Promotion of Cancer Research in Japan and by a grant from the Children's Cancer Association, Japan.

REFERENCES

1. Foon KA, Todd RF: Immunological classification of leukemia and lymphoma. Blood 68:1–31, 1986
2. Kjeldsgerg CR, Wilson JF: Malignant lymphoma in childhood, in Finegold MF (ed): Pathology of Neoplasia in Children and Adolescents, Philadelphia, W.B. Saunders Co. 1986, 87–125
3. Callihan TR, Berard CW: Childhood non-Hodgkin's lymphomas in current histologic perspective, in Rosenberg HS, Bernstein J. (eds): Perspectives in Pediatric Pathology, Vol. 7, New York, Masson Publishing Inc. 1982, 259–277
4. Poppema S, Hollema H, Visser L, Vos H: Monoclonal antibodies (MT1, MT2, MB1, MB2, MB3) reactive with leukocyte subsets in paraffin-embedded tissue sections. AM J Pathol 127:418–429, 1987
5. Ishii Y, Takami T, Yuasa H, et al: Two distinct antigen systems in human B lymphocytes: Identification of cell surface and intracytoplasmic antigens using monoclonal antibodies. Clin Exp Immunol 58:183–192, 1984
6. Stein H, Mason DY, Gerdes J, et al: The expression of the Hodgkin's disease associated antigen Ki-1 in reactive and neoplastic lymphoid tissue: Evidence that Reed-Sternberg cells and histiocytic malignancies are derived from activated lymphoid cells. Blood 66:848–858, 1985
7. Kadin ME, Sako D, Berliner N, et al: Childhood Ki-1 lymphoma presenting with skin lesions and peripheral lymphadenopathy. Blood 68:104–1049, 1986
8. Reinherz EL, Kung P, Goldstein G, et al: Discrete stage of human intrathymic differentiation: Analysis of normal thymocytes and leukemic lymphoblasts of T-cell lineage. Proc Natl Acad Sci, 77:1588–1592, 1980
9. Weiss LM, Bindl JM, Picozzi VJ, et al: Lymphoblastic lymphoma: An immunophenotype study of 26 cases with comparison to T cell acute lymphoblastic leukemia. Blood 67:474–478, 1986
10. Gregory CD, Trusz T, Edward CF, et al: Identification of a subset of normal B cells with a Burkitt's lymphoma (BL)-like phenotype. J Immunol, 139:313–318, 1987
11. Showe LC, Croce CM: The role of chromosomal translocations in B- and T-cell neoplasia, in Paul WE, Fathman CG, Metzger H (eds), Annual Review of Immunology, Vol. 5, Palto Alto, Annual Reviews Inc, 1987, 253–277
12. Fujimoto J, Hata J, Ishii E, et al: Ki-1 lymphomas in childhood: Immunohistochemical analysis and the significance of epithelial membrane antigen (EMA) as a new marker. Virchows Archiv A, 412:307–314, 1988

24

Lymphotropic Viruses Interacting with Epstein-Barr Virus in the Pathogenesis of Immunodeficiency and Lymphoproliferative Diseases

D. T. Purtilo
M. Okano
G. Thiele
J. Davis
H. Grierson

Abstract

Human lymphocytes can be infected with a variety of DNA and RNA viruses. Each virus, in its own special way, is capable of tranforming or lysing the infected target cell. Often the destruction of the virus-infected cell results from cytotoxic immune responses to viral antigens. Concurrently, the infection evokes an immunosuppressive response due to elaboration of viral products and activation of suppressor T cells. Among the DNA viruses infecting lymphocytes are EBV, cytomegalovirus, varicella-zoster, herpes simplex, hepatitis B virus, human B lymphotropic virus (herpesvirus VI), and adenovirus. Transforming retroviruses including human lymphotropic viruses-I and II, and the non-transforming human immunodeficiency viruses are being intensively investigated. When these viruses simultaneously infect a person, an enormous challenge is presented for the immune system. Understanding the pathogenesis of newly emerging diseases associated with coinfection by these agents is also challenging to investigators. Here the focus is on EBV and assessing the impact of coinfection with the other lymphotropic viruses in selected individuals with immune deficiency.

Diverse viruses that infect lymphocytes and monocytes (Fig. 24-1) often induce temporary immune suppression, especially during acute infection from intrinsic or extrinsic mechanisms.[1] When various lymphotropic viruses infect a person, a variety of unique diseases can emerge simultaneously. For example, human immunodeficiency virus (HIV) and Epstein-Barr virus (EBV) usually coinfect patients who develop acquired immune deficiency syndrome (AIDS).

Most manifestations of EBV infection in AIDS patients come about from proliferation of the target cells. Herein, we summarize several of these lesions in AIDS patients. Purtilo et al conclude the report by describing another type of dual viral interaction, namely, EBV coinfecting with adenovirus.[2]

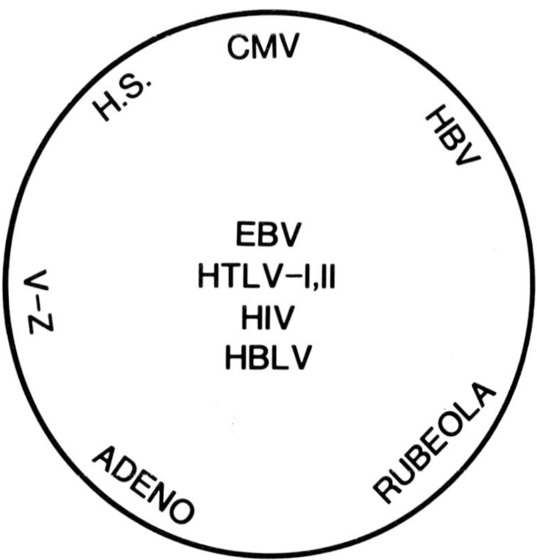

Fig. 24-1. Selected lymphotropic viruses are displayed in this figure. Abbreviations: CMV = cytomegalovirus; HBV = hepatitis B virus; Adeno = adenovirus; V-Z = varicella-zoster; H.S. = herpes simplex; EBV = Epstein-Barr virus; HTLV-I,II = human T lymphotropic virus I and II; HIV = human immunodeficiency virus; HBLV = human B lymphotroic virus.

EBV AND AIDS

Clearly, HIV is the major etiologic agent responsible for AIDS. However, various cofactors, especially infectious agents such as EBV may be responsible for progression from asymptomatic infection with HIV to AIDS. Supporting this hypothesis is the prolonged incubation time from infection with HIV to the emergence of AIDS, which is estimated to range from one to 15 years with a mean of approximately 10 years. Well known is the markedly enhanced production of retroviruses within murine lymphocytes, which have been stimulated during a mixed lymphocytic response *in vitro* or graft versus host disease *in vivo*.[3] Growing evidence suggests that multiple infectious agents could contribute to the emergence of AIDS.[4] By stimulating T cells they could increase productivity of HIV and cause immune suppression.

Patients with AIDS in North America and Africa are all infected with various infectious agents that could act as cofactors along with HIV in the induction of AIDS.[5] An extremely high prevalence rate of antibody to cytomegalovirus (range 92% to 100%), herpes simplex virus (range, 90% to 100%), hepatitis B virus (range, 78% to 82%), hepatitis A virus (range, 82% to 95%), and EBV capsid antigen (100%) prevails in the patients. Other epidemiologic studies have identified that a prior history of infectious mononucleosis is an important risk factor for the development of AIDS in homosexual men.[6] Studies performed in our laboratory during 1983–1984 revealed that 396 consecutive homosexual men from Greenwich Village were seropositive for EBV. Generally, about 90–95% would be expected to be seropositive for EBV. Lymph node biopsy specimens from 6 of these homosexual patients with persistent lymphadenopathy revealed mixed T and B cell proliferations and EBV genome was found in 3 of the specimens.[7] It is well known that EBV is a polyclonal activator of B cells. Similarly, HIV can activate and induce polyclonal proliferation of B cells. Moreover, HIV is capable of dually infecting EBV infected transformed lymphoblastoid cell lines.[8] Described below are 5 EBV-related lesions recently described in HIV seropositive patients.

Hairy Leukoplakia

Greenspan et al[9] have described a gray-white, shaggy lesion on the lateral surfaces of the tongue of homosexual men in San Francisco. Electron microscopy studies have revealed EBV virions and DNA hybridization studies have confirmed the presence of EBV genome in these lesions. When hairy leukoplakia occurs in HIV seropositive homosexual men, it can herald the onset of AIDS. The lesion is very uncommon in other risk group members. It is not surprising that EBV should infect the epithelium of the tongue as the virus normally infects salivary glands.[10] EBV is shed in a very high proportion of individuals infected with HIV.

Persistent Generalized Lymphadenopathy

As noted above, persistent generalized lymphadenopathy is a manifestation of AIDS-related complex, especially in homosexual males. This lesion is due to the expansion of both T and B cell populations within the lymph nodes. Lipscomb et al have demonstrated EBV genome is approximately one-half of these lesion.[7] Many of the patients with persistent lymphadenomegaly go on to develop AIDS.[11]

Eventually, lymphoid tissue in HIV-infected persons become depleted due to destruction of infected T cells. In addition, Hassall's bodies in the thymus gland are frequently destroyed.[12] Similar lesions have been observed in young males infected with EBV who have the X-linked lymphoproliferative syndrome (XLP).[13] The finding in patients with XLP of EBV-infected cells in the thymus gland suggests that infection of the thymus gland either by HIV or EBV may be pivotal in the destruction of the thymus. Alternatively, immune responses to the p27 core protein of HIV that cross-react with thymosin α-1 may destroy the epithelium. Loss of thymic control of immune regulation might ensue.

Malignant B-Cell Lymphoma

Early during the AIDS epidemic, Burkitt-like lymphomas were identified that carried EBV in homosexual males in San Francisco.[14] During October 1987, 2–3 new patients were being encountered in San Francisco with EBV carrying B-cell lymphomas.* Curiously, malignant lymphomas are not prominent in other high risk groups such as intravenous drug users, their children, and hemophiliacs. The extranodal Burkitt-like lymphomas or large-cell lymphoma often involved the central nervous system and gastrointestinal tract. Fewer T-cell tumors and Hodgkin's disease cases have been identified. EBV is found in the vast majority of B-cell tumors. As for endemic Burkitt lymphoma, translocations involving chromosome 8 at the c-MYC locus and immunoglobulin loci involving chromosomes 2, 14, and 22 are found.[15]

The roles of EBV in the induction of Burkitt lymphoma and the translocation involving c-MYC have been widely studied. Recently, amplification and deregulation of MYC expression have been shown following EBV infection of the human B cell line (BJAB).[16] Comparison of the EBV-negative BJAB and several EBV-transformed infected sublines derived from it have altered the expression and copy number of MYC in the cell lines. The MYC expression remained elevated even as cells entered a stationary phase of their growth. Since the homogeneously staining region in chromosome 8q24 expanded in the infected karyotyped BJAB cells this finding prompted the investigators to speculate that the chromosomal rearrangement in the region of the MYC locus in BL may potentially be caused by EBV infection.

The loss of T cell surveillance against EBV results from infection of T4 cells by HIV. This leads to reactivation of EBV in the homosexual males. Thus, an ever increasing polyclonal B cell proliferation can occur when the virus reactivates in these individuals. The

---

*personal communication—Jay Levy, M.D.

pathogenesis of the malignant lymphomas likely occurs in a fashion analagous to immune deficient individuals in the regions of Africa endemic for BL.

Colonic Lymphoid Hyperplasia

Recently, Kotler et al[17] have described lymphoid lesions in colorectal biopsies of homosexual males. Damaged colonic epithelium show apoptotic cells in the base of the colonic crypts and the underlying lamina propria often contains hyperplastic lymphoid tissue. EBV genome is found in many of these lesions. Moreover, frozen sections of lymphoid tissue have revealed an EBV determined nuclear-associated antigen in the lymphoid cells confirming the presence of the virus. It is not surprising to us that an EBV transformed B cell should expand in this site: the loss of T cell surveillance against EB viral antigens occurs in the patients and reactivation of EBV is observed. Harrington et al described malignant lymphomas induced by EBV in patients with XLP that were located primarily in the ileocecal region.[18] Whether exposure to sperm introduced during anal intercourse evokes B cell proliferation and contributes to the development of the colonic lymphoid lesion is unclear.[19]

Interstitial Lymphoid Infiltrate in Children

Rubinstein et al[20] proposed involvement by EBV in the development of pediatric AIDS. Within a few years following the description of pediatric AIDS, investigators had noted a patchy lymphoid infiltrate within the interstitium of the lung of children born of intravenous drug abusers. EBV has been detected by Southern blot hybridization in 8 of 10 lung biopsy specimens in children with AIDS.[21] The authors' collaborative studies[22] with Joshi[23] have confirmed the presence of EBV in the lymphoproliferative lesions in children dying with AIDS. Moreover, using the J_H probe, they have identified oligoclonality of the B cells in these lesions.[22]

As stated above, malignant lymphoproliferative diseases are more uncommon in intravenous drug abusers and hemophiliacs than in homosexual males. These former patients frequently succumb to opportunistic infections owing to very profound defects in immunity. The development of malignant lymphoma and the lymphoproliferative diseases in homosexual males probably requires a longer incubation period for the cytogenetic and molecular events to take place. Patients who develop opportunistic infections have more profound immune defects. These patients succumb to such infections before malignant lymphoma can develop. The lymphoproliferative lesions in the lungs of the pediatric AIDS cases are very reminiscent of fatal infectious mononucleosis in males with XLP.[24] The latter group of patients die on an average of 32 days following onset of infectious mononucleosis. Whether EBV-induced lymphoproliferative diseases will occur at a higher frequency in all risk groups for AIDS in the future remains to be seen. This may transpire if drugs improve the immune competence of HIV-infected individuals sufficiently to prevent lethal opportunistic infections. Residual low-grade immune deficiency might permit a malignant lymphoma driven by EBV to emerge. Purtilo et al predict that malignant lymphomas may, along with the devastating central nervous system infection by HIV, become major problems in these patients.

CHRONIC ACTIVE EBV INFECTION

During the past several years, a growing number of patients have been diagnosed with chronic fatigue syndrome/chronic mono/post viral syndrome/ or chronic active EBV infection (CAEBV). Although these patients were initially considered to have a chronic EBV infection,[25,26] recent studies reveal that EBV may not be involved in the majority of adults showing chronic persistent fatigue with mental confusion.[27]

Nevertheless, within young adults and children following primary infection with EBV, one may rarely encounter CAEBV. Features of these patients include fever, lymphadenopathy, hepatosplenomegaly, polyclonal gammopathy, pancytopenia, extremely high EBV titers, and the presence of EBV genome in tissue. Okano et al[28] noted an inability to culture EBV from throat washings or from peripheral blood. Alfieri et al[29] suggested that this results from an infection with a lytic strain of EBV. Recent patient studies conducted by Purtilo et al suggest that interactions between EBV in a patient dually infected with adenovirus (Ad-2) might have been responsible for hemorrhagic colonic ulcers in a young man whose disease was initiated following acute infectious mononucleosis.

Okano et al's failure to develop spontaneous lymphoblastoid cell lines from peripheral blood of this patient heavily infected with EBV was likely due to coinfection of B cells with EBV and Ad-2.[2] Supporting this postulated mechanism is the report that two small molecular weight RNAs designated virus-associated (VA) 1 and 2 of Ad-2 and 5 are strikingly similar to the low molecular weight RNAs of EBV (EBER 1 and EBER 2). These two small RNAs encoded by EBV can functionally substitute for the virus-associated RNAs responsible for the lytic growth of adenoviruses.[30] When normal B cells are infected by EBV in vitro, the cells are immortalized in continuously dividing permanent cells. On the other hand, infection of human cells by adenovirus always leads to a lytic event.

ACKNOWLEDGEMENTS

This work was supported in part by PHS CA30196, awarded by the National Cancer Institute, DHHS, the NIH Research Grant number CA36727 from the National Cancer Institute, the State of Nebraska Department of Health, LB506, and the Lymphoproliferative Research Fund.

REFERENCES

1. McChesney MB, Oldstone MBA: Viruses perturb lymphocyte functions: Selected principles characterizing virus-induced immunosuppression. Ann Rev Immunol 5:279–304, 1987
2. Okano M, Thiele G, Davis JR, et al: Adenovirus type-2 in a patient with lethal hemorrhagic colonic ulcers and chronic active Epstein-Barr virus infection. Ann Int Med 108:693–699, 1088
3. Schwartz JA, Schwartz RS, Hirsh MS, et al: Activation of leukemia viruses by graft-versus-host and mixed lymphocyte-culture reactions: Electron microscopic evidence of C-type particles. J Natl Cancer Inst 51:507–518, 1973
4. Sonnabend J, Witkin S, Purtilo DT: Acquired immunodeficiency syndrome, opportunistic infections, and malignancies in male homosexuals. A hypothesis of etiologic factors in pathogenesis. J Am Med Assoc 249:2370–2374, 1983
5. Quinn TC, Piot P, McCormick JB, et al: Serologic and immunologic studies in patients with AIDS in North American and Africa. J Am Med Assoc 257:2617–2621
6. Marmor M, Friedman-Kien AE, Laubenstein L, et al: Risk factors for Kaposi's sarcoma in homosexual men. Lancet 2:1084–1087, 1982
7. Lipscomb H, Tatsumi E, Harada S, et al: Epstein-Barr virus, chronic lymphadenomegaly, and lymphoma in male homosexuals with acquired immunodeficiency syndrome (AIDS). AIDS Res 1:59–83, 1983
8. Montagnier L, Gruest J, Chamaret S, et al: Adaptation of lymphadenopathy associated virus (LAV) to replication in EBV-transformed B lymphoblastoid cell lines. Science 225:63–66, 1985
9. Greenspan JS, Greenspan D, Lennette ET, et al: Replication of Epstein-Barr virus within the epithelial cells of oral "hairy" leukoplakia, an AIDS-associated lesion. N Engl J Med, 313:1564–1571, 1985
10. Wolf H: Biology of Epstein-Barr virus, in Purtilo DT (ed): Immune Deficiency and Cancer: Epstein-Barr Virus and Lymphoproliferative Malignancies, New York, Plenum Press, 1985, 233–242
11. Abrams DI, Kaplan LD, McGrath MS, Volberding PA: AIDS-related benign lymphadenopathy and malignant lymphoma: Clinical aspects and virologic interactions. AIDS Research: 2:131–140, 1986
12. Seemayer TA, Laroche AC, Russo P, et al: Precocious thymic involution manifest by epithelial injury in the acquired immune deficiency syndrome. Human Path 15:469–474, 1984
13. Mroczek E, Seemayer T, Grierson HL, et al: Thymic lesions in fatal infectious mononucleosis. Clin Immunol Immunopathol 43:243–255, 1987
14. Ziegler JL, Miner RC, Rosenbaum E, et al: Outbreak of Burkitt's-like lymphoma in homosexual men. Lancet 2:631, 1982
15. Magrath I, Erikson J, Whang-Peng J, et al: Synthesis of kappa light chains by cell lines containing an 8:22 chromosomal translocation derived from a male homosexual with Burkitt's lymphoma. Science 222:1094–1098, 1983

16. Lacey J, Summers WP, Watson M, et al: Amplification and deregulation of MYC following Epstein-Barr virus infection of a human B cell line. Proc Natl Acad Sci 84:5838–5842, 1987
17. Kotler DP, Sinangil F, Scholes JV, et al: Epstein-Barr virus-associated lymphoproliferation in rectal mucosa of patients with acquired immune deficiency syndrome. Gastroenterology (submitted for publication)
18. Harrington DS, Weisenburger DD, Purtilo DT: Malignant lymphomas in the X-linked lymphoproliferative syndrome. Cancer 59:1419–1429, 1987
19. Witkin SS, Sonnabend J, Richards JM, Purtilo DT: Induction of antibody to asialo GM_1 by spermatozoa and its occurrence in the sera of homosexual men with the acquired immune deficiency syndrome. Clinical Exptl Immunology 54:346–350, 1983
20. Rubinstein A: Acquired immunodeficiency syndrome in infants. Am J Dis Child 137:825–827, 1983
21. Andiman WA, Eastman R, Martin K, et al: Opportunistic lymphoproliferation associated with Epstein-Barr viral DNA in infants and children with AIDS. Lancet 2:1390—1393, 1985
22. Brichacek B, Davis J, Joshi V, et al: Development of B- and T-cell oligoclonality and alterations in c-myc and c-Ha-ras in immunodeficient patients. Cancer Detection and Prevention (in press)
23. Joshi VV, Kaufman S, Oleske JM, et al: Polyclonal polymorphic B-cell lymphoproliferative disorder with prominent pulmonary involvement in children with acquired immune deficiency syndrome. Cancer 15:1455–1462, 1987
24. Mroczek E, Weisenburger DD, Grierson HL, et al: Fatal infectious mononucleosis and virus-associated hemophagocytic syndrome. Arch Path Lab Med 111:530–535, 1987
25. Straus S, Tosato G, Armstrong G, et al: Persisting illness and fatigue in adults with evidence of Epstein-Barr virus infection. Ann Int Med 102:7–16, 1985
26. Jones J, Ray C, Minnich L, et al: Evidence for active Epstein-Barr virus infection in patients with persistent unexplained illness: Elevated anti-early antigen antibodies. Ann Int Med 102:1–6, 1985
27. Holmes GO, Kaplan JE, Stewart JA, et al: A cluster of patients with a chronic mononucleosis-like syndrome: Is Epstein-Barr virus the cause? JAMA 257:229–2302, 1987
28. Okano M, Sakiyama Y, Matsumoto S, et al: Unusual lymphoproliferation associated with chronic active Epstein-Barr virus infection. AIDS Res 2:121–123, 1986
29. Alfieri C, Joncas JH: Biomolecular analysis of a defective nontransforming Epstein-Barr virus (EBV) from a patient with chronic active EBV infection. J Virol 61:3306–3309
30. Bhat RA, Thimmappaya B: Two small RNAs encoded by Epstein-Barr virus can functionally substitute for the virus-associated RNAs in the lytic growth of adenovirus 5. Proc Natl Acad Sci 80:4789–4793, 1983

25

Malignant Lymphomas in Non-Endemic Areas of ATLL, Particularly on B-Cell Lymphoma

Haruki Wakasa
Masafumi Abe
Shigeyuki Asano
Hiroshi Hojo
Kunihiko Tominaga
Yoshihiro Nozawa

Abstract

Of 302 cases with malignant lymphomas obtained from the non-endemic area of Japan, several key points were concluded as follows:
1. Mantle-zone lymphocytes express SIgM, SIgD and alkaline phosphatase, and a small number of those are positive for IL-2R and CD 5 (Leu 1). Ki-67 is negative for mantle-zone lymphocytes.
2. B lymphoma is histogenetically divided into 3 forms: pre-follicle center cell, follicle center cell, and post-follicle center cells.
3. B lymphoma of the medium-sized cell type is derived from mantle-zone lymphocytes or small cleaved cells of follicle center cell.
4. Based on the DNA content measured with MSP and the reactivity of Ki-67 in different cell types, diffuse large-cell lymphoma has the most aggressive growth.
5. A new $EBNA^-$ cell line was established from lymphoma cells of pleural effusion and a monoclonal antibody positively selected for large cell of follicle center and large cell lymphoma was made.
6. The $EBNA^-$ cell line is now being utilized to distinguish the immunoblastic type from large cell lymphoma by using this monoclonal antibody.

During the past two decades, remarkable progress has been observed in the pathology of malignant lymphomas. Particularly, the development of monoclonal antibodies has made it possible to define the characters of lymphoma cells (T and B cells), and the stage of differentiation of those tumor cells.

The present paper will be report on the features of malignant lymphomas observed in non-endemic area of ATL in Japan.

Frequencies of T and B cell Lymphomas in the Northeastern District of Japan

Fresh materials were obtained from surgical specimens to examine cellular characteristics in detail. For this purpose, commercial monoclonal antibodies were used. Table 25-1 shows the T or B frequencies of the cases obtained for 9 years from 1979 to 1987. The cases were mainly obtained from Fukushima Prefecture, where our school is located, and there were 302 cases in total, consisted of 262 cases of non-Hodgkin lymphoma and 40 cases of Hodgkin's disease. Among 262 cases of non-Hodgkin's lymphoma, 198 were of B-cell lymphomas, 58 were of T-cell lymphomas, and 6 were of an undetermined type. The frequencies of T or B lymphomas were quite different from the data reported from Kyushu, almost opposite in results.[1] It also indicates histologic subtypes of non-Hodgkin lymphomas according to LSG classification[2] proposed by Japanese pathologists as the most appropriate classification for Japanese lymphomas.

With regard to histologic subtypes, follicular lymphomas were encountered as 18% in all B-cell lymphomas. This may be the highest frequency of those previously reported in Japan.[3,4] In diffuse lymphomas, large-cell lymphomas containing cleaved or noncleaved nuclei with abundant cytoplasm were the most frequently observed in this series.

TABLE 25-1
Immunologic Phenotypes of B Cell Lymphomas, Medium-sized Cell Type

I. Non-Hodgkin		262	
	B (76%)	T (22%)	Und. (2%)
(1) Follicular lymphoma			
medium-sized	9	0	0
mixed	17	0	0
large	10	0	0
	36	0	0
(2) Diffuse lymphoma			
small	10	0	1
medium	32	5	1
mixed	32	8	2
large	80	8	2
lymphoblastic	0	7	0
pleomorphic	0	9	0
Burkitt	7	0	0
ATL	0	8	0
IBL-like T	0	4	0
Cut. T	0	9	0
Signet cell 1.	1	0	2
	162	58	6
II. Hodgkin's disease		40	

IMMUNOREACTIVITY OF FOLLICLE-FORMING CELLS

The primary follicle of a 24-week-fetus and the component cells bear IgM + D, though IgM^+ cells were more numerously observed.[6] In adult tonsils, IgM + D cells are present in the mantle-zone. Next, alkaline-phosphatase positive lymphocytes were also observed in the lymphocytes of the primary follicle of the fetus and in those of the mantle zone of adult tonsillar tissue. No positive cells for IgD or alkaline phosphatase were observed in the germinal center. Therefore, based on these findings, it might be possible to differentiate mantle-zone lymphocytes from germinal center cells (Table 25-2). Furthermore, double-staining for IgD and alkaline phosphatase produced an interesting finding that alkaline phosphatase-positive cells were found in outer layer of the mantle-zone and IgD positive cells were present in inner layer of it. It is, however, still unclear what relation may exist between alkaline phosphatase and lymphocyte differentiation.

TABLE 25-2
Characterization of Mantle Zone and Follicular Center Cells

	Mantle Zone	Follicular Center
SIg	IgM + D	IgM (A, G)
B1	+	+
AlPase	+	−
CALLA	−	+

HISTOGENESIS OF B-CELL LYMPHOMAS

If Koepke's shema[6] concerning B lymphocyte maturation in the lymph node is applied for histogenesis of B cell lymphomas (Fig. 25-1), there will be at least 3 steps: pre-follicle center cell, follicle center cell, and post-follicle center cell, as the occurrence site of malignant lymphomas. It is said that B lymphocytes may arrive around the medullary area first. B-CLL or malignant lymphoma consisting of small lymphocytes might occur at this stage in accord with the maturation stage of early B. In Japan, B-CLL is remarkably low in frequency in comparison to that of the western country. It is rather difficult to obtain fresh lymph node. However, a typical B-CLL cell distinctly contain IgM + D, though IgD positivity is usually low. It is unclear that the occurrence site of B-CLL is from a primary follicle or in another area.

In 1982, Weisenburger[7] proposed the concept of "Mantle-zone lymphoma" from a morphologic basis showing wide neoplastic growth of mantle-zone lymphocyte with preservation of the reactive germinal center. He added some immunologic data 2 years later,[8]

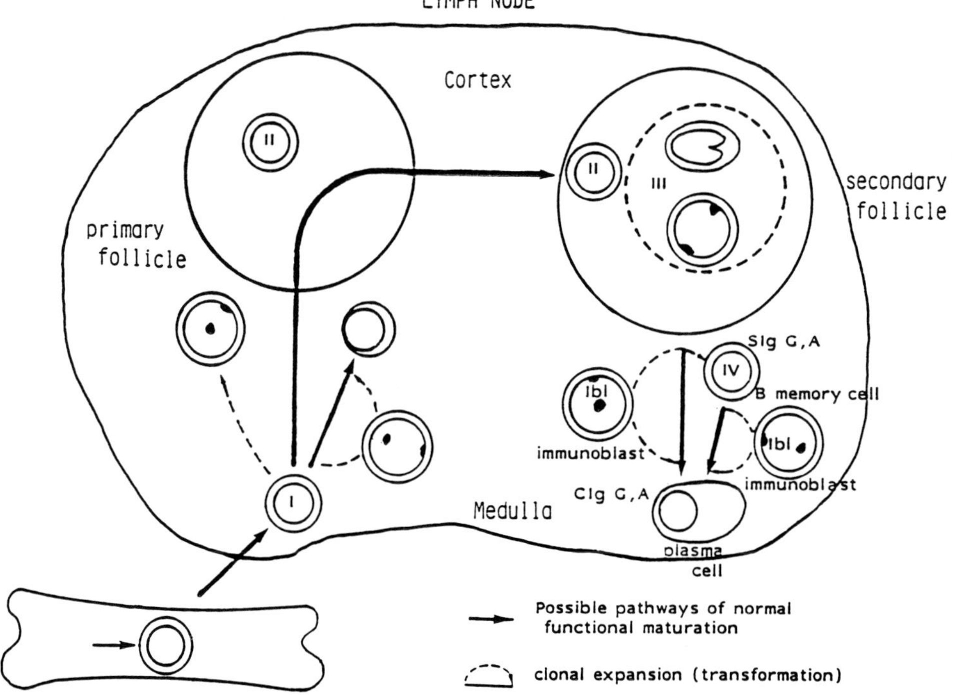

Fig. 25-1. Schema of B lymphocyte differentiation of the lymph node (modified from Koepke's schema).

but no description of IgD and alkaline phosphatase[9] was shown at that time. At present, there are still controversial discussions on the nature of such a lymphoma: if it is a distinct subtype or if it should be included in follicle center cell lymphomas.[10–12] The authors have studied 20 cases of B-cell lymphomas consisting of medium-sized cells. Growth pattern of these lymphoma cells were follicular, vaguely nodular, or diffuse. The result of immunologic and alkaline phosphatase staining was indicated in Table 25-3.

In the case showing neoplastic nodules limited in the mantle-zone with a reactive germinal center, alkaline phosphatase[9] positive cells were observed in neoplastic areas, but staining was absent in the remaining germinal center (Figures 25-2, 25-3, 25-4). Moreover, these cases showed medium-sized neoplastic cells positive for Leu 1 or IL-2R. Ki-67 antibody was applied for mantle-zone lymphoma, but positive cells were found in quite a low percentage. It was concluded that in cases of the medium-sized cells with both IgD and alkaline phosphatase positivity or only one of those might be termed mantle-zone lymphoma.[5]

Malignant lymphomas originating from the next stage of B lymphocyte maturation in the lymph node are classified as follicular lymphomas,[13] composed of medium-sized, mixed and large cells. In our series, the mixed type was the most frequently observed. All cases of this type were positive for B1 and contained DRC-1 positive networks, suggesting that these lymphomas originated from follicle center cells. There were 7 cases with Burkitt type positive for B1, NUB1, and CALLA. Since the positive reactivity for CALLA was observed in one-third of follicular lymphoma cases, the origin of the Burkitt type might be considered to be follicle center cells.

B-cell lymphomas originating from the last stage of B lymphocyte maturation in the

TABLE 25-3

Case No.	Histologic Type	SIgM	SIgD	B1 (CD 20)	IL-2R (CD 25)	Leu 1 (CD 5)	ALPase
		Phenotypic Expression					
1	FL	+	−	+	−	−	−
2	FL	+	−	+	−	−	−
3	FL	+	+	+	+	−	−
4	FL	+	−	+	+/−	−	+
5	FL	+	−	+	−	−	−
6	DL	−	+	−	−	−	−
7	DL	+	+	+	−	−	−
8	DL	+	−	+	+	−	−
9	DL	+	+/−	+	+/−	−	−
10	DL	+	+	+	+	−	−
11	DL	+	+	+	−	−	+
12	DL	+	−	+	−	+	−
13	DL	+	−(SIgA$^+$)	+	−	+	−
14	DL	+	+	+	−	+	−
15	DL	+	+	+	+	−	−
16	DL	+	−	+	−	+	−
17	DL	+	+	+	+	+	+
18	DL	+	−	+	−	−	−
19	MZL	+	+	+	+	−	+
20	MZL	+	+	+	−	+/−	+/−

FL: Follicular Lymphoma DL: Diffuse Lymphoma MZL: Mantle Zone Lymphoma

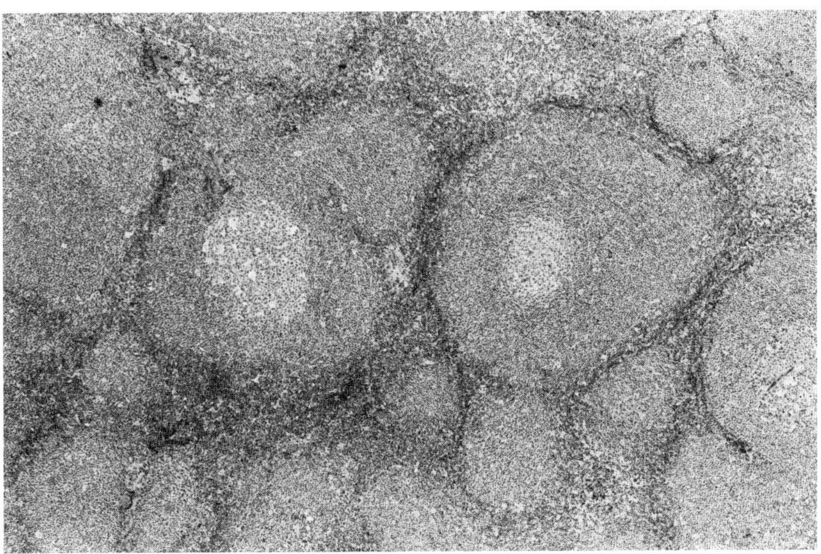

Fig. 25-2. Mantle-zone lymphoma, showing follicular growth with normal appearing germinal center (H&E × 40).

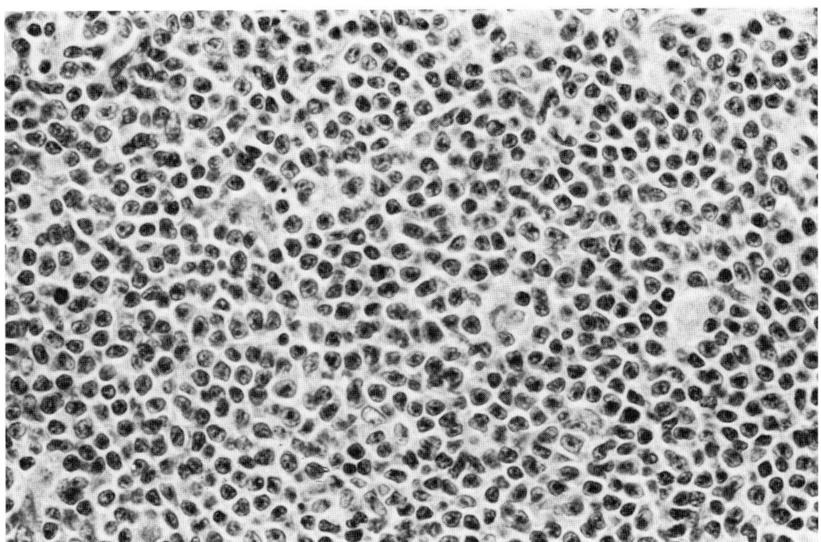

Fig. 25-3. Mantle-zone lymphoma: Neoplastic cells are rather uniform in size and show a slight nuclear irregularity (H&E × 436).

lymph node are called immunoblastic or lymphoplasmacytoid type. It is considered that macroglobulinemia Waldenström might be included in post-follicle center cell origin revealing immunoglobulin production and secretion. However, at present, there has been no appropriate indicator in distinguishing the last stage of B lymphoma from other subtypes. Further effort is needed in this aspect.

Next, studies were conducted to determine the capacity of the growth fraction of B-cell lymphomas according to different cell types.

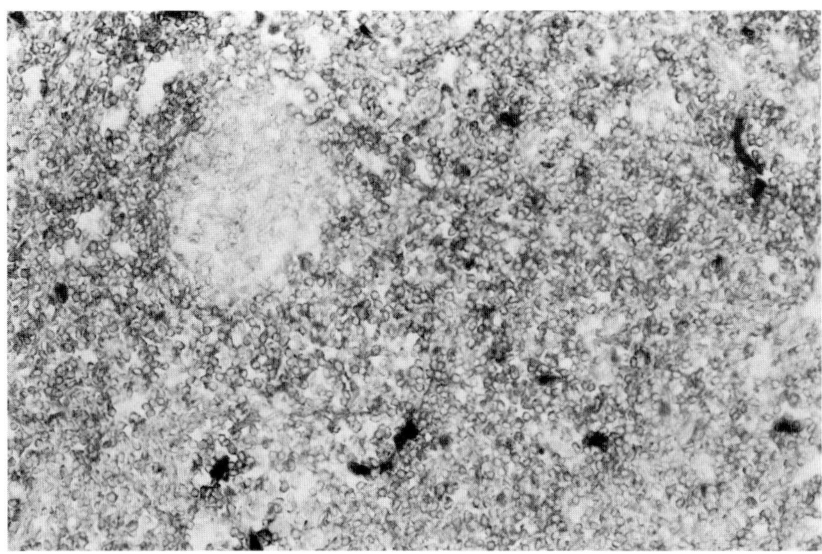

Fig. 25-4. Mantle-zone lymphoma: Neoplastic cells positive for alkaline phosphatase and germinal center negative for alkaline phosphatase. (× 218).

For this purpose, the DNA content of lymphoma cells was measured using smears made from free cells separated from thick-cut paraffin section preserving whole nuclei. The smears were stained with Feulgen and analyzed with computerized microspectrophotometer (Olympus, Japan). The DNA content of diffuse lymphoma was usually higher than that of follicular lymphoma cells, and the highest DNA content was found in the large-cell type of diffuse lymphomas.[14] These data were also confirmed by an analysis of the use of Ki-67, which detects growth fraction of proliferating cells. For the measurement of Ki-67 positive cells in B-cell lymphomas, frozen sections cut from PLP-fixed tissues were doubly stained with B1 and Ki-67 in order. The stained sections were photographed and the ratio of Ki-67 positive lymphoma cells among B1 positive lymphoma cells was calculated. The data showed a rather wide variation from case to case, but a similar tendency to that of DNA measurement was confirmed (Fig. 25-5). These findings suggest that the large cell type of diffuse lymphomas has the most aggressive growth in comparison to all other cell types of B-cell lymphomas.[14]

A NEW MONOCLONAL ANTIBODY

A new type of monoclonal antibody reactive with large B cells was developed by the use of established B lymphoma cell line.[15] During the past decade, the authors have been developing a B lymphoma cell line derived specifically from lymphoma cells. At present, Wakasa et al have five B lymphoma cell lines of different cell types and differentiation stages. The sources of lymphoma cells were pleural effusion, lymph nodes, and bone marrow, and the usual culture technique was employed.

Monoclonal antibodies were developed using a B lymphoma cell line established from pleural effusion of a 65-year-old male with large cell lymphoma.[16] Immunologic and chromosomal analysis revealed that the established cell line had the same phenotypic feature to that of original lymphoma cells includ-

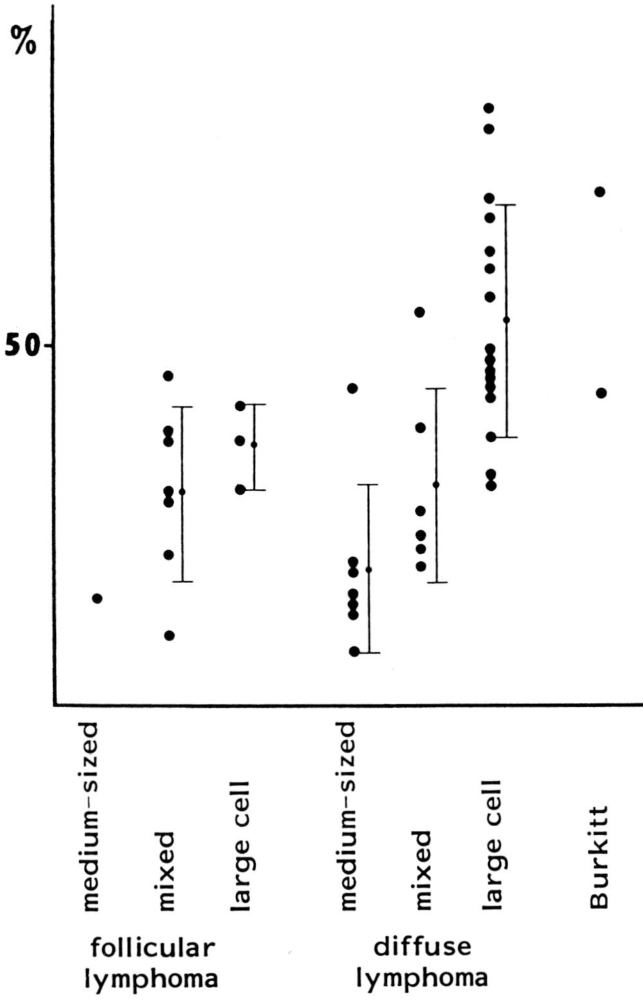

Fig. 25-5. The ratio calculated from Ki-67 positive lymphoma cells among B1 positive lymphoma cells.

ing $14q^+$ chromosome in both original and established cells. The heterotransplantation to nude mice was positive in about 60% success. A new monoclonal antibody termed as N6 showed 78 kd molecular weight and reacted mainly with the follicle center cell, particularly with large cell. Wakasa et al applied this monoclonal antibody (N6) to lymphoma cases.

The result was shown in Table 25-4, revealing the different reactivity compared with that of B1. It is very interesting that a new monoclonal antibody (N6) showed an intense staining on the cell membrane of large lymphoma cells and did not react with medium-sized lymphoma cells and myeloma cells. During the course of the study, only one case of malignant lymphoma with the large-cell type showed negative staining in comparison to the reactivity of B1. Neoplastic cells of this case were indicated as immunoblasts from cytologic basis.

TABLE 25-4
Reactivity of N6 for B Lymphoma
—Comparison with B1—

Pattern	Cell type	B1	N6
Follicular	Medium	2/2 (100%)	0/2 (0%)
	Mixed	3/3 (100%)	3/3 (100%)
lymphoma	Large	3/3 (100%)	3/3 (100%)
Diffuse	Small	0/1 (0%)	0/1 (0%)
	Medium	8/8 (100%)	0/8 (0%)
	Mixed	2/2 (100%)	2/2 (100%)
lymphoma	Large	17/17 (100%)	16/17 (94%)

This work will be extended to confirm that a new monoclonal antibody is possible to inhibit the growth of established cells and also possible to distinguish lymphomas occuring from the follicle center cell and post-follicle center cell.

Acknowledgment

This work was supported by a Grant-in-Aid from the Ministry of Health and Welfare of Japan for Cancer Research (61–2), and a Grant-in-Aid for Cancer Research (63010035) from the Ministry of Education, Science and Culture of Japan.

REFERENCES

1. The T- and B-cell Malignancy Study Group: Statistical analysis of immunologic, clinical and histologic data on lymphoid malignancies in Japan. Jpn J Clin Oncol 11:15–38, 1981
2. Suchi T, Tajima K, Nanba K, et al: Some problems of the histopathological diagnosis of non-Hodgkin's malignant lymphoma. A proposal of a new type. Acta Pathol Jpn 29:755–776, 1979
3. Nanba K, Itagaki T: Geographic pathology of follicular lymphoma. J Jap Soc RES 19:311–316 1979 (in Japanese)
4. Wakasa H, Abe M Nozawa Y: Nodal B-cell lymphomas in Japan—particularly in Tohoku district—. Jpn J Clin Oncol 13:577–590, 1983
5. Wakasa H: Malignant lymphomas and related disorders—A pathological study—. Acta Haematol Jpn, 49:1475–1490, 1986
6. Dick FR: Plasma cell myeloma and related disorders with monoclonal gammopathy, in Koepke JA (ed): Laboratory Hematology, Vol. 2, New York, Churchill Livingstone, 1984, 445–481
7. Weisenburger DD, Kim H, Rappaport H: Mantle-zone lymphoma: A follicular variant of intermediate lymphocytic lymphoma. Cancer 49:1429–1438, 1982
8. Weisenburger DD: Mantle-zone lymphoma. An immunologic study. Cancer 53:1073–1080, 1984
9. Nanba K, Jaffe ES, Braylan RC, et al: Alkaline phosphatase-positive malignant lymphoma: A subtypes of B cell lymphomas. Am J Clin Pathol 68:535–542, 1977
10. Harris NL, Bhan AK; mantle-zone lymphoma. A pattern produced by lymphomas of more than one cell type. Am J Surg Pathol 9:872–882, 1985
11. Samoszuk MK, Epstein AL, Said J, et al: Sensitivity and specificity of immunostaining in the diagnosis of mantle-zone lymphomas. Am J Clin Pathol 85:557–563, 1986
12. Pileri S, Rivano T, Gobbi M, et al: Neoplastic and reactive follicles within B-cell malignant lymphomas. A morphological and immunological study of 30 cases. Hematol Oncol 3:243–260, 1985
13. Kojima M, Imai Y, Mori N: A concept of follicular lymphoma—A proposal for the existence of a neoplasm originating from the germinal center. GANN Monogr. Cancer Res 15:195–208, 1973
14. Tominaga K: Nuclear DNA amount and fraction of proliferating cells of non-Hodgkin's lymphoma. J Jap Soc RES 27:249–261, 1987 (in Japanese)
15. Abe M, Nozawa Y, Wakasa H: EBNA-negative cell lines established from B-cell lymphoma. J Jap Soc RES 25:348, 1986 (in Japanese)
16. Nozawa Y: The establishment of B lymphoma cell line and its application—particularly on the production of monoclonal antibody—. J Jap Soc RES 26:273–292, 1987 (in Japanese)

Part IV

New Concepts of Non-Neoplastic Lymphoproliferative Disorders

26

Follicular Dendritic Cells in Lymphoid Malignancies—Morphology, Distribution, and Function

Yutaka Imai
Mikio Matsuda
Kunihiko Maeda
Masaru Narabayashi
Atsuko Masunaga

Follicular dendritic cell (FDC) is one of non-lymphoid, nonphagocytic cells in the primary and secondary follicles of the peripheral lymphoid tissues. Microscopically, it has uniquely entangled dendritic cytoplasmic processes and desmosome-like junctional structures at the plasma membrane.[1–4] Besides, it is capable of trapping and retaining immune-complexes on the extensive cell surface.[5–7] These suggest that FDCs constitute the dense reticular framework and maintaining the follicular structure and play some important roles in germinal center reactions. These results were principally from the examination of physiologic or reactive follicles, and FDCs of lymphoid malignancies have been described in only a few papers.[8–10] Therefore, behavior and contribution of FDCs in pathological situations are not clarified fully yet.

Imai et al investigated the FDCs in 33 cases of lymphoid malignancies immunohistochemically and ultrastructurally. DRC-1$^+$ FDCs in the mature type, bearing an immune complex trapping ability, were recognized densely apparent in the neoplastic follicles of follicular lymphomas, which became focal or only vestigial in diffuse B cell lymphomas. CD35$^+$ reticulum cells were distributed in relatively wider areas. These findings were also revealed in diffuse lymphomas that had been diagnosed as follicular lymphoma previously, or that showed some residual vague follicular patterns in a part of biopsied lymph nodes. In IBL-like T-cell lymphomas and lymphocytic predominance (LP) type of Hodgkin's disease, FDCs presented irregularly, widespread distributions closely attached to fibrous bundles. In clear cell lymphomas and in other types of Hodgkin's diseases, Imai et al could recognize only solitary DRC-1$^+$ cells, or there were no DRC-1 positive cell. FDCs might have transformed to CD35$^+$ reticulum cells and lost their DRC-1 positivity as the development of the lymphoma, so their distribution pattern and morphology are closely related to the histologic features of the lymphoid malignancies.

LYMPHOID MALIGNANCIES

Thirty-six lymph nodes from 33 patients with malignant lymphomas (7 follicular lymphomas, 13 diffuse B-cell lymphomas, 6

TABLE 26-1
Lymphoic Maligancies

Case	Age	Sex	Histological Dx	Markers
1	29	F	Follicular lymphoma, large cell	IgM-κ
2	79	F	small cleaved	IgM-λ
3	40	F	mixed	ND
4	76	F	mixed	IgM-λ
5	68	F	mixed	IgG-κ
6	46	F	mixed	ND
7	62	M	mixed	IgM-λ
8	70	F	Diff. B cell lymphoma, small cleaved*	IgM-λ
9	81	F	small cleaved	IgM-λ
10	47	M	small cleaved*	IgM-κ
11	75	F	small cleaved	IgM-λ
12	77	F	small cleaved	ND
13	65	M	small cleaved	IgA-κ
14	66	F	small cleaved	ND
15	53	M	small cleaved	IgG-κ
16	55	M	mixed	IgM-κ
17	51	M	large cell	IgG-κ
18	59	F	large cell**	IgM-λ
19	77	M	large cell	IgM-κ
20	79	M	large cell	IgM-κ
21	64	M	IBL-like T cell lymphoma	$CD5^+,CD5^+,CD8^-$
22	71	M		$CD5^+,CD4^+,CD8^-$
23	58	M		$CD5^+,CD4^+,CD8^-$
24	53	F	Clear cell lymphoma	$CD5^+,CD4^+,CD8^-$
25	70	M		$CD5^+,CD4^+,CD8^-$
26	24	M	Lymphoblastic lymphoma	$CD5^+,OKT9^+,OKT10^+$
27	63	M	Hodgkin's disease, LP	
28	73	M	LP	
29	63	M	MC	
30	79	M	MC	
31	69	F	NS	
32	51	F	NS	
33	56	M	LD	

* with some petty vague nodular patterns in parrafin section
** with previously diagnosed follicular lymphoma

T-cell lymphomas, and 7 Hodgkin's diseases) were examined (Table 26-1). Nine reactive lymph nodes served as control. Two cases of diffuse B cell lymphomas (Cases 1, 3) showed some petty, vague nodularities only in the paraffin sections and one case (Case 18) had a history of previously diagnosed follicular lymphoma, large cell type. IBL-like T-cell lymphoma[11,12] was restricted to T-cell malignancy showing unique histological pattern resembling IBL. Clear cell lymphoma was the name assigned to the cases showing intense diffuse or clustering proliferation of clear tumor T cells, exclusively.

Paraffin sections were susceptible to immunohistochemical stainings using peroxidase-antiperoxidase (PAP) method and freshly frozen sections were stained by the indirect immuno-peroxidase method. Polyclonal and monoclonal antibodies employed in this study are given in Table 26-2. Conventional electron microscopical observations were also made.

TABLE 26-2
Panels of Antibodies

	Reactivity	Source
Monoclonal antibodies		
Leu1 (CD5)	pan T cells (some B cells but not normal B cells)	B-D (Becton-Dickinson)
Leu2a(CD8)	suppressor/cytotoxic T cells	B-D
Leu3a(CD4)	helper/inducer T cells, some hitiocytes	B-D
LeuM1(CD15)	myeloid/histioctic cells, Hodgkin's cells, some epithelial neoplasms	
LeuM3(CD14)	macrophages/histiocytes	B-D
LeuM5(CD11c)	macrophages/histiocytes, some B cells	B-D
Leu7	natural killer cells, some T cells	B-D
B1(CD20)	pan B cells	Coulter Clone
DRC-1(R14/23)	follicular dendritic cells	DAKO
Anti CR-1(CD35)	human C3b receptor	B-D
Anti CR-2, B2 (CD21)	human C3d receptor	B-D Coulter Clone
Anti CR-3, OKM1 (CD11)	human C3bi receptor	B-D Ortho Diagnostics
H107(CD23)	human Fc-E receptor	Nichirei Inc.
HLA-DR	human HLA-DR	DAKO
Polyclonal antibodies		
IgG	human gamma heavy chain	DAKO
IgA	alpha	DAKO
IgM	mu	DAKO
IgD	delta	DAKO
IgE	epsilon	DAKO
κ	kappa light chain	DAKO
λ	lambda	DAKO
Lysozyme	human lysozyme	DAKO
α_1-antitrypsin	α_1-antitrypsin	DAKO
α_1-antichymotrypsin	α_1-antichymotrypsin	DAKO
Ferritin	human ferritin	DAKO
S-100 protein	S-100 protein	Original
Cla	human Clq component	DAKO
C3d	C3d	DAKO
C5	C5	DAKO

IMMUNOHISTOCHEMICAL EXAMINATION

DRC-1

In reactive lymph node, there was revealed an intense meshwork positive pattern throughout almost entire reactive germinal centers and their mantle-zone (Fig. 26-1A). In all cases of follicular lymphoma, DRC-1 also revealed dense meshwork-like or partially disrupted positive figures within neoplastic follicles (Fig. 26-2A). In contrast, diffuse B-cell lymphomas showed scattering focal or only vestigial positivity in their tumor tissues (Fig. 26-3A). Imai et al could not recognize the diffuse growth pattern of DRC-1$^+$ cells in any cases of diffuse B-cell lymphoma. In

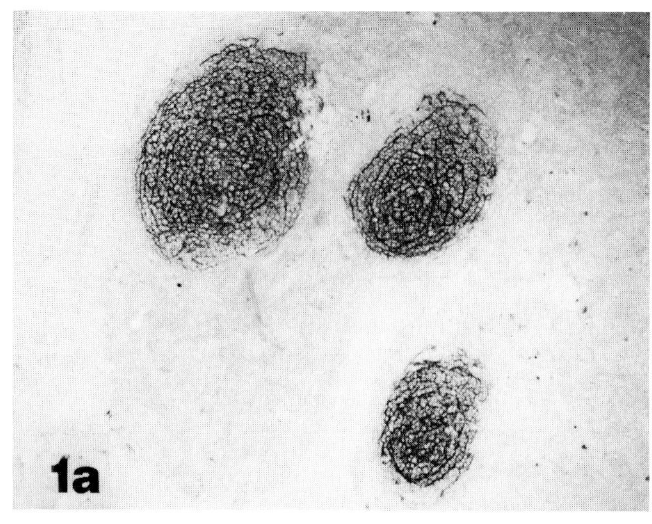

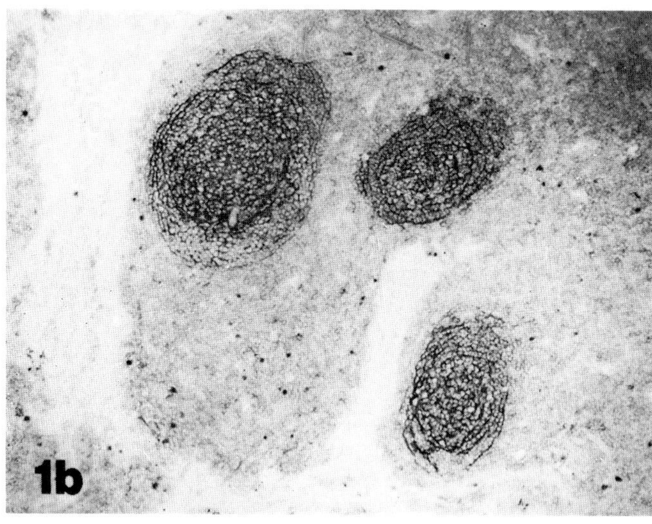

Fig. 26-1. Immunostaining of reactive lymph node with DRC-1(a) and CR-1(b), Positive follicles for both antibodies (X 75).

T-cell lymphomas, there were two distinct types of staining patterns. One was irregularly shaped, ill-defined reticular positivity in relatively wide areas (Fig. 26-4A), which was observed in IBL-like T-cell lymphoma, and another was only vestigial or solitary positivity in clear cell lymphoma. In Hodgkin's diseases, the cases of LP type showed the wide irregularly shaped reticular positivity (Fig. 26-5A) and in other types, including NS, MC, and LD, there were shown only solitary or no positivity. There was no distinct positivity for DRC-1 on the surface of lymphoma cells of all cases examined.

Complement Receptors (CR-1, CR-2, and CR-3)

The monoclonal antibodies against CR-1 (human C3b receptor) or CR-2 (human C3d receptor) revealed intense meshwork-like pos-

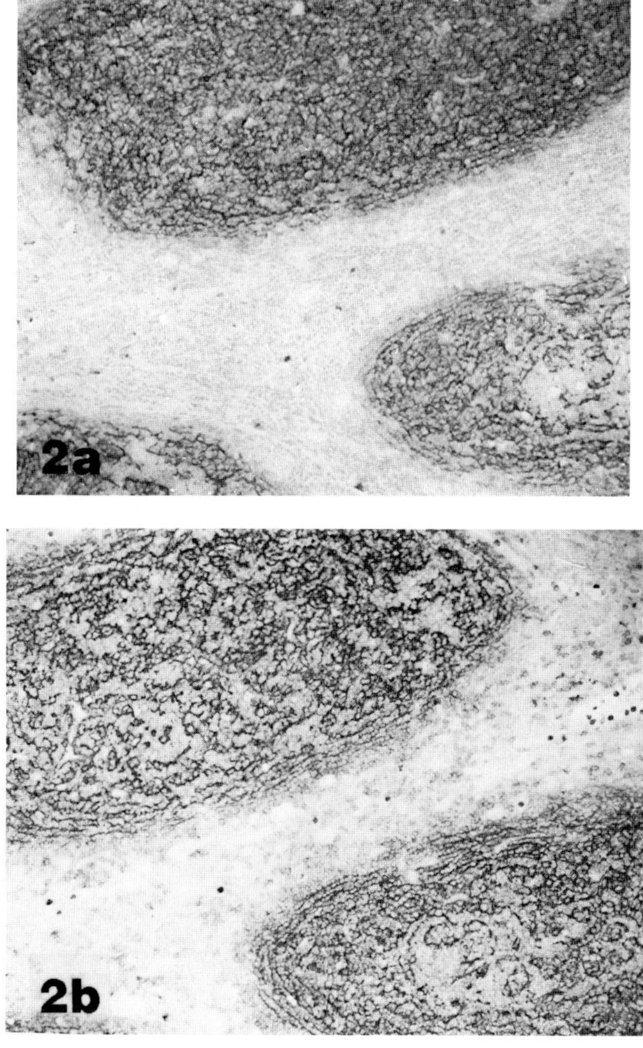

Fig. 26-2. Follicular lymphoma (small cleaved cell type). Neoplastic follicles were positive for DRC-1(a), and CR-1(b). Positive areas were wider (X 75).

itive figures within the reactive follicles and neoplastic follicles consistent with DRC-1 (Figs. 26-1B, 26-2B). There was only weak positive reaction for CR-1 And CR-2 on the surface of germinal center cells, mantle-zone lymphocytes, and follicular lymphoma cells, whereas the almost identical staining pattern and distribtuion were obtained with DRC-1, CR-1, and CR-2 in the reactive hyperplasia and follicular lymphoma. A distinct discrepency of the staining results was found in diffuse B-cell lymphoma, T-cell lymphoma, and Hodgkin's disease. In diffuse B-cell lymphoma, anti CR-1, CR-2, and especially CR-1, showed rather wide, reticular positivity overlapping above mentioned focal or vestigial DRC-1^+ positive area (Fig. 26-3B). In T-cell lymphoma, CR-1^+ and CR-2^+ areas were also wider than DRC-1^+ areas (Fig. 26-4B). The discrepancy became

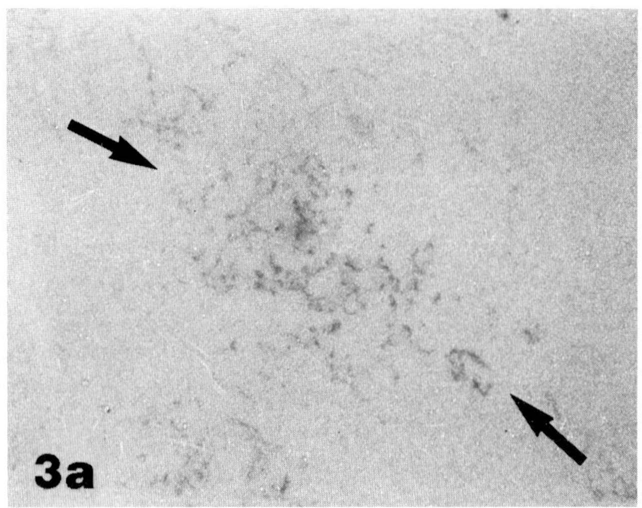

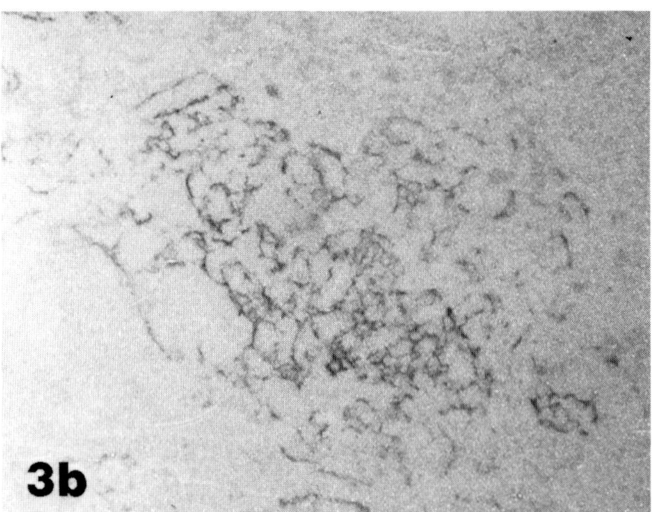

Fig. 26-3. Diffuse B-cell lymphoma (small cleaved cell type). Focal reticular reaction with DRC-1(a, arrow), and wider and more distinct deposition with CR-1(b) (X 75).

remarkable especially in clear cell lymphoma. In the LP type of Hodgkin's disease, the same staining pattern as in T-cell lymphoma was recognized (Fig. 26-5B) and in other types, especially NS type, the spindle cells constituting the sclerosing background revealed CR-1 positive. Positive reaction for CR-3 (human C3bi receptor) was not confirmed on the surface of FDCs.

H107 (Human Fc-epsilon Receptor)

This showed the dense meshwork positivity within the germinal center, especially in the light zone, of reactive follicles, and within the neoplastic follicles of follicular lymphoma (Fig. 26-6A). In the diffuse B-cell lymphoma, T-cell lymphoma, and Hodgkin's disease, this antibody showed focal or vestigial positivity

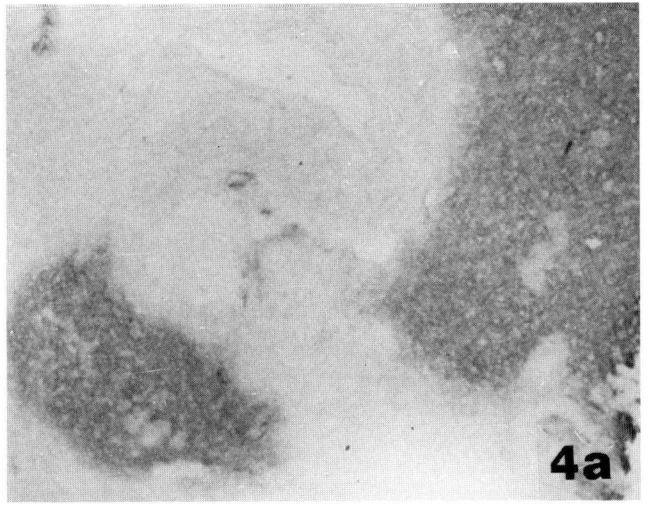

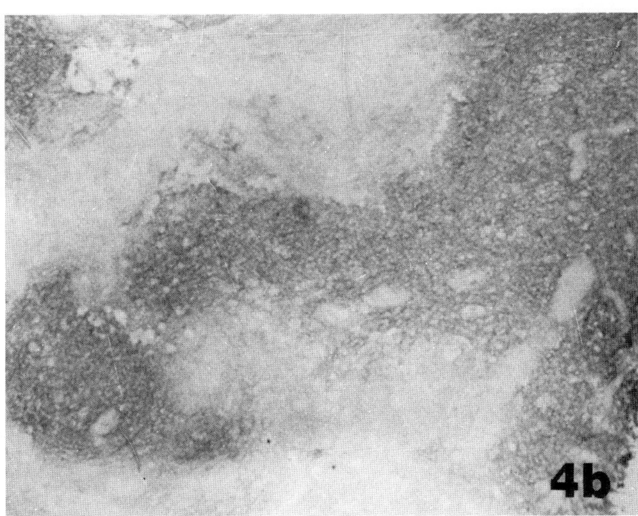

Fig. 26-4. IBL-like T cell lymphoma. Positive for DRC-1(a) and wider for CR-1(b) (X 30).

almost consistent with DRC-1, or in wider areas.

Immunoglobulins

In the reactive lymph nodes, the reticular deposition of each heavy and light chains other than IgD, especially of IgM, were detected in the light zone of the germinal center. And the similar reticular deposition of IgM or IgE were also detected in the neoplastic follicles of follicular lymphoma (Fig. 26-6B). Such distinct reticular deposition of immunoglobulins could not be observed in the diffuse B-cell lymphoma, T-cell lymphoma, and Hodgkin's disease except for one case of

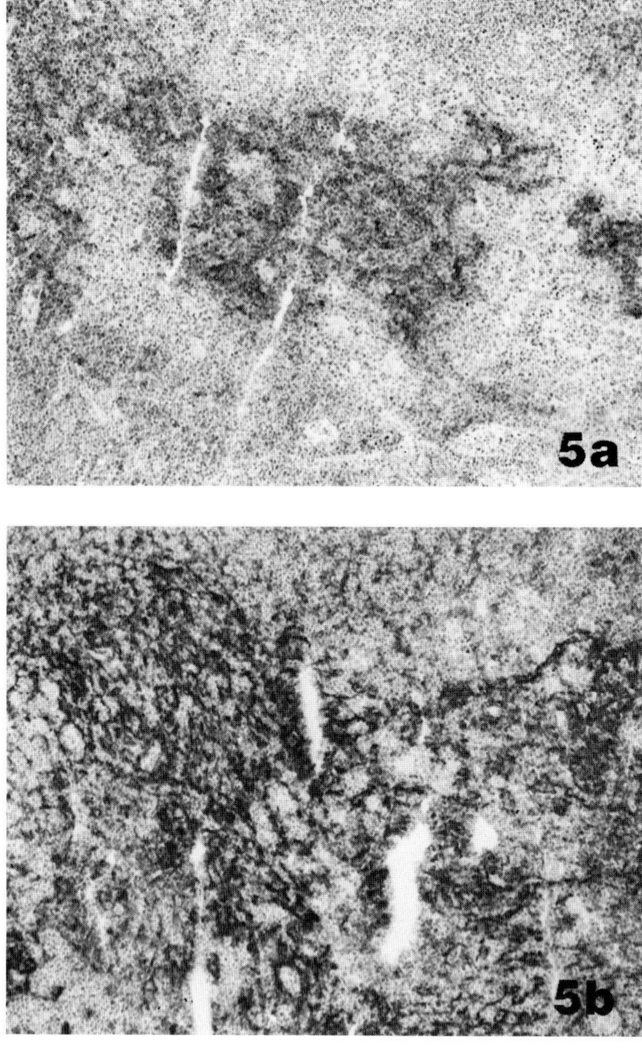

Fig. 26-5. Hodgkin's disease (LP) with irregular positive pattern for DRC-1(a) and CR-1(b) (X 30).

IBL-like T-cell lymphoma, in which some focal reticular deposition of IgE was detected.

Complement Components

Some complement components (C1q, C3d, C5) showed the reticular deposition as immunoglobulins seen in the light zone of the reactive greminal centers and in the neoplastic follicles of follicular lymphoma. Any distinct deposition of complement components could not be detected in the lymph nodes involved with diffuse B-cell lymphoma, T-cell lymphoma, and Hodgkin's disease.

Myelo/Macrophage Markers

Myelo/macrophage markers (LeuM1, LeuM3, LeuM5, OKM1, or CR-3, lysozyme, α-1-antitrypsin, α-1-antichymotrypsin and

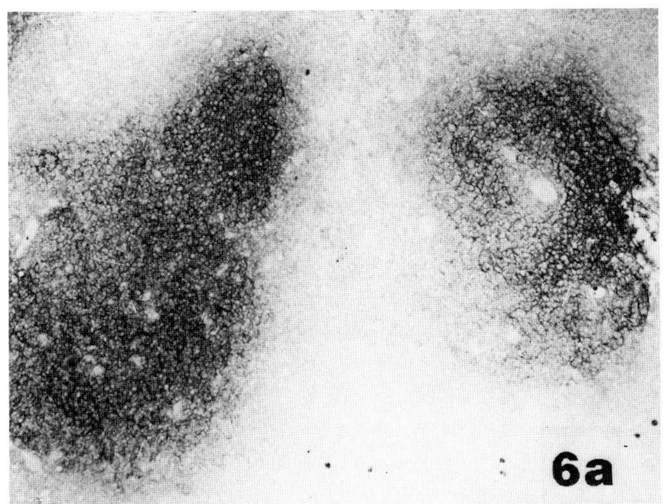

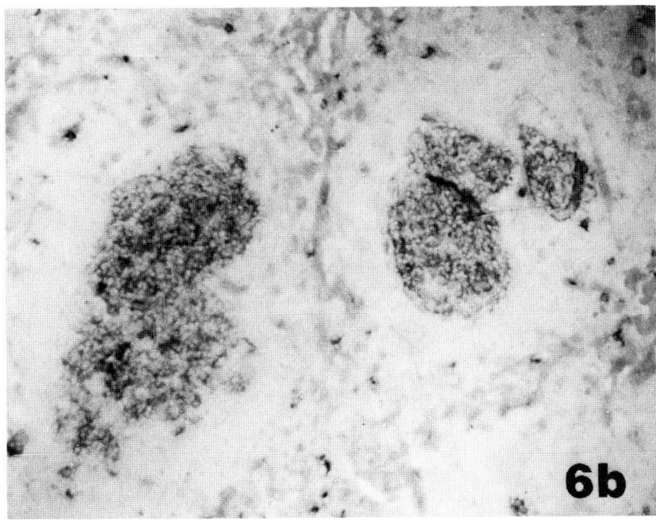

Fig. 26-6. Follicular lymphoma (mixed type) revealed nodular positivity for H107(a) and for IgE(b) in neoplastic follicles (X 80).

human ferritin) did not show positive staining patterns corresponding with DRC-1, except for Leu M5, which revealed the weak reticular positivity within the reactive and/or neoplastic follicles.

S100 Protein

In some reactive lymphoid hyperplasias, FDCs were positive in nucleus and cytoplasm for S100 protein. On the other hand, interdigitating cells in T-cell zone were always positive. In the lymph nodes of follicular lymphoma, diffuse B-cell lymphoma, T-cell lymphoma, and Hodgkin's disease, the distinct positivity for S100 protein corresponding to DRC-1 could not be recognized.

T-cell Markers and Leu7

Special attention was given to the localization of Leu3a^{+} lymphocytes (helper/inducer

T-lymphocytes) and Leu7^{+} cells (natural killer cells) within the reactive follicles, especially in the light zone, and in the neoplastic follicles. However, any positive FDCs and the specific distribution of T cells in relation to the FDCs were not confirmed in either reactive or neoplastic lymph nodes.

ELECTRONMICROSCOPICAL EXAMINATIONS

In the reactive follicles, FDCs had more intricate dendritic cytomplasmic processes that were entangled with surrounding germinal center cells and were constituting the "labyrinthine structure." Desmosome-like junctional structures between dendritic processes and neighboring cells or between opposing dendritic processes were often observed (Fig 26-7). In the neoplastic follicles of all follicualr lymphomas, the dendritic cells morphologically resembling the FDC in the reactive follicles could be seen, in lesser degree of the intrication of their dendritic processes (Fig. 26-8). In diffuse B-cell lymphoma, we could not observe these dendritic cells, and the spindle-shaped reticulum cells were seen that did not have the intricated dendritic cytoplasmic processes and showed the morphology resembling so-called fibroblastic reticulum cell. Immunoelectron-microscopically, some of these cells revealed the positivity for DRC-1 or CR-1 on their surface (Fig. 26-9). In T-cell lymphoma, especially in IBL-like T-cell lymphoma which showed the wide positive area for DRC-1, the reticulum cells with branching cytoplasmic processes were observed among the clear lymphoma cells. In particular, these cells often closely attached the dense collagenous bundles (Fig. 26-10).

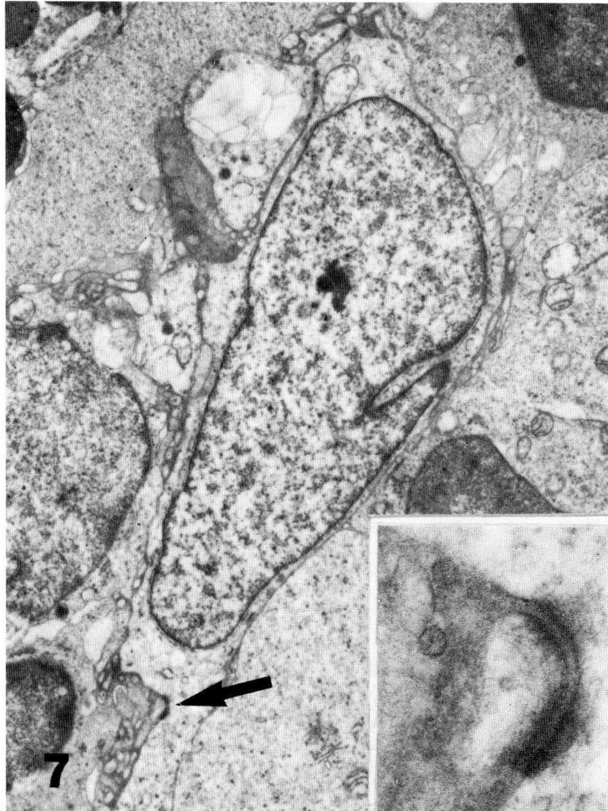

Fig. 26-7. Electron microscopy of FDC in reactive follicle with labyrinthine structure on extending cell membrane. (X 5,300, arrow and inset: desmosome-like junction, X 60,000).

Fig. 26-8. FDC in follicular lymphoma, reserving labyrinthine structure (X 9,500).

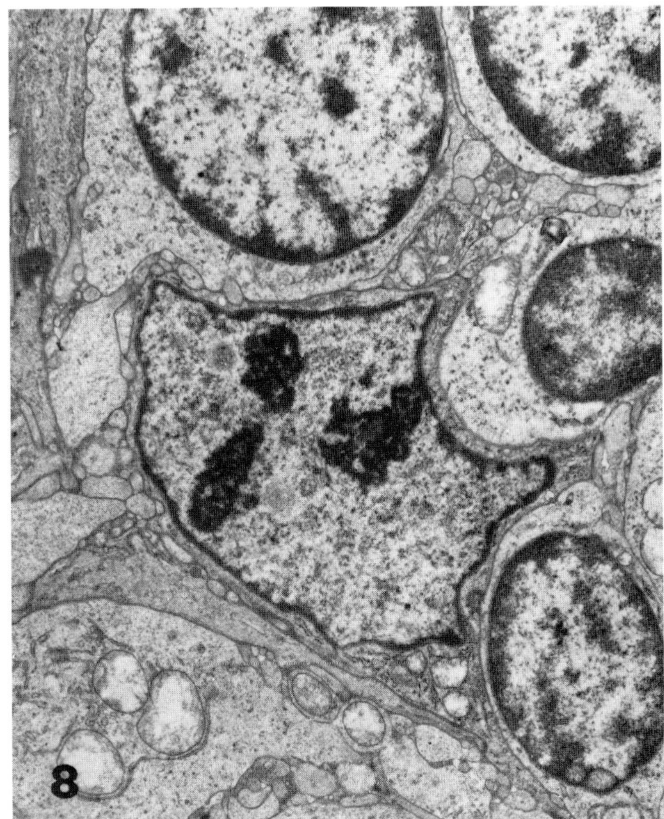

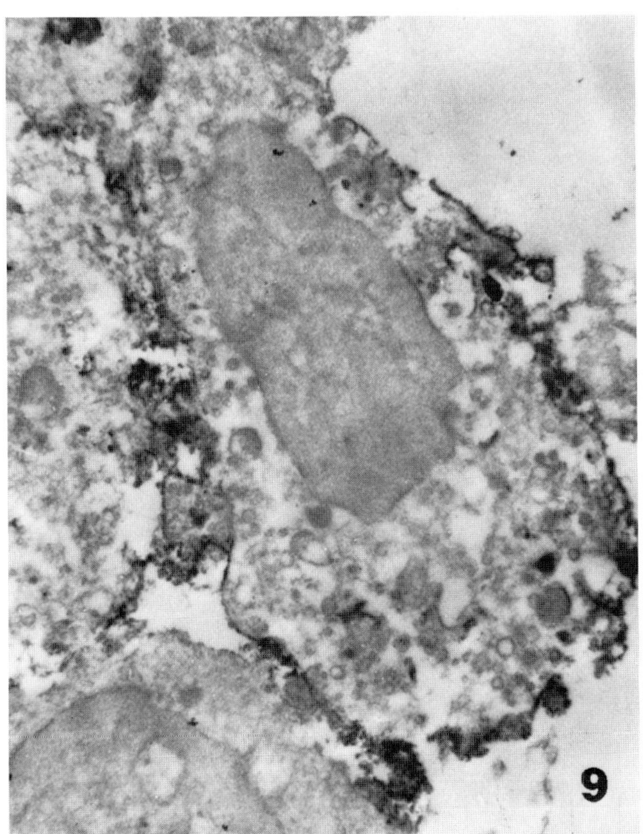

Fig. 26-9. CR-1 positive dendritic cell in diffuse B-cell lymphoma (X 12,000).

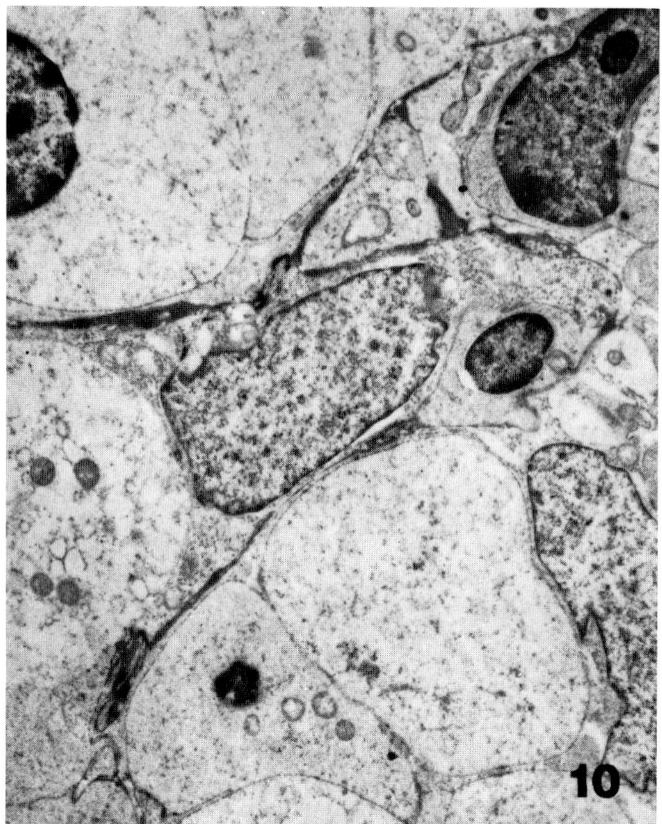

Fig. 26-10. Dendritic cell in IBL-like T cell lymphoma, without complicated cell surface (X 8,000).

GENERAL CONSIDERATIONS AND SUMMARY

From these results, an attempt was made to give an immunohistochemical definition of FDC in the reactive follicle as a mature type (Fig. 26-11). Indeed, as described,[13–15] it revealed the intense positivity for DRC-1, CR-1, CR-2, H107, some immunoglobulins, and some complement components. Opposed to the observations of Gerdes et al[13] or Parwaresch et al,[16] however, distinct positivity of FDC for myelo/macrophage markers could not be confirmed. More cases must be examined on this point since it is very pertinent to the nature of FDC.

In neoplastic follicles of follicular lymphoma, there were FDCs recognized that represented almost the same immunohistochemical properties and ultrastructural features as mature FDCs in the reactive follicles. In addition, the coarse reticular deposition of some immunoglobulins (especially IgM and/or IgE) and some complement components (C3d and/or C5) within the neoplastic follicles indicated that the FDC of follicular lymphoma may also have the immune-complex trapping ability and this functionally mature FDC may play inportant roles in the appearance and maintenance of follicular structure, even in the neoplasm. In diffuse B-cell lymphoma, only the focal or vestigial distribution of DRC-1^+ cells was observed. In contrast, the CR-1^+ reticulum cells were distributed in relatively wide areas overlapping DRC-1^+ areas. Such discrepancy of distribution of DRC-1^+ cells and CR-1^+ cells was also recognized in Case 18 that had been diagnosed as follicular lymphoma in the previous biopsy, and in Cases 8 and 10, which were including some vague follicualr patterns in a part of the biopsied lymph nodes. These results suggest that the FDC might have transformed to a (fibroblastic) reticulum cell bearing C3b receptor (CR-1^+) and lost the DRC-1 positivity as the development of the lymphoma (Fig. 26-12).

Reactive follicle

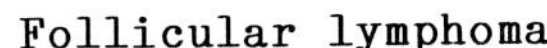

Follicular lymphoma

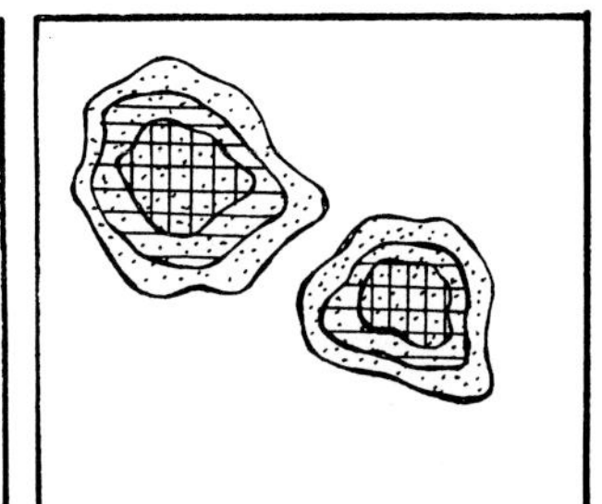

Diffuse B cell lymphoma

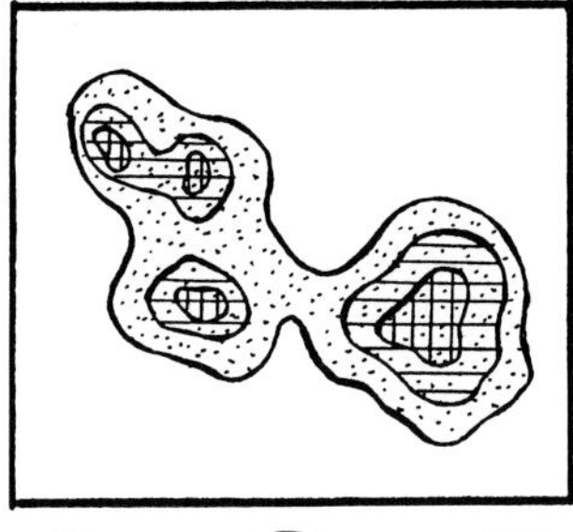

T cell lymphoma and Hodgkin's disease

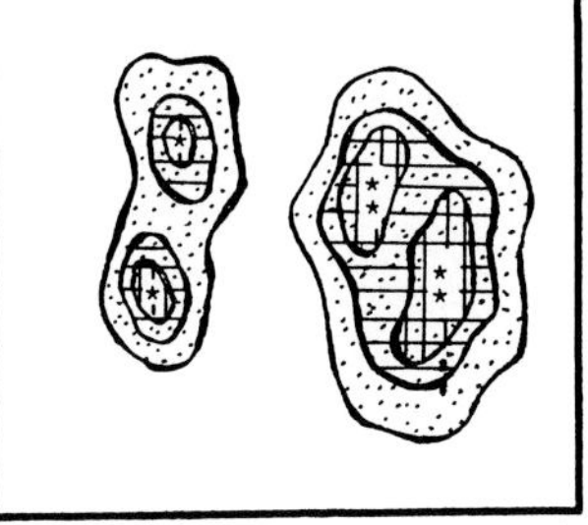

* Clear cell lymphoma & Hodgkin's disease (MC,NS,LP)

** IBL-like T cell lymphoma & Hodgkin's disease (LP)

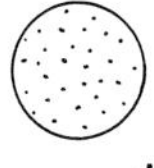

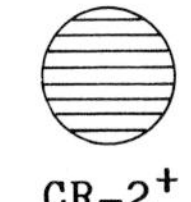

DRC-1+ CR-1+ CR-2+

Fig. 26-11. Distribution patterns of DRC-1, CD-1, and CR-2 positive cells.

Reactive follicle

DRC-1	++
CR-1	++
CR-2	++
Ig	++
Compl.	++
Fc-εR	++

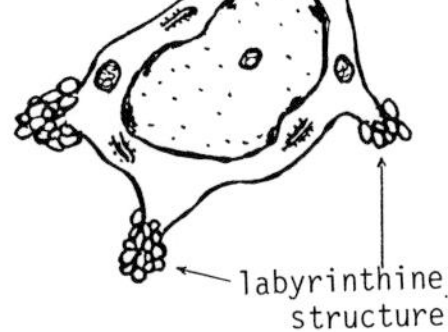

Neoplastic follicle
(Follicular lymphoma)

DRC-1	++
CR-1	++
CR-2	++
Ig	+/-
Compl.	+/-
Fc-εR	++

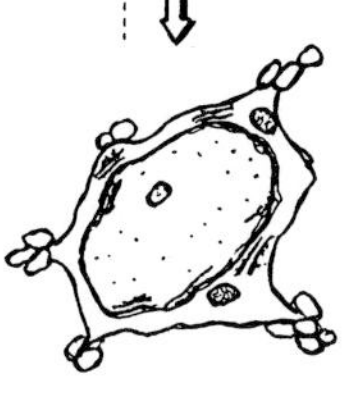

Diffuse lymphoma

DRC-1	-/+
CR-1	+
CR-2	+/-
Ig	-
Compl.	-
Fc-εR	+/-

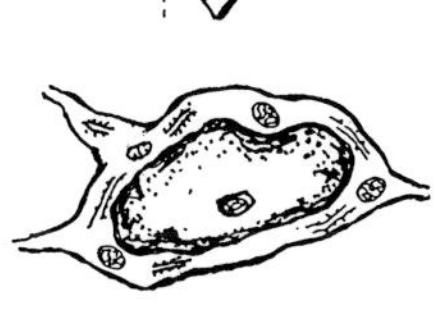

Fibroblastic reticulum cell

DRC-1	-
CR-1	+/-
CR-2	-
Ig	-
Compl.	-
Fc-εR	-

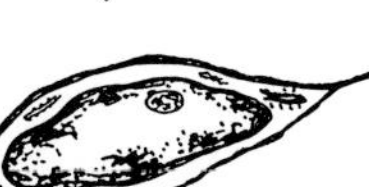

Fig. 26-12. Hypothetical schema of transformation of FDC in the progression of lymphoid malignancies.

DRC-1^+ cells distributed reticularly in the rather wide area in IBL-like T-cell lymphoma and LP type of Hodgkin's disease. In contrast, in clear cell lymphoma, which showed more monotonous and diffuse proliferation of clear lymphoma cells than in IBL-like T-cell lymphoma, and in MC type, NS type, and LD type of Hodgkin's disease, DRC-1^+ cells localized focally or vestigially (Fig. 26-11). These results suggest that distribution of FDCs (DRC-1^+ cells) is relative to histologic development of the lymphoma. In the early stage of lymphomas, such as folicular lymphomas before diffuse evolution, IBL-like change prior to development of distinct T-cell lymphomas, or in LP type of Hodgkin's disease, FDC were distributed in a wide and meshwork pattern. Therefore, the examination of the distribution pattern of the FDCs may be useful to understand the condition of progress and development of lymphoma and to estimate its prognosis.

REFERENCES

1. Kojima M: Macrophages, reticuloendothelial system and mononuclear phagocyte system. Recent Adv RES 16:1–25, 1978
2. Lennert K: Malignant Lymphomas Other Than Hodgkin's Disease. Handbuch der speziellen pathologischen Anatomie und Histologie. Verlin, Springer-Verlag 1978, 1–71
3. Groscurth P: Non-lymphatic cells in the lymph node cortex of the mouse. I, Morphology and distribution of the interdigitating cells and the dendritic reticulum cells in the mesenteric lymph node of the adult ICR mouse. Path Res Pract 169:212–234, 1980
4. Imai Y, Terashima K, Matsuda M, et al: Reticulum cell and dendritic reticulum cell; Origin and function. Recent Adv RES 22:51–81, 1983
5. Nossal GJV, Abbot A, Michell J, Lummus Z: Antigen in immunity. XV Ultrastructural features of antigen capture in primary and secondary lymphoid follicles. J Exp Med 127:277–290, 1968
6. Chen LL, Frank AM, Adams JC, Steinman RM: Distribution of horseradish peroxidase (HRP)-anti HRP immune complexes in mouse spleen with special reference to follicular dendritic cells. J Cell Biol 79:184–199, 1978
7. Imai Y, Dobashi M, Terashima K: Postnatal development of dendritic reticulum cells and their immune complex trapping ability. Histol Histopath 1:19–26, 1986
8. Gerdes J, Stein H: Complement (C3) receptors on dendritic reticulum cells of normal and malignant lymphoid tissue. Clin Exp 48:348–352, 1982
9. Peters JPJ, Rademakers LHPM, Roelofs JMM, et al: Distribution of dendritic reticulum cells in follicular lymphoma and reactive hyperplasia. Light microscopic identification and general morphology. Virchow Arch Cell Pathol 46:215–228, 1984
10. Carbone A, Manconi R, Poletti A, et al: S100 protein, fibronectin and laminin immunostaining in lymphomas of follicular center cell origin. Cancer 58:2169–2176, 1986
11. Shimoyama M, Minato K, Saito H, et al: Immunoblastic lymphadenopathy (IBL)-like T-cell lymphoma. Jpn J Clin Oncol 9:347–356, 1979
12. Shimoyama M, Tobinai K, Minato K, Watanabe S: Immunoblastic lymphadenopathy (IBL)-like T-cell lymphoma. GANN Monograph on Cancer Research 28:121–134, 1982
13. Gerdes J, Stein H, Mayson DY, Ziegler A: Human dendritic reticulum cells of lymphoid follicles: Their antigenic profile and their identification as multinucleated giant cells. Virchows Arch Cell Pathol 42:161–172, 1983
14. Kasajima T, Yamakawa M, Imai Y: Immunohistochemical study of intrathyroidal lymph follicles. Clin Immunol Immunopathol 43:117–128, 1987
15. Imai Y, Yamakawa M, Masuda A, et al: Function of the follicular dendritic cell in the germinal center of lymphoid follicles. Histol Histopath 1:341–353, 1986
16. Parwaresch MR, Radzun HJ, Feller AC, et al: Peroxidase positive mononuclear leukocytes as possible precursors of human dendritic reticulum cells. J Immunol 131:2719–2725, 1983

27

Nodal Inflammatory Pseudotumor

G. Frizzera
T. Perrone
C. De Wolf-Peeters

Abstract

Reported here is a previously undescribed, distinctive pattern of nodal reaction, characterized by: (1) predominant involvement of the connective tissue framework of the node (hilum, trabeculae, capsule): (2) storiform pattern; (3) rich vascularity with evidence of vasculitis and microthrombosis; and (4) a polymorphous inflammatory cell component. This needs to be distinguished not only from other reactive processes but, more importantly, from malignancies such as Hodgkin's disease, peripheral T-cell lymphoma, and histiocytic and reticulum cell tumors, in order to avoid overtreatment. Clinically, the process may be asymptomatic or be associated with systemic symptoms and a chronic, at times relapsing course. This nodal process is histologically and clinically similar to the inflammatory pseudotumor of the lung and other organs and tissues. Most of its features can be explained as effects of mediators of inflammation.

By making use of correlations with clinical and immunologic data, modern hematopathology has come a long way in identifying histologic features that define specific lympho-reticular disorders. However, it is still not uncommon in practice to encounter nodal reactions whose histologic characteristics do not fit into any of the previously recognized categories. Of particular concern are those that produce a marked distortion of the normal nodal architecture or other features usually associated with malignancy: overinterpretation of these processes, variously called "atypical lymphoproliferations" or "pseudolymphomas," may result in overtreatment of patients.

In this report a distinctive pattern of nodal reaction will be described, which has been recognized from a larger group of ill-defined nodal processes, and which has not been previously described. Histologically, it closely resembles the inflammatory pseudotumor or plasma cell granuloma of other organs, especially the lung. Its recognition is important because, in addition to other reactive processes, it may mimick malignant ones, such as malignant lymphomas and sarcomas.

Clinical Findings

The clinical characteristics of 7 patients are summarized as follows. Four were males and 3 females; their ages ranged from 16 to 62 years, with a median age of 33. Relevant past family histories included recent local trauma in one patient, previous malignancies in 2 and a familial history of auto-immune diseases and lymphoma in one. The onset of signs and symptoms was acute in 3, and chronic in 4. At presentation, constitutional symptoms were present in 5, lymphadenopathy was the relevant finding in all, and spleno- or hepatomegaly was observed in only 3. Laboratory findings included elevated ESR (5 patients), mild anemia and hypergammaglobulinemia (2 patients each). At lymph node biopsy, the surgeon described the nodes as being large (≥3 cm) in 5 cases, matted together in 2 or adherent to adjacent structures in 2. The histologic diagnoses returned by the original pathologists varied from reactive process (nonspecific, atypical, possible Castleman's disease), to reactive versus malignant (Hodgkin's or non-Hodgkin's lymphoma), to Hodgkin's disease, mixed cellularity. Treatment varied consequently from surgery only (4 patients), to chemotherapy (2) to radiotherapy (1). The disease resolved in 4 cases, and relapsed in 3. At last follow-up, all patients were alive, 5 off and 2 on therapy.

While these raw data do now tell much by themselves, there are in fact correlations among them. Once one excludes a patient in whom the evolution of the nodal disease cannot be evaluated due to early aggressive chemotherapy for a diagnosis of T-cell lymphoma, 2 patterns emerge. Two patients had an asymptomatic disease only manifested by localized peripheral adenopathy, were given no therapy and had spontaneous continuous remission (9 and 36 month follow-up). Another 4 patients had a symptomatic disease, which was protracted (3–5 years) in 3 of them, and manifested with more extensive lymphadenopathy, which was, in contrast, mostly visceral. In all of these patients, laboratory abnormalities were present and the disease persisted for a long time (12–60 months), before therapy was instituted. Treatment was diverse (Table 27-1), with slow or modest

TABLE 27-1
Treatment and Evolution of Disease in Clinical Pattern 2*

Therapy	Response	Relapse	Follow-up (months)
#4 CVP	Resolution of adenopathy, later of symptoms	No	A & W (40)
#5 Radiotherapy, predn., AZT	Modest improvement	Progressive disease	
Indomethacin		Remission	A on RX (29)
#6 Excision of nodes	Remission	3 (9,16,22 months) Spontaneous remission	A & W (23)
#7 Indomethacin	Modest improvement		
Splenectomy, steroids	Improvement	No	A on RX (7)

* CVP: cytoxan, vincristine, prednisone; AZT: azathioprine; A & W: alive and well; RX: therapy.

resolution of signs and symptoms, and 2 patients had relapses. All patients are alive (at 7–40 months from diagnosis), but 2 are still on therapy.

Histopathologic Findings

The histology of the nodal lesions was similar in all of our patients, with no appreciable differences between those with asymptomatic and those with symptomatic disease. The lesions were characterized by a complex of four features: predominant involvement of the connective tissue framework (hilum, trabeculae and capsule); storiform pattern of growth; rich vascularity with evidence of vasculitis and microthrombosis; and a polymorphous cellular composition, which included fibroblasts, polymorphonuclears, lymphocytes, immunoblasts, plasma cells, histiocytes, and rarely, eosinophils.

At low power, frequently one discrete focus was observed in the node, centered in the hilar region (Fig. 27-1). In continuity with it, the trabeculae also appeared thickened and prominent and the adjacent paracortex became hypervascular and hypercellular (Fig. 27-2). Edematous (Fig. 27-3), hypercellular (Fig. 27-4), or sclerotic (Fig. 27-5) areas may represent different phases of the process: all demonstrated a more or less prominent storiform pattern (Fig. 27-5) and abundant vascularity. Lesions, such as perivascular cuffing with lymphocytes and immunoblasts, perivascular fibrosis, and microthrombosis were consistently seen in capillaries or small vessels, while medium-sized vessels showed a proliferative and obliterative vasculitis, best evidenced by the broken muscular coat and near-obliteration of the lumen in sections stained for actin or desmin (Fig. 27-6). The cellular infiltrate was more or less florid and, as mentioned, polymorphous (Fig. 27-4): plasma cells predominated in the cellular areas, and spindle cells in the sclerotic ones. Mitotic figures were rare and no atypia or necrosis was observed. Nor were micro-organisms detected with stains for bacteria, fungi or viruses.

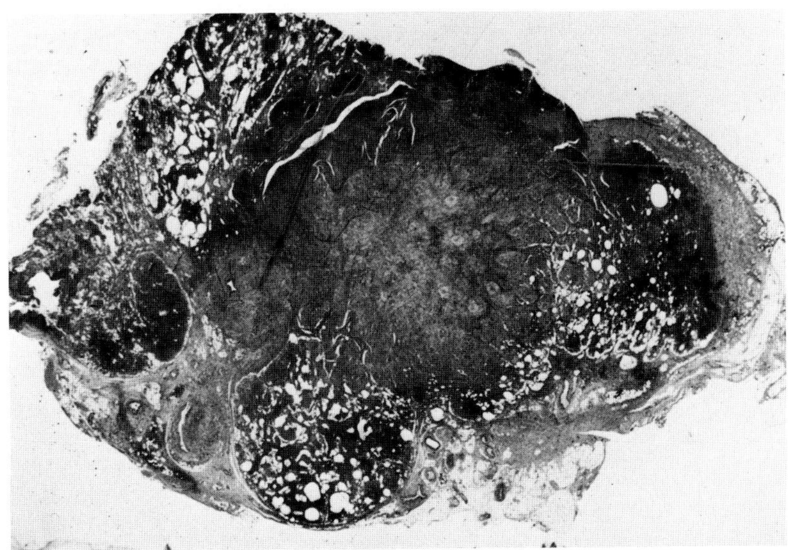

Fig. 27-1. Central focus of IPT, with lymphangiographic changes at the periphery.

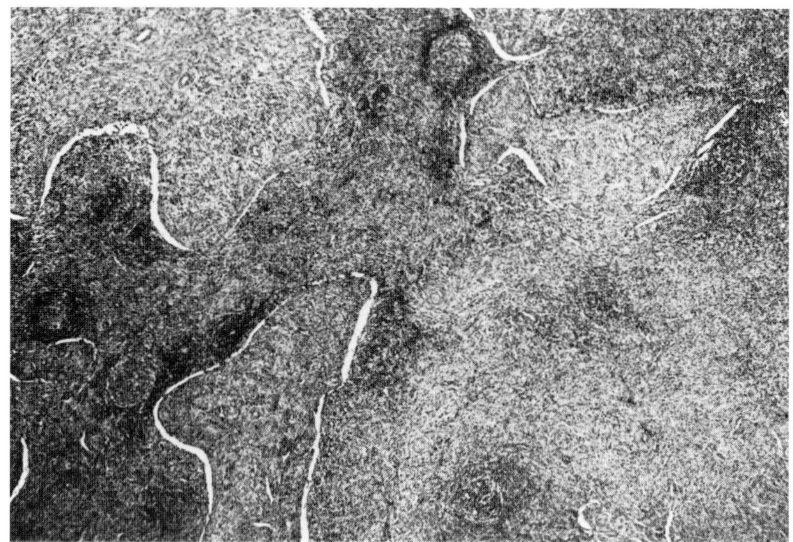

Fig. 27-2. Expansion of the trabeculae, lined by open sinuses.

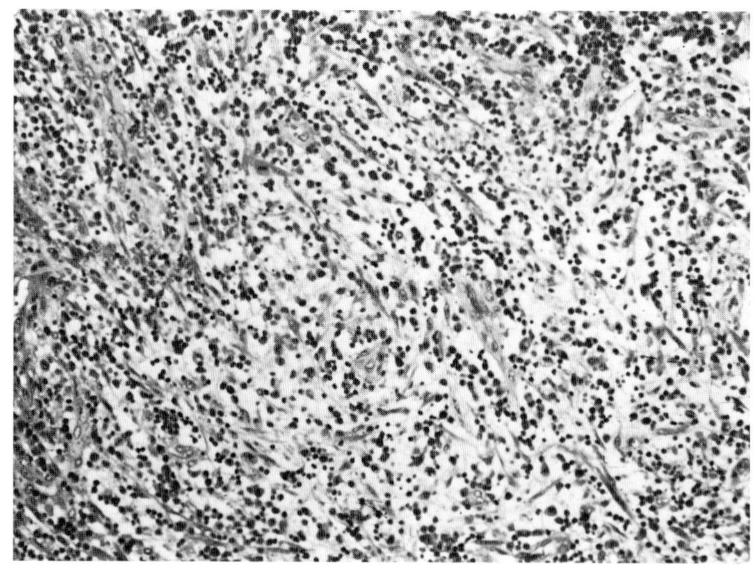

Fig. 27-3. Edematous area.

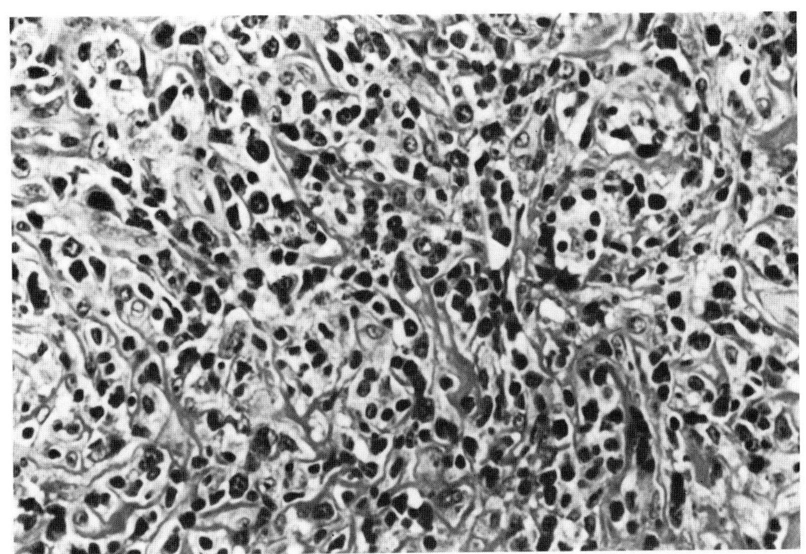

Fig. 27-4. Hypercellular area, with polymorphous composition.

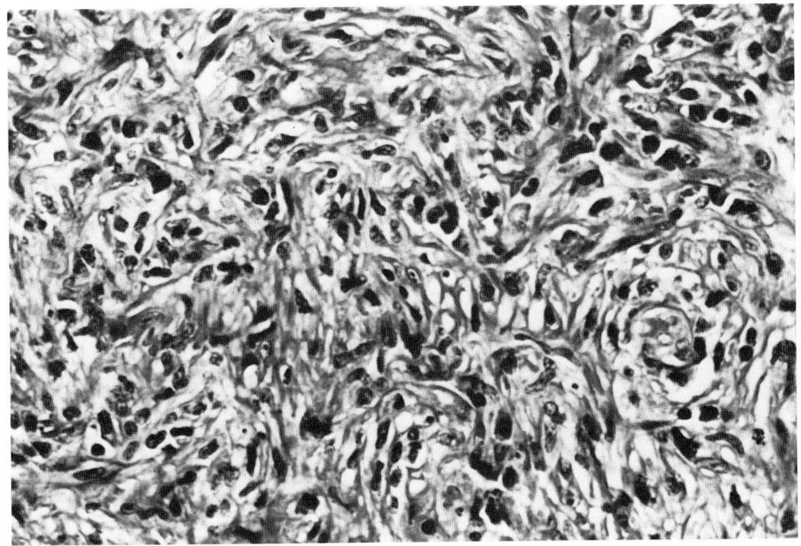

Fig. 27-5. Sclerotic area, with prominent storiform pattern.

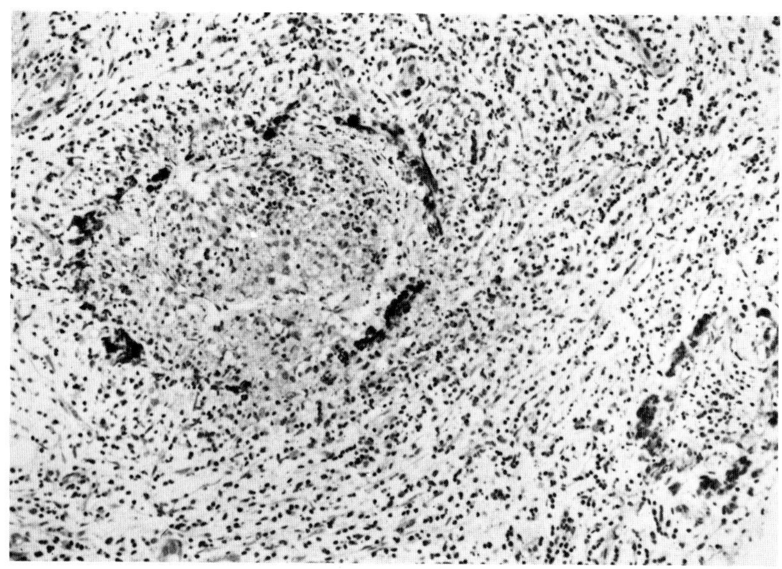

Fig. 27-6. Obliterative vasculitis. The broken muscular coat is evidenced by the anti-desmin immunoperoxidase stain.

Differential Diagnosis

Depending on the predominance of one or another of the above features, this process may be reminiscent of other reactive or malignant nodal lesions. In fact, it shares with Castleman's disease[1] the interfollicular vascularity and plasma cell infiltration, but does not have hyaline-vascular germinal center changes. It shares with drug lymphadenopathies the paracortical involvement, polymorphous infiltrate, and vasculitic lesions, but it does not have either necrosis or granulomas. Similarly, the paracortical involvement, cellular polymorphism, fibrosis or hypervascularity may suggest Hodgkin's disease or peripheral T-cell lymphoma, but other features of these diseases, such as, respectively, Reed-Sternberg cells and necrosis or lymphoid cell atypia and mitoses, are missing. Finally, when the storiform pattern and the spindle-cell component are conspicuous, the process may be reminiscent of malignant fibrous histiocytoma or dendritic reticulum cell tumors,[2] but it differs from these since it lacks cytologic atypia, mitoses, and necrosis.

Most of all, this lesion may be distinguished from all others listed above by relying on the very characteristic low-power view of an expansion of the nodal connective-tissue framework by a hypervascular storiform tissue. This impression is confirmed at higher magnifications, by the presence of vascular lesions and polymorphous cell infiltrate.

Pathogenesis

The above features are very similar to those of s.c. inflammatory pseudo-tumor (IPT) or plasma cell granuloma, originally described by Bahadori and Liebow in the lung,[3] and then reported in a host of other organs and tissues such as soft tissues of the mediastinum, retroperitoneum and extremities,[4,5,6] stomach,[7] appendix,[8] pancreas,[9] liver,[10] spleen,[11] urinary tract,[12] thyroid,[13] and meninges.[14] Such processes have been attributed to an infection,[15] a reaction to adjacent necrosis[11] or neoplasia,[7] or an immunologically mediated reaction.[3,9,13,16] A rather different interpretation sees them as part of the spectrum of myofibroblastic tumors, akin to nodular fasciitis, at one end, and to malignant fibrous histiocytoma, at the other.[5,12] As for the authors' cases, the negativity of cultures and special stains for microorganisms makes an infectious etiology unlikely. In two cases, local trauma and auto-immunity might have been etiologically relevant.

In fact, when considering on one hand, all the etiologies suggested for IPT and, on the other hand, the histologic consistency of the lesions, a common reaction pattern rather than a common etiology may better explain this lesion. Most of the clinical and histopathologic features of IPT may be accounted for by the production of mediators of inflammation, especially interleukin-1 (IL-1): proliferation of fibroblasts, extravasation of neutrophils, activation of T cells, with release of lymphokines, activation of B cells, with plasma cell accumulation, angiogenesis and microthrombosis, acute phase reactants in the serum, fever, and anorexia.[17,18]

Other features, such as the characteristic involvement of the nodal framework and vessels and the protracted and progressive course in some cases, are more difficult to explain. The vasculitis might be either the primary event[19] or a consequence of inflammation, as suggested in Kawasaki's disease,[20] or structural components of vessels and stroma may be a common target of an immunologic insult. The chronic and progressive evolution of this process may be an expression of the variations of the inflammatory response, based on diverse forms of IL-1 or altered regulation of mediators' production or activity.[17]

REFERENCES

1. Frizzera G, Banks PM, Massarelli G, Rosai J: A systemic lymphoproliferative disorder with morphologic features of Castleman's disease. Pathological findings in 15 patients. Am J Surg Pathol 7:211–231, 1983
2. Monda L, Warnke R, Rosai J: A primary lymph node malignancy with features suggestive of dendritic reticulum cell differentiation. A report of 4 cases. Am J Pathol 122:562–572, 1986
3. Bahadori M, Liebow AA: Plasma cell granulomas of the lung. Cancer 31:191–208, 1973
4. Day DL, Sane S, Dehner LP: Inflammatory pseudotumor of the mesentery and small intestine. Pediatr Radiol 16:210–215, 1986
5. Dehner LP: Extrapulmonary inflammatory myofibroblastic tumor: The inflammatory pseudotumor as another expression of the fibrohistiocytic complex. Lab Invest 54:15A, 1986
6. Turina J, Maurer R, Hollinger A, et al: Abdominaler entzundlicher Pseudotumor (Plasmazellgranulom) mit Anamie und Hypergammaglobulinamie. Schweiz Med Wochenschr 116:473–478, 1986
7. Tada T, Wakabayashi T, Kishimoto H: Plasma cell granuloma of the stomach. A report of a case associated with gastric cancer. Cancer 54:541–544, 1984
8. Narasimharao KL, Malik AK, Mitra SK, Pathak IC: Inflammatory pseudotumor of the appendix. Am J Gastroenterol 79:32–34, 1984
9. Abrebanel P, Sarfaty S, Gal R, et al: Plasma cell granuloma of the pancreas. Arch Pathol Lab Med 108:531–532, 1984
10. Anthony PP, Telesinghe PV: Inflammatory pseudotumor of the liver. J Clin Pathol 39:761–768, 1986
11. Cotelingam JD, Jaffe ES: Inflammatory pseudotumor of the spleen. Am J Surg Pathol 8:375–380, 1984
12. Nochomovitz LE, Orenstein JM: Inflammatory pseudotumor of the urinary bladder. Possible relationship to nodular fasciitis. Two case reports, cytologic observations, and ultrastructural observations. Am J Surg Pathol 9:366–373, 1985
13. Yapp R, Linder J, Schenken JR, Karrer FW: Plasma cell granuloma of the thyroid. Hum Pathol 16:848–850, 1985
14. Eimoto T, Yanaka M, Kurosawa M, Ikeya F: Plasma cell granuloma (inflammatory pseudotumor) of the spinal cord meninges. Report of a case. Cancer 41:1929–1936, 1978
15. Berardi RS, Lee SS, Chen HP, Stines GJ: Inflammatory pseudotumors of the lung. Surg Gynecol Obstet 156:89–96, 1983
16. Vitali C, Tavoni A, Simi U, et al: A plasma cell granuloma in a patient with Sjogren's syndrome. J Rheumatol 12:1212–1214, 1985
17. Beisel WR: Evolving concepts of the role of interleukin-1 (IL-1) and cortisol in stress: Similarities and differences, in Klueger MJ, Oppenheim JJ, Powanda MC (eds): The Physiologic, Metabolic and Immunologic Actions of Interleukin-1, New York, Alan R Liss, Inc., 1985, 3–12
18. Powanda MC: The role of interleukin-1 in homeostasis, in Kleuger MJ, Oppenheim JJ, Powanda MC (eds): The Physiologic, Metabolic and Immunologic Actions of Interleukin-1. New York, Alan R Liss, Inc., 1985, 535–546
19. Libby P. Ordovas JM, Auger KR, et al: Endotoxin and tumor necrosis factor induce interleukin-1 gene expression in adult human vascular endothelial cells. Am J Pathol 124: 179–185, 1986
20. Leung DYM, Geha RS, Newburger JW, et al: Two monokines, interleukin 1 and tumor necrosis factor, render cultured vascular endothelial cells susceptible to lysis by antibodies circulating during Kawasaki syndrome. J Exp Med 164:1958–1972, 1986

28

Histiocytic Necrotizing Lymphadenitis: Clinicopathologic, Immunologic, and HLA Typing Study

Masahiro Kikuchi
Morishige Takeshita
Tadaaki Eimoto
Hiroshi Iwasaki
Youichi Minamishima
Yoshiaki Maeda

Abstract

Histiocytic necrotizing lymphadenitis (HNL) affects primarily young women causing swelling of cervical lymph nodes, leukopenia, occasional skin rashes, and an elevation of LDH and transaminase. Recurrence occurs sometimes. Lesion can be divided into 4 subtypes on the basis of histology: lymphohistiocytic, phagocytic, necrotic and foamy cell types, but the lymphohistiocytic type that shows a proliferation of T lymphocytes and histiocytes with nuclear debris in the paracortex or cortex is an essential feature. Proliferating lymphocytes in the foci are composed mainly of both CD4 and CD8 cells, with a predominance of CD8 in the early stage. Early elevation of 2′,5′, oligoadenylate synthetase in serum, as well as a high incidence of tubuloreticular structures in lymphocytes, histiocytes, and endothelial cells in affected foci suggest a viral etiology for these lesions. A significantly higher frequency of HLA antigens A11 and DR12 ($p<0.01$) and a lower frequency of A24 ($p<0.05$) than in controls suggests an association of an immunologic response and a genetic basis for occurrence of this lesion.

HISTIOCYTIC NECROTIZING LYMPHADENITIS

In 1972 Kikuchi[1] reported a kind of lymphadenitis showing focal proliferation of reticular cells with nuclear debris and histiocytes in 26 patients. Following their report, many similar cases of this type of lymphadenitis have been demonstrated, mainly from Japan and some from other countries (Table 28-1).[2–12] The lymphadenitis is characterized by a proliferation of transformed large T cells with many histiocytes and nuclear debris, mainly in the paracortex, usually in cervical lymph nodes of young people.[10] The nature of the lesion is not yet certain, but viral infection is suspected. This paper describes the clinicopathologic and immunologic findings of this lesion and an activity of 2′,5′, oligoadenylate synthetase, which is elevated at acute phase of viral infection. HLA antigens were also investigated to detect the association of the lesion with HLA antigens.

Histopathology

The diagnosis of HNL was made by histology. The cases of this paper were obtained from the file of lymph node registry at the Department of Pathology, Fukuoka University, School of Medicine, Japan.

Histologic criteria of HNL were as follows: (1) Focal, well circumscribed lesions with aggregation of large lymphocytes, histiocytes with or without phagocytosis, and karyorrhectic nuclear debris, mainly in the paracortex or cortex; (2) absence of significant numbers of neutrophils, eosinophils, and plasma cells; (3) Occasional prominent individual cell necrosis, eosinophilic fibrin deposits, foamy cells and necrotic foci. The criteria are the same in previous reports.[1,4,11]

The essential histology is the proliferation of transformed large lymphocytes with histiocytes and nuclear debris, in association with an absence of neutrophils in paracortex or cortex (Fig. 28-1). The authors have subdi-

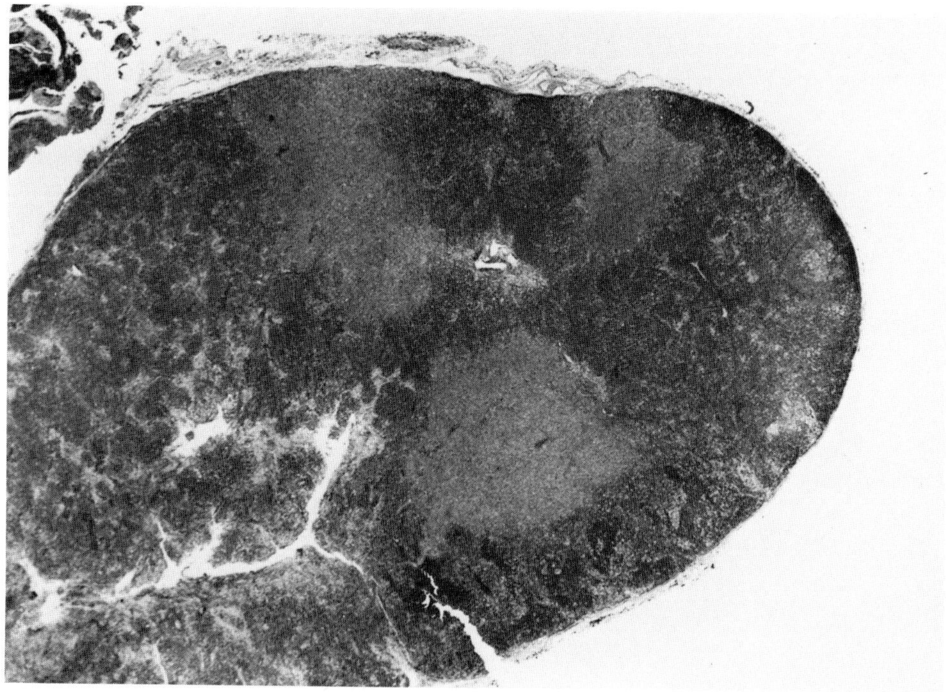

Fig. 28-1. Several well circumscribed lesions in the cortex and paracortex. Lymph follicles are diminished.

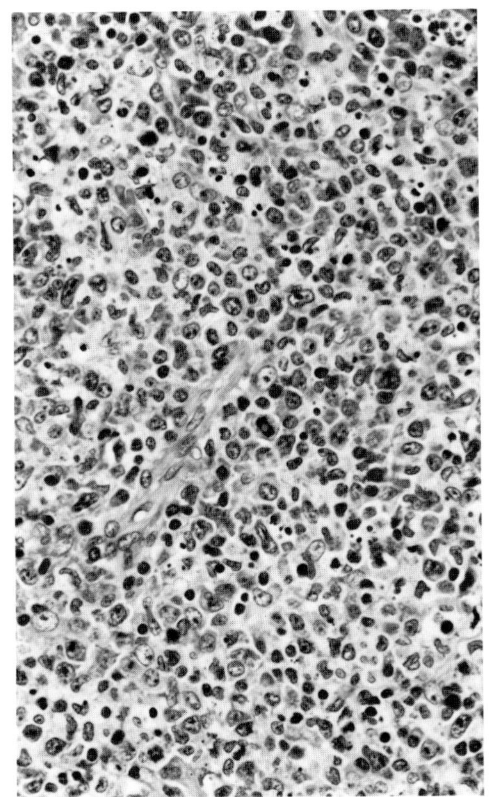

Fig. 28-2. Lymphohistiocytic type is characterized many transformed lymphocytes and macrophages, accompanied by some nuclear debris.

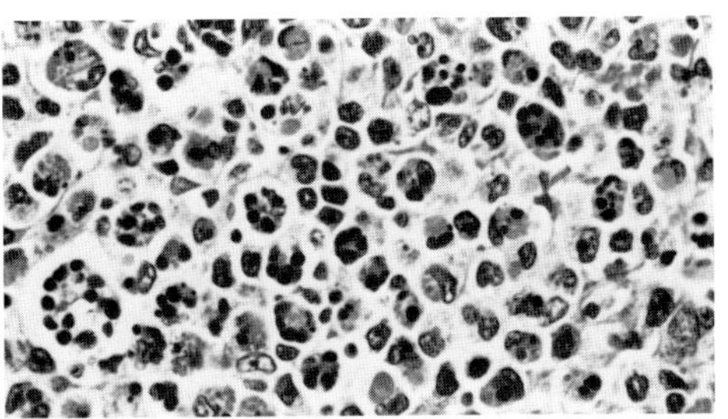

Fig. 28-3. Phagocytic type is characterized by proliferated lymphocytes with numerous histiocytes containing nuclear debris.

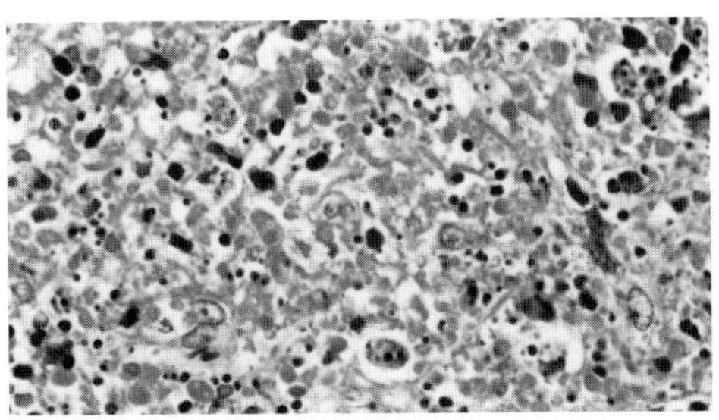

Fig. 28-4. Necrotic type is characterized by karyorrhectic nuclear materials associated with fibrin deposits.

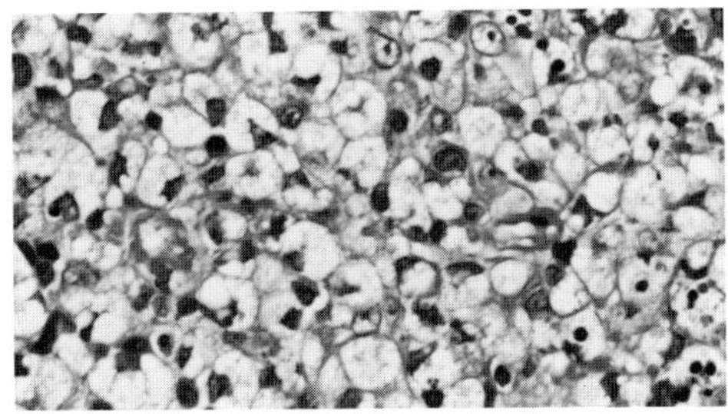

Fig. 28-5. Foamy-cell type is characteized by aggregates of foamy histiocytes.

Lymphohistiocytic type (*LH*) (*114 cases, 50.7%*): The main and essential type. The affected foci show a proliferation of transformed lymphocytes with considerable histiocytes. Usually nuclear debris are scattered among them (Fig. 28-2).

Phagocytic type (*P*) (*81 cases, 29.3%*): In addition to the features of the LH type, numerous phagocytes contain nuclear debris and red cells. Occasionally individual cell necrosis is present (Fig. 28-3).

Necrotic type (*N*) (*66 cases, 23.9%*): Individual cell necrosis of proliferating cells and eosinophilic fibrin deposits are obvious and occasionally focal necrosis in affected areas are demonstrated (Fig. 28-4).

Foamy cell type (*F*) (*15 cases, 5.4%*): Aggregates of foamy histiocytes are found, usually surrounding necrotic foci in the affected foci (Fig. 28-5).

The LH type is constant and in three other types are variably present.

Clinical Findings and Laboratory Findings

The age range of the patients was distributed between 4 and 53 years old with a mean age of 26.9. The ratio of female to male was 1.56 with a gradual increase of the ratio in older age groups (Fig. 28-1). The main clinical manifestations and laboratory data are tabulated in Tables 28-1 and 28-2. Lymphadenopathy of the neck was most common (97.5%) and other superficial lymph nodes were occasionally involved. Generalized adenopathy was found in 11.3%. Visceral lymph nodes were involved in only one case. Fever over 38°C was found in 30.2%. The entire clinical course was less than 2 months in 79.8% and 11 patients had recurrence between 6 months and 5 years after the resolution of the first symptom. Leukopenia below 4,000/cmm was noted in 58.3% and leukocytosis over 10,000/cmm was present only in 2.1%. Some atypical lymphocytes, less than 3% of all lymphocytes, were found in 31.1%.

TABLE 28-1
Synonyms for Histiocytic Necrotizing Lymphadenitis

Lymphadenitis showing reticulum cell hyperplasia with debris and phagocytes (Kikuchi, 1972)
Subacute necrotizing lymphadenitis (Fujimoto et al, 1972)
Necrotizing lymphadenitis (Wakasa et al, 1975)
Pseudolymphomatous hyperplasia in lymph node (Michaelek, 1977)
Xanthogranulomatous lymphadenitis (Cozzutto et al, 1979)
Histiocytic-necrotizing lymphadenitis (Kikuchi et al, 1981)
Histiocytic necrotizing lymphadenitis without granulocytes (Pileri et al, 1982)
Kikuchi disease (Dorfman, 1984)

Increase of transaminase and elevation of LDH were 23.6% and 61.8%, respectively. The results were early the same as the previous reports.[1,4,11]

TABLE 28-2
Hematological and Laboratory of Histiocytic Necrotizing Lymphadenitis (%)

	LH	P	N	F	Total
No. of Cases	114	81	66	15	276
CRP	23.6(10/38)	16.7(2/12)	50.0(11/22)	50.0(2/4)	32.9(25/76)
WBC (mm^3)					
below 4000	54.3(38/70)	66.7(20/30)	58.3(21/36)	62.5(5/8)	58.3(84/144)
4000–10000	42.9(30/70)	30.0(9/30)	41.7(15/36)	37.5(3/8)	39.6(57/144)
10000–	2.8(2/70)	3.3(1/30)	0.0(0/36)	0.0(0/8)	2.1(3/144)
Atypical Lymphocytes in PB	25.5(14/55)	26.7(4/15)	37.0(10/27)	66.7(4/6)	31.1(32/103)
Increase of transaminase	16.7(6/36)	0.0(0/9)	40.9(9/22)	40.0(2/5)	23.6(17/72)
Elevation of LDH	39.5(15/38)	66.7(6/9)	91.3(21/23)	83.3(5/6)	61.8(47/76)
Autoantibodies positive titers	2.7(1/37)	4.4(1/15)	7.1(2/28)	0.0(0/6)	4.7(4/86)
Toxoplasma	1 case	2 cases	0	1 case	4 cases
Rubella	1 case	1 case	0	0	2 cases
Measles	0	0	1 case	0	1 case
Influenza	1 case	0	0	0	1 case

Autoantibodies: RA test (+); 3 cases and LE test (+); 1 case

The LH type was found in early biopsies and the F type was often detected in cases biopsied after 2 months. P and N types were not temporally associated with the biopsy.

Fever, skin rashes, and appearance of typical lymphocytes were most common in the F type and an increase of trans-amylase and elevation of LDH were frequent in both N and F types. Other clinical and laboratory findings such as affected sites, durations, recurrernce rate, and blood pictures were similar in each type.

Electronmicroscopy

Electron microscopic examination was performed in 15 cases. Frequent appearance of tubuloreticular structures and intracytoplasmic rodlets in transformed lymphocytes, histiocytes, and vascular endothelial cells in the affected foci were characteristic findings in the examined cases as in previous reports.[13,14]

Immunohistochemistry

Affected foci showed proliferation of histiocytes (positive for lysozyme, alpha 1 antichymotrypsin, CD11) as well as CD3, DC4, and CD8 positive T lymphocytes with a predominance of CD8 cells in the early stage and an increase of CD4 cells in the later phase. Interleukin II receptor (CD25) was positive in a few T cells, and OKT 9 for proliferating cells was positive in about 30% of lymphocytes. However, markers for B cells, NK cells, complement proteins and receptors, and neutrophils were scanty or absent in the foci. Details of the results were reported previously.[11] In addition Ki67 was examined for proliferating cells and Kil for activated lymphocytes. The lymphocytes in the affected foci showed a slightly higher positivity of Ki67 than lymphocytes in the surounding tissue. Few Kil positive cells were found in affected areas. The findings were similar to those found in delayed type hypersensitivity reactions.[15]

2′5′ oligoadenylate acetate synthetase

Among several speculations, the viral nature of the lesion has been suggested by the clinical features of acute onset with an appearance of atypical lymphocytes, skin rash, and fever. A frequent appearance of tubuloreticular structures in proliferating T cells, which is thought to be related to activity of interferon alpha[16] and viral infection was also suggestive of a viral origin for HNL. Kikuchi et al therefore investigated activity of 2′5′ oligoadenylate synthetase, which becomes elevated in the acute phase of viral infection and relates to alpha interferon.[17] Elevation of this synthetase over 100 pmol/dl (cut of value is 100 pmol/dl) was found in 12 of 30 examined patients as shown in Fig. 28-6. The results strongly supported the possibility of acute viral infection of the lesion.

Typing of HLA Antigens

HNL is usually found in Japanese. Reported patients except Japanese were 47 in Caucasian, 8 in Asian, 3 in Arabian, and 1 in African. The variance of occurrence rate in different races suggested the genetic association of HNL, and immunologic histologic factors were also considered. HLA typing of the patients was also examined. Typing of HLA antigens was examined by the standard methods, recommended by the NIH and the 9th International Histocompatibility Workshop. Antigen frequencies for HLA were examined in 11 patients for A, B, C, and in 10 patients for DR and DQ. The results are shown in Table 28-3. A11 (63.6%) and DR12 (40.0%) has a significantly higher association for the etiologic factor than controls ($p<0.01$) and A24 (36.4%) was significantly lower ($p<0.05$).[18] A11 and A24 are found near the same gene locus. The results suggested that the occurence of HNL might relate to the

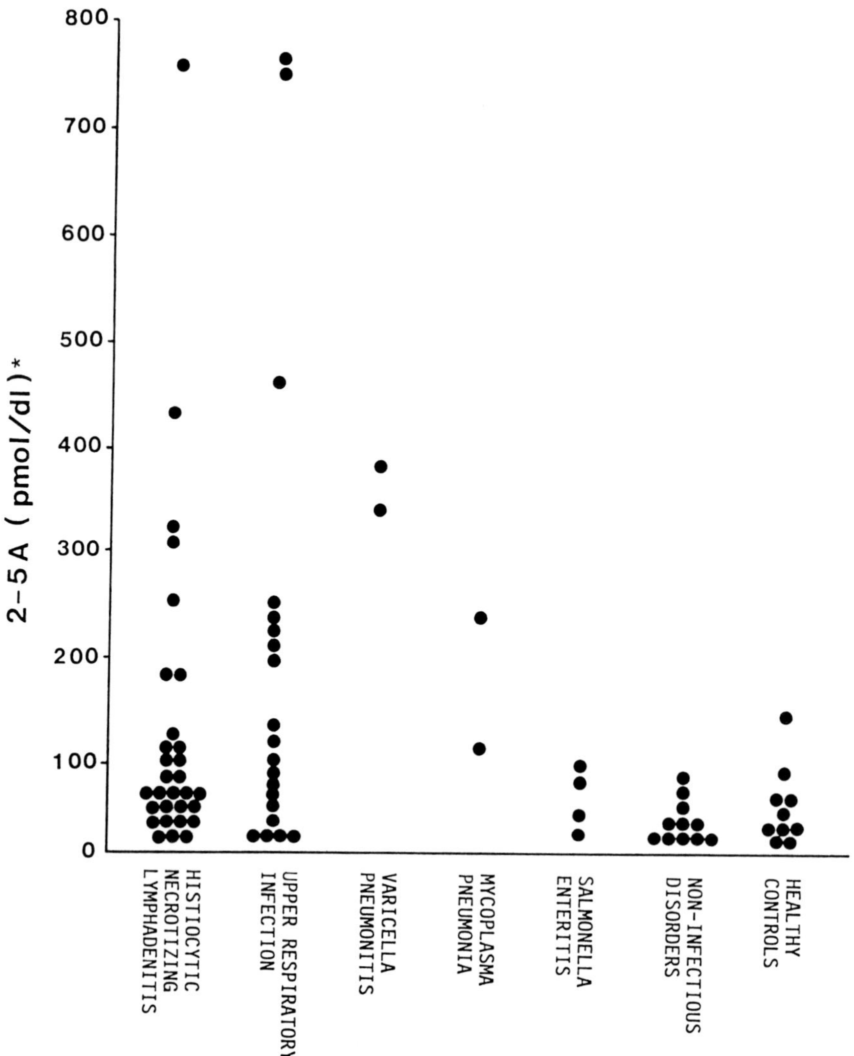

Fig. 28-6. Activity of 2′5′ oligoadenylate synthetase (2–5A) in sera of various diseases and healthy controls.

TABLE 28-3
Antigen Frequencies for HLA in Histiocytic Necrotizing Lymphadenitis

Antigens	Patients (A,B,C:n = 11) (DR,DQ:n = 10)	Controls[18] (n = 236)	R.R.	EF†	PF§	Pc value
A11	63.6%	16.0%	9.12	0.57		p<0.01
A24	36.4%	69.2%	0.26		0.51	p<0.01
DR12	40.0%	6.2%	10.16	0.36		p'0.01

Other following antigens were not significant
A 2, 26, 31
B 7, 13, 35, 39, 48, 51, 54, 59, 60, 61, 62
C 1, 3, 4, 7
DR 2, 4, 8, 9, w52, w53
DQ w1, 13

† Etiologic Factor
§ Preventive Factor

immunologic response. Antigen frequency of A11 is 17.2% in Japanese; 12.5% in Caucasian, North America; 11.5% in Caucasian, Europe; 7.1% in Mexican; and 1.1% in Negro. High frequency of HNL in Japanese, occasionally in Caucasian and few in Negros seems related to the frequency of HNL to the frequency of this antigen in different races. Concerning DR12, the accuracy of the examination method was not yet complete, so the date is problematic. Further studies on many cases are necessary to establish the association of HNL with HLA types.

REFERENCES

1. Kikuchi M:Lymphadenitis showing focal reticulum cell hyperplasia with nuclear debris and phagocytes: A clinicopathological study. Acta Hematol Jpn, 35:379–380, 1972 (in Japanese)
2. Fujimoto Y, Kojima Y, Yamaguchi K: Cervical subacute necrotizing lymphadenitis. Naika 30:920–927, 1972 (in Japanese)
3. Kikuchi M, Yoshizumi M, Nakamura H: Necrotizing lymphadenitis: Positive acute toxoplasmi infection. Virchow Arch (Pathol Anat) 376:247–253, 1977
4. Kikuchi M: Lymphadenopathy due to toxoplasmic infection and anti-convolsant. Recent Adv RES 18:97–124, 1978
5. Fujimori F, Shioda K, Sussman EB, et al: I. Subacte necrotizing lymphadentiis. A clinicopathologic study. Acta Pathol Jpn 31:791–797, 1981
6. Pileri S, Kikuchi M, Helbron K, Lennert K: Histiocytic necrotizing lymphadenitis without granulocytic infiltration. Virchow Arch (Pathol Anat) 395:257–271, 1982
7. Turner RR, Martin J, Dorfman RF: Necrotizing lymphadenitis: A study of 30 cases. Am J Surg Pathol 7:115–123, 1983
8. Feller AC, Lennert K, Stain H, et al: Immunohistology and aetiology of histiocytic necrotizing lymphadenitis. Report of three instructive cases. Histopathol 7:825–839, 1983
9. Ali MH, Horton LWL: Necrotizing lymphadenitis without granulocytic infiltration (Kikuchi's disease). J Clin Pathol 38:1252–1257, 1985
10. Kikuchi M, Takeshita M, Tashiro K, et al: Immunohistological study of histiocytic necrotizing lymphadenitis. Virchow Arch (Pathol Anat) 409:299–311, 1986
11. Carbone A, Mancon R, Volpe R, et al: Enzyme- and immunohistochemical study of a case of histiocytic necrotizing lymphadenitis. Virchows Arch (Pathol Anat) 408:637–647, 1986
12. Kuo TT, Shih LY: Surgical pathology of lymph node biopsy specimens in Taiwan with a report of adult T cell leukemia/lymphoma.
13. Eimoto T, Kikuchi M, Mitsui T: Histiocytic necrotizing lymphadenitis. An ultrastructural study in comparison with no other types of lymphadenitis. Acta Pathol Jpn 33:868–879, 1983
14. Imamura M, Ueno H, Masuura A, et al: An ultrastructural study of subacute necrotizing lymphadenitis. Am J Pathol 107:292–299, 1982
15. Platt JL, Grant BW, Eddy AA, Michael AF: Immune cell populations of cutaneous delayed-type hypersensitivity. J Exp Med 158:1227–1242, 1983
16. Kuyama J, Kanayama Y, Mizutani H, et al: Formation of tubuloreticular inclusions in mitogen-stimulated human lymphocyte cultures by endogenous or exogenous alpha-interferon. Ultrastr Pathol 10:77–85, 1986
17. Fujioka K, Ohashi T, Minamishima Y: Activity of 2'5' oligoadenylate synthetase in sera of patients with viral infection Igaku to Yakugaku 16:1123–1125, 1986 (in Japanese)
18. Tanaka K, Sato H, Okochi K: HLA antigens in patients with adult T-cell leukemia. Tissue Antigens 23:81–83, 1984

29

Angioimmunoblastic Lymphadenopathy with Dysproteinemia (AILD)—Its Clinicopathologic and Genetic Aspects

Shigeo Mori
Haruo Sugiyama

Abstract

Angioimmunoblastic lymphadenopathy with dysproteinemia (AILD) is a clinicopathologically defined disease entity. Previously, hematopathologists tried to separate this disease from malignant lymphomas (MLs). Recent research, however, revealed a close relationship between AILD and ML, especially of the T-cell type. It is becoming more and more difficult to place a demarcation between these two entities. To know further the nature of AILD, 21 cases were studied clinicopathologically, immunopathologically, and on molecular biology. These 21 cases included 13 AILDSs that satisfied the criteria of AILD, termed in this article as typical AILD, and 8 atypical AILDs that in a part differed from the typical AILD. Typical cases were characterized by the infiltration of polymorphous lymphocytes, presence of clear cells, plasma cells, and histiocytes, together with proliferation of postcapillary venules. Seven of 13 typical cases showed hyperimmunoglobulinemia. Typical cases favored better natural history when compared to atypical cases. On immunopathologic study, 10 out of 11 typical cases showed helper/inducer type T cell dominancy. Atypical cases included those that represented heavy histiocytic reaction, preservation of follicles, or poor vascular proliferation. They showed worse natural history. Some such cases showed suppressor/cytotoxic T cell dominancy. Molecular biological study showed monospecific Tcβ gene rerarrangement in 3 out of 7 cases, among which 2 in 3 were typical and one of 4 belonged to atypical cases. Thus, the data show that a large part of typical AILDs are the T-cell malignancy of the helper-inducer type, while atypical cases were composed of a heterogenous group.

* This paper was presented at a symposium of 49th Japan Hematological Society meeting.[13]

THE CONCEPT OF ANGIOIMMUNOBLASTIC LYMPHADENOPATHY:

Angioimmunoblastic lymphadenopathy (AILD, Frizzera et al., 1974)[1] was defined from clinicopathologic viewpoint. This particular disease was first described by Suchi under the term atypical lymphoid hyperplasia with fatal outcome.[2] It is also called as immunoblastic lymphadenopathy. The existence of this disease has been widely accepted. Prognostically, one half of the patients eventually developed overt malignant lymphomas (MLs), while a large part of the remainder died of opportunistic infections attributable to oncostatic chemotherapy.[3]

The nature of AILD has been a puzzle. The concept of the ''pre-neoplastic state'' was introduced to explain AILD. This is a quite an ambiguous word and does not make sense in modern biology.

In 1979, Shimoyama and his group first described a specific type of T-ML that was characterized by hyperimmunoglobulinemia and histiolgic vascular proliferation.[4] Even though their cases were the apparent lymphoma and somehow different from the classical definition of AILD, it has brought up the assumption that AILD, at least in part, may be included in this specific type of ML.

Thereafter, many papers appeared from the field of immunology, genetics, and molecular biology. Many of these indicated that some of angioimmunoblastic lymphadenopathy (AILD) belong to the T-cell malignancy. They were based on: the first is the demonstration of monophenotypic T cells in AILD lesions,[3] the second is the demonstration of chromosomal aberration,[5–7] and the third is the demonstration of the T-cell receptor gene rearrangement.[8,9]

If some of the AILDs are accepted to be the real T-cell malignancy, the succeeding research subject would be to determine if all the AILDs were the T cell malignancy, and if not, how the T-cell malignancies can be demarcated from other groups. This is the very problem hematopathologists are now facing: we must struggle further to solve this problem.

One of the problems relying on further AILD study is that we are still uncertain as to what is considered typical AILD. Hematopathologists are still using, without confidence, the classical clinicopathologic definition of 1974 that may include a different group of diseases or may pick up a limited portion of a distinct disease entity under the term AILD. The second problem that somehow overlaps the first is the presence of a gap in understanding of this disease among hematologists. This is a serious problem as there is no way to exchange information and achievements if two groups study different group of patients under the same disease name, AILD. Many of Japanese hematopathologists realized this gap at a meeting which was held in Tokyo in 1984 under the title of ''International Colloquium on AILD and Related Disorders.'' In this meeting, the slides brought from US were mostly categolized as malignant lymphomas by Japanese patholgoists. The American cases contined much more large blasts and histiocytic cells when compared to the Japanese cases, while they lacked the clear (pale) cells which is commonly seen in Japanese AILDs. This experience showed that we still are not sure about what is the typical AILD. We have to be careful in referring reports with the caution that ''what is the AILD of these authors?''

CLINICOPATHOLOGIC ASPECTS OF AILD

Because of the limited knowledge the classical clinicopathologic definition will be used to describe this disease. Clinically, patients suffer from fever, skin rash, hepatosplenomegaly, and lymphadenopathy. Laboratory data show polyclonal hyperimmunoglobulinemia. Histopathology of the lymph node shows total effacement of the basic structure with proliferation of arborizing vessels and histiocytic cells, accumulation of eosinophilic PAS-positive amorphous mass around blood vessels, and infiltration of polymorphous lymphocytes, including large lymphoid cells, immunoblasts, and plasma cells. Shimoyama's group, as well as other Japanese hematopathologists, stress the existence of clear cell, or pale cell lymphoma.[2,4]

Most of Mori's and Sugiyama's cases have 80%, or even 90% of these clinicopathologic characteristics. Cases that show all of these characteristics are, however, exceedingly rare. Rather common are cases that do not show hyperimmunoglobulinemia. There are also cases in which vascular proliferation, although present, is not extensive. It has to be stressed that there are no cases that show the famous ''eosinophilic amorphous material around blood vessels'' in this series.

There are 21 cases that were diagnosed or highly suspected as AILD. Included were the cases with total effacement of nodal structure by proliferation of the polymorphous, large and small cells, and arborizing blood vessels. Apparent non-Hodgkin's lymphomas, characterized by monotonous proliferation of lymphoid cells, Hodgkin's disease characterized by the presence of Reed-Sternberg giant cells, and cases with intact nodal structure were excluded. These 21 cases could be divided further into two groups: the typical cases that satisfy most of the classical criteria of AILD, termed as AILD lesion, and atypical cases that lack a part of the items in the criteria. The latter included cases with less developed blood vessels, heavy histiocytic reactions, or partially remaining follicles (Figs. 29-1, and 29-2).

Under these criteria for selection, the cases consisted of 18 males and 3 females. Ages ranged between 30 and 70 years of age with the peak on 50. All patients showed generalized lymphadenopathy. Other findings included fever (7/10), skin rash (5/11), and hypergammaglobulinemia (9/21). The prognosis of patients were listed on Table 29-1 and Fig. 29-3).

A histopathologic review of slides revealed 13 typical cases and 8 atypical cases. Typical cases were further divided into those with

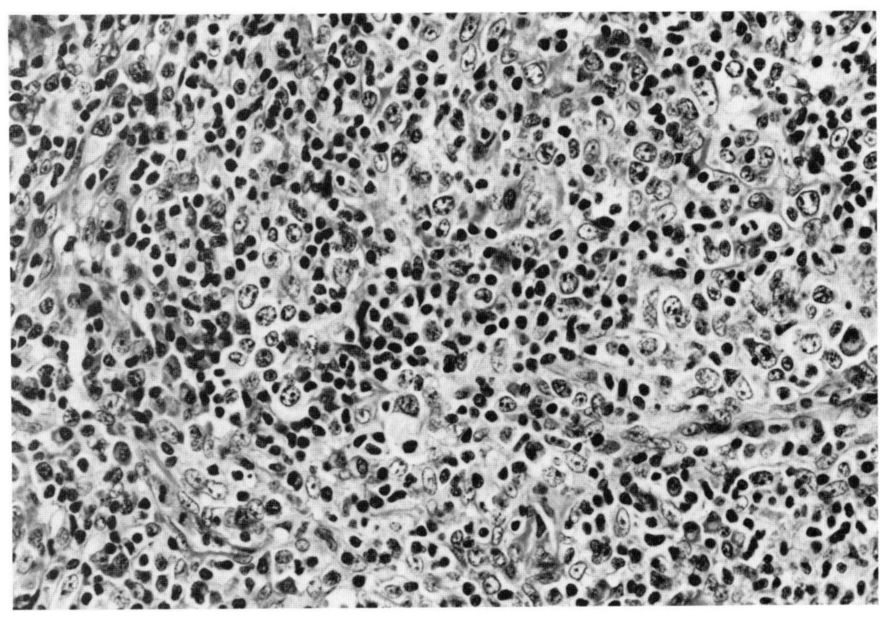

Fig. 29-1. Typical AILD lesion (H and E stain, × 220)

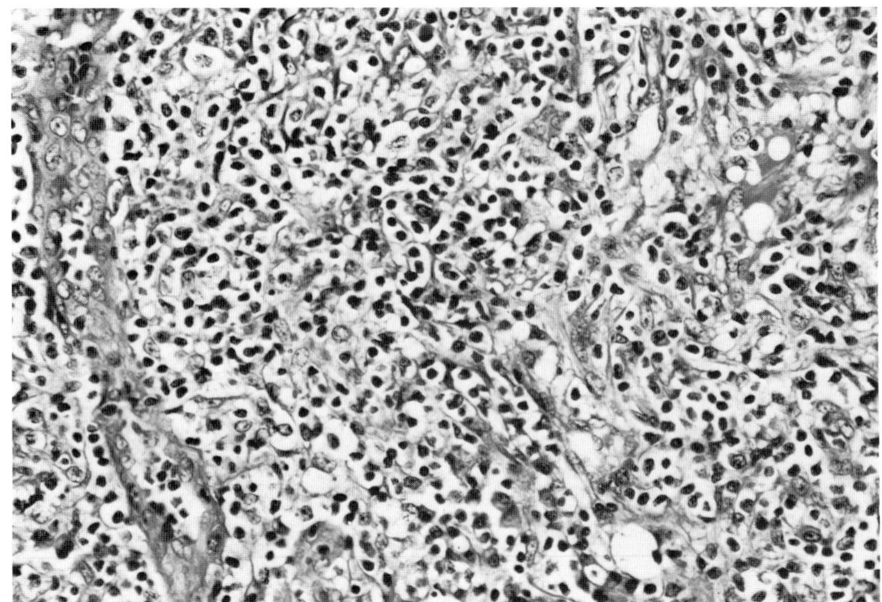

Fig. 29-2. Typical AILD, small lymphocyte dominant (H and E stain, × 220)

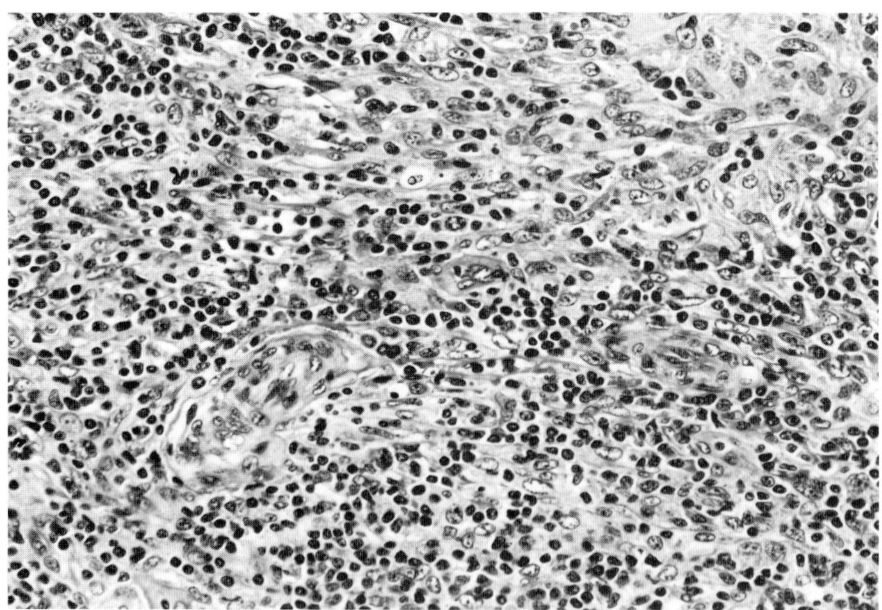

Fig. 29-3. Atypical AILD lesion with poorly developed blood vessels.

TABLE 29-1
Follow-up Data of Typical and Atypical AILDs.

Prognosis	Number of Cases
Alive	10
Under chemotherapy	5
Under observation without chemotherapy	3
New patient	2
Dead	11
Tumor proliferated in spite of chemotherapy	2
Tumor disappeared by chemotherapy	8
Death with secondary diseases	1
Unknown	1

many large lymphocytes (blasts): 5 cases; and those with fewer blasts: 8 cases. Atypical cases consisted of heavy histiocytic reaction: 4; partial preservation of follicles: 2; and poor vascular development: 2.

IMMUNOPATHOLOGICAL ASPECTS

Immunopathologic marker study[10] has been used widely as a powerful methodology in modern hematopathology. Actually, a large part of the recent information in lymphoma research was brought from this technic, however, it has not contributed much on AILD research. The difficulty resides mainly in that monoclonal proliferation of specific lymphocyte lineage, which is the very characteristic finding of malignant lymphoma, but is not observed on AILD theoretically and practically: This difficulty has two confusing aspects: (1) in a large number of AILD cases, the lesion is composed of heterologous lymphocytes and monoclonal proliferation can hardly be observed; (2) meanwhile, when a monoclonal proliferation is observed in the lesion, pathologists are tempted to call such cases AILD-like T-cell lymphoma, even though other clinicopathologic features might satisfy the criteria of AILD.

In the Mori/Sugiyama cases, all 19 cases studied immunopathologically, showed prominent T cell dominancy. Among these, the helper/inducer type T cell was dominant in 16, and the suppressor/cytotoxic T cell was greater or equal to 3. The correlation of immunopathologic findings with morphology was shown on Table 29-2.

It is a common agreement that the marker of AILD-like T-cell lymphoma is the helper/inducer type T cell, although a small number of reports stress the dominancy of suppressor/cytotoxic T cells.[4] Data showed that a large part of AILD also represents helper/inducer type T cell dominancy. It is thus far practically and theoretically impossible to differentiate AILD from AILD-like ML on immunopathologic examination.

TABLE 29-2
Correlation of Lymphocyte Marker and Histology

Histopathological findings	Dominant marker	
	Th/i	Ts/c
Typical AILDs	11	1
Large lymphocyte dominant	4	1
Small lymphocyte dominant	7	0
Atypical AILDs	5	2
Heavy histiocytic reaction	2	2
Follicles remaining	2	0
Blood vessels not developed	1	0

MOLECULAR BIOLOGICAL ASPECT

Molecular biology has been introduced recently in lymphoma study. One advantage of this method is that it can demonstrate the presence of a small number of monospecific cells, or clonally proliferating cells,[11] which can not be detected by immunologic methods. Its main strategy is to show the presence of uniform rearrangement of marker genes. By the introduction of this method, a small number of clonal T cells was demonstrated in

TABLE 29-3
Correlation of Genetic Data and Histology

Histopathological findings	Rearrangement of TC gene	
	yes	no
Typical AILDs	2	1
Large lymphocyte dominant	1	1
Small lymphocyte dominant	1	0
Atypical AILDs	3	1
Heavy histiocytic reaction	2	0
Follicles remaining	1	0
Blood vessels not developed	0	1

AILD that could not be detected by the immunopathologic method. Bertness et al[8] first reported the existence of clonal T cells in AILD, which was followed by several groups.[9] In this series, 7 cases were studied for their DNA rearrangement. Rearrangement of genes encoding immunoglobulin heavy chain (JH) and T-cell receptor chain Tcβ) was studied by the introduction of a southern blot assay. Hind III and EcoRI were used as the restriction enzymes. The methods were described previously. As the result, 3 out of 7 cases showed rearrangement of T-cell receptor β chain gene (Tcβ). Not a case showed rearrangement of immlunoglobulin JH chain gene. The correlation of DNA analysis with morphology was shown on Table 29-3. This result correlates with the former reports that at least a part of AILD showing monoclonal proliferation of T lymphocytes.

NEXT STEP OF AILD RESEARCH

Our experiences showed that cases with typical AILD lesions have the following clinical, pathologic, immunologic, and molecular-biological characteristics (Table 29-4).

The most convincing evidence that tells the nature of AILD so far seems to be brought from DNA analysis. Even though the reported data are still fragmental, at least a large portion of typical AILDs seem to bear monoclonally rearranged T-cell receptor gene. It is natural to assume now that most, if not all, typical AILDs are the neoplasm of T cells. Further accumulation of data on this line, with the cooperation of hematopathologists, will confirm this problem. It is worth to review here the paper by Watanabe et al[12] published in 1986. They regarded AILD, IBL and IBL-like T-cell lymphoma as a spectrum of histologic changes of a single disease entity. Weiss et al,[9] on molecular biology level, supported this view. There of course remains a question as to if the AILD without clonal proliferation of the T cell exists. This question will be settled soon by the accumulation of cases studied by the modern methods used in these studies. It might be worth adding that all the reported clonally proliferating cells in AILD are T cells and not B cells.

Such findings as hyperimmunoglobulinemia, proliferation of blood vessels or the histiocytic reaction are commonly found but not the universal findings. Undoubtedly, these are the associated findings and not critically essential. It will be tempting to speculate that these changes are the para-neoplastic changes induced by some chemical factors, lymphokines namely, which are produced by neoplastic T cells. This lymphokine cannot be defined at present. Monoclonal antibodies that demonstrate as yet unclarified lymphokines or that associated products may be found and introduced in revealing new aspects of this disease and conclusive diagnosis. The ambiguity of the disease concept of AILD, which was discussed in the above section of this report,

TABLE 29-4
The Morphology of a Typical AILD Lesion

1. Found in aged group.
2. Hypergammaglobulinemia is seen in most, but not all, of the patients.
3. Much more helper/inducer type T cells are found in the lesion.
4. Many cases show Tcβ gene rearrangement. None shows immunoglobulin gene rearrangement.

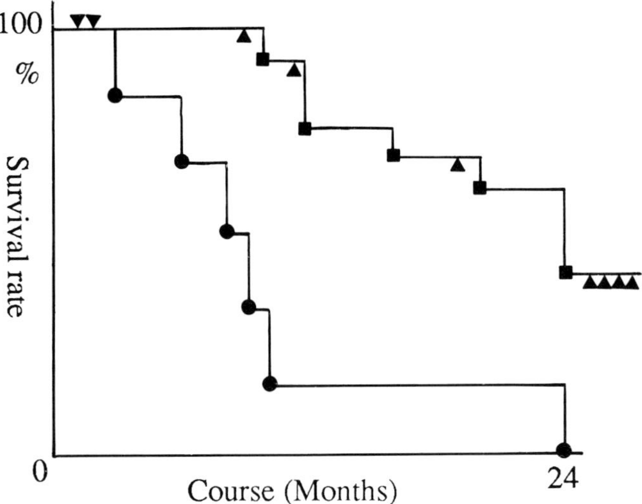

Figure 29-4. Survival curve of typical and atypical AILDs (Kaplan Meyer method)

can only be overcome by the introduction of such pathogenesis-related chemicals.

There remains a disagreement in the nature of clonally proliferating cells in AILD. Watanabe et al.[12] stressed the dominancy of suppressor/cytotoxic T cells, while other groups regard helper/inducer type T cells as the neoplastic cells of AILD. Any difficulties in settling this problem, can be resolved by simply collecting properly studied cases. The next step here is to further characterize the nature of neoplastic T cells in terms of their functions, including lymphokine production, as described above.

REFERENCES

1. Frizzera G, Moran EM, Rappaport H: Angioimmunoblastic lymphadenopathy with dysproteinemia. Lancet 1:1070–1073, 1974
2. Suchi T: Atypical lymph node hyperplasia with fatal outcome. A report on the histological, immunological and clinical investigation of the cases. Recent ADV RES Res 14:13–34, 1974
3. Nathwani BN, Rappaport H, Moran EM, et al: Malignant lymphoma arising in angioimmunoblastic lymphadenopathy. Cancer 41:578–606, 1978
4. Shimoyama M, Minato K, Saito H, et al: Immunoblastic lymphadenopathy (IBL) like T-cell lymphoma. Jpn J Clin Onc 9:347–356, 1979
5. Volk SL, Monteleone PL, Knight WAK: Chromosome abnormalities in AILD. N Engl J Med 292:975, 1975
6. Hossefeld DK, Hoeffken K, Schmidt CG, et al: Chromosome abnormalities in angioimmunoblastic lymphadenopathy. Lancet 1:198, 1976
7. Kaneko Y, Richard AL, Larson DV, et al: Nonrandom chromosome abnormalities in angioimmunoblastic lymphadenopathy. Blood 60:877–887, 1982
8. Bertness V, Kirsch I, Hollis G, et al: T cell receptor gene rearrangements as clinical markers of human T cell lymphomas. N Engl J Med 313:534–538, 1985
9. Weiss LM, Strickler JG, Dorfman RF, et al: Clonal T cell populations in angioimmunoblastic lymphadenopathy and angioimmunoblastic lymphadenopathy-like lymphoma. Am J Pathol 122:392–397, 1986
10. Hsu SM, Raihe L, Fanger H: Use of avidin-biotin-peroxidase complex (ABC) in immunoperoxidase techniques. J Histochem Cytochem 29:577–580, 1981
11. Southern EM: Detection of specific sequences among DNA fragments separated by gel electrophoresis. J Mol Biol 98:503–517, 1975
12. Watanabe S, Sato Y, Shimoyama M, et al: Immunoblastic lymphadenopathy, angioimmunoblastic lymphoadenopathy, and IB1 like T-cell lymphoma. A spectrum of T cell neoplasia. Cancer 58:2224–2232, 1986
13. Mori S, Sugiyama H: Angioimmunoblastic lymphadenopathy, its position in T cell proliferative disorder. Acta Hematol Jpn 50:208–212, 1978

30

Proliferating Cell Population in Angioimmunoblastic Lymphadenopathy with Dysproteinemia

Ryuzo Ueda
Reiko Namikawa
Hirotaka Suzuki
Yuichi Obata
Taizan Suchi
Masahiro Kikuchi
Toshitada Takahashi

Abstract

The nature of the proliferating cell population in angioimmunoblastic lymphadenopathy with dysproteinemia (AILD) was analyzed by double immunoenzymatic staining and Southern blotting. Double immunoenzymatic staining was carried out using the combination of a monoclonal anatibody against lymphocyte membrane antigen and that against human DNA polymerase α (pol α), present in the nucleus of cells in G1, S, and G2 phases, while Southern blot analysis was conducted with T cell receptor (TCR) β, and immunoglobulin heavy chain (IgH) gene probes. Double immunoenzymatic staining revealed that the pol α - positive proliferating cells had a single peripheral T-cell phenotype in most cases. The majority of AILD cases showed CD4-positive phenotypes, while a few were CD8-positive phenotypes. By Southern Blot analysis, clonal T cell populations were observed in most lesions. The results suggest that a substantial proportion of AILD lesions were mature T-cell malignancies.

One of the characteristic features of angioimmunoblastic lymphadenopathy with dysproteinemia (AILD)[1,2] lesions is a polymorphic cellular infiltration, including small lymphocytes, plasma cells, and immunoblasts. Central questions about these lesions concern which subsets of lymphocytes are proliferating and whether the proliferating cells are malignant or not. Thus, this study was conducted with double immunoenzymatic staining to determine the subset of proliferating lymphocytes and by Southern blotting to see the cell lineage and monoclonal proliferation of lymphocytes.

DISEASE ENTITY OF AILD

AILD also referred to as immunoblastic disease, immunoblastic lymphadenopathy (IBL)[3] or lymphogranulomatosis X[4], is a systemic disease characterized by generalized lymphadenopathy, hepatosplenomegaly, and immunologic abnormalities. The morphologic features in lymph nodes are diffuse effacement of nodal architecture, polymorphic cellular infiltration, and proliferation of arborizing small vessels. In spite of its fatal outcome, the disease was originally considered to be a non-neoplastic, reactive process of a B cell system. After the proposal of these new disease entities, malignant lymphomas arising in AILD, angioimmunoblastic lymphadenopathy plus immunoblastic lymphoma (AILD + IL), were reported by Nathwani et al.[5] In addition, IBL-like T-cell lymphoma (IBL-like T), which had atypical lymphoid elements in addition to the features originally described as AILD, was reported by Shimoyama et al, and they reported that tumor cells in this lesion had a T suppressor/killer (S/K) phenotype.[6,7] Thus, the differential diagnosis between AILD without any histologic manifestations of malignancy and T-cell lymphoma with the features of AILD turned out very important. Recently, a few papers demonstrated that the some AILD lesions showed rearrangements of TCRβ gene by Southern Blot analysis.[8–10] In this paper AILD lesions were morphologically subdivided into AILD and AILD-like T-lymphoma (AILD-T). AILD-T was diagnosed for lesions with a zonal proliferation of various transformed cells including clear cells atypical lymphocytes, and immunoblasts, in addition to the morphologic features of AILD. The term of AILD-T was considered to be a synonym of IBL-like T by Drs. Shimoyama[6] and Watanabe,[7] or of AILD-IL by Dr. Nathwani.[5]

TABLE 30-1
Cell Composition of Lymph Node with AILD Lesions Studied by Membrane Immunofluorescence

	surface phenotype (% positive*)					
	T cell			B cell		
Case No	CD3† Leu4	CD4 T4	CD8 T8	CD20 B1	κ‡	λ‡
1	64%	48%	17%	35%	16%	19%
2	44	45	4	9	7	2
3	56	37	12	28	14	10
5	50	39	18	18	10	3
6	61	49	24	20	14	11
7	64	53	6	15	9	16
8	43	10	35	17	3	2
9	66	44	25	16	6	2

* The percentage of positive cells was estimated by counting at least 200 cells by indirect immunofluorescence.
† CD; cluster of differentiation.
‡ Light chain of Ig.

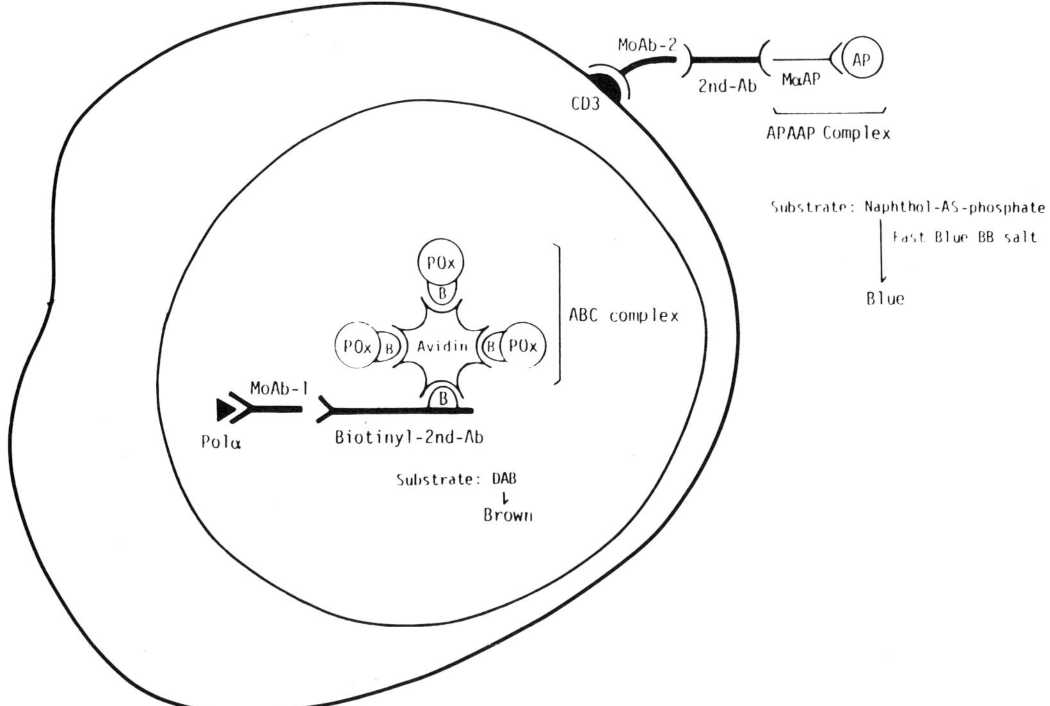

Fig. 30-1. Schematic diagram of double immunoenzymatic staining. Nucleus was stained with MoAb-1 (anti-poly α) by ABC method and then membrane antigen was stained with MoAb-2 (antilymphocyte differentiation antigen) by APAAP method.

This procedure was carried out on periodate-lysine-paraformaldehyde (PLP) fixed frozen section as follows; first, the immunoperoxidase staining against pol α in the nucleus using avidin-biotin-peroxidase complex (ABC) method was performed with Vectastain ABC Kit (Vector, Burlingame, CA), and then the immunoalkaline phosphatase monoclonal anti-alkaline phosphatase (APAAP) method was conducted with an APAAP Kit (Zymed Laboratories, San Francisco, CA). Consequently, the nucleus of proliferating cells was stained brown, while the lymphocyte membrane antigen was stained blue.

Cell Composition Analysis by Membrane Immunofluorescence Assay

Cell suspensions were prepared from biopsied lymph nodes with AILD lesions and stained with various monoclonal antibodies reactive with lymphocyte differentiation antigens to study cell surface antigens.[11] The percentage of cells showing surface fluorescence is summarized in Table 30-1. The predominant cell population isolated from AILD lesions were CD2- and CD3- positive peripheral T cells in all cases examined. Although 10 to 35% of CD20-positive B cells were also found, monoclonality of immunoglobulin (Ig) was not observed. As for T-cell subset antigens, the number of T cells with a CD4-positive phenotype was greater than that of the CD8- positive phenotype in all but Case 8, wherein the ratio of CD4-and CD8-positive cells was reversed. These data obtained from cell suspension analysis were not sufficient to determine the phenotype of the proliferating cells in these lesions.

Immunohistological Analysis of Diseased Lymph Node by Double Immunoenzymatic Staining

To determine the surface phenotype of proliferating lymphocytes, Namikawa et al developed a double immunoenzymatic staining technique[11] (Fig. 30-1). A monoclonal antibody against human DNA polymerase α(pol α) was used. Pol α is known to be present in cells capable to DNA replication, and it remains in the nuclei during G_1, S and G_2 phases of the cell cycle, but is not found in G_0 phase.[12] This enzyme molecule should be, therefore, a suitable marker for detecting the proliferating cells in tissues. Thus, the same specimen was stained with anti-pol α together with monoclonal antibodies (MoAb) detecting lymphocyte membrane antigens.

Surface Phenotype of Proliferating Lymphocytes in Non-neoplastic Lymph Node

In the lymph nodes with reactive hyperplasia, pol α positive cells were rich in germinal centers. They were also scattered in the mantle zone of the follicle and interfollicular area. Double immunoenzymatic staining demonstrated the percentage of pol α-positive cells as well as that of membrane antigen-positive cells among the pol α-positive cells in the cortical area of reactive lymph nodes. As shown in Table 30-2, pol α -positive cells were generally less than 17% in 10 lymph nodes with reactive changes.

Surface Phenotype of Proliferating Lymphocytes in Neoplatic Lymph Node

In contrast to the results with reactive lymph nodes as described above, the percentage of proliferating cells was more than 40% in malignant lymphomas, except for 2 cases of B-lymphomas, one case each of small lymphocytic (SL) type and diffuse small cleaved cell (DSC) type (Table 30-3). Although most of the proliferating cells were CD20- positive B-cells in diffuse B-lymphomas, small num-

TABLE 30-2
Surface Phenotype of Proliferating Lymphocytes in Reactive Lymphoid Hyperplasia

		pol α and			
		T cell			B cell
Diagnosis (No. cases)	pol α	CD3 Leu4	CD4 T4	CD8 T8	CD20 B1
Follicular hyperplasia (4)	14%*	84%†	69%	14%	15%
	14	88	79	20	10
	8	67	58	9	15
	9	64	72	13	14
Predominantly interfollicular hyperplasia with immunoblast (3)	17	81	73	19	6
	13	52	59	15	26
	6	86	72	8	1
Suggestive of toxoplasmosis (2)	15	62	56	32	3
	14	71	56	16	10
Suggestive of cat scratch disease (1)	12	89	71	23	7

* The percentage of polymerase α-positive cells was estimated in representative parts of the interfollicular area by counting at least 200 cells.
† The percentage of membrane antigen-positive cells was estimated by counting at least 300 polymerase α-positive cells.

TABLE 30-3
Surface Phenotype of Proliferating Lymphocytes in Non-Hodgkin's Lymphoma Studied by Double Immunoenzymatic Staining

		pol α and			
		T cell			B cell
Diagnosis (No. cases)	pol α	CD3 Leu4	CD4 T4	CD8 T8	CD20 B1
B cell lymphoma*					
SL (1)	15%†	1%‡	1%	0%	90%
DSC (1)	28	11	11	2	88
DL (2)	74	8	7	1	84
	65	10	13	1	90
IBL (1)	41	1	1	0	85
SNC (2)	64	0	0	0	72
	47	1	1	1	61
Peripheral T cell lymphoma§					
diffuse (3)					
	63	86	86	1	1
	54	9	25	1	1
	74	44	28	12	1
pleomorphic(1)	41	34	52	4	3
	40	80	89	1	1
	46	69	57	40	1
	42	74	88	68	2

* B-cell lymphoma were classified according to the description of a working formulation of classification of non-Hodgkin's lymphoma.[13] SL; small lymphocytic, DSC; diffuse small cleaved cell, DL; diffuse large cell, IBL; large cell immunoblastic, SNC; small noncleaved cell.
† The percentage of polymerase α-positive cell was estimated in representative area by counting at least 300 cells.
‡ See footnote to Table 30-2.
§ Peripheral T-cell lymphomas were classified according to Kadin and associates.[14]

bers of CD4- positive helper T-cells were also found to proliferate in some cases. Most of the proliferating cells in peripheral T-cell lymphomas were positive for CD3 molecules by monoclonal antibody Leu-4. The proliferating T-cells had mainly a CD4- positive helper phenotype in 7 out of 11 cases, but those in 2 cases of pleomorphic type had both CD4 and CD8 antigens defined by Leu-3a and Leu-2a, respectively.[13,14] Most CD20- positive B-cells were negative for pol α.

Surface Phenotype of Proliferating Lymphocytes in AILD Lesions

The surface phenotype in nine AILD lesions analyzed by double-staining[15] is summarized in Table 30-4. The percentage of pol α -positive cells is more than 30% except for one case (Case 3a). It was noteworthy that the cases analyzed did not show a monoclonal proliferation of B cells, although a polyclonal elevation of serum Ig was observed in 5 of

TABLE 30-4
Surface Phenotype of Proliferating Lymphocytes in Lymph Node with AILD Lesion Studied by Double Immunoenzymatic Staining

		pol α and			
		T cell			B cell
Case No	pol α	CD3 Leu4	CD4 T4	CD8 T8	CD20 B1
1	49%*	74%‡	80%	6%	4%
2	63	27	37	0	7
3a	12	50	49	8	8
b‡	54	9	25	1	1
4a	31	66	42	52	6
b‡	27	64	10	61	14
5	66	51	74	6	4
6	53	56	51	5	5
7	53	49	64	1	3
8	89	74	23	61	0
9	49	25	24	10	9

* The percentage of polymerase α-positive cells was estimated in representative parts by the lesion by counting at least 300 cells.
† See footnote to Table 30-2.
‡ Malignant lymphoma.

8 cases examined. Another important finding regarding the phenotype of the proliferating cell population is that 7 of 9 cases were of CD4- positive phenotype, whereas 2 cases were of CD8-positive phenotype.

It is also noted that in the CD8-predominant cases such as case 4a and 8, a considerable number of CD4- positive proliferating cells were also recognized, although only a small number of CD8- positive cells were observed in CD4-dominant lesions. Thus, lymph node lesions with the features of AILD may be considered as a neoplastic disease of periheral T cells of both CD4 and CD8 subtypes based on the data of double-immunoenzymatic staining.

SOUTHERN BLOT ANALYSIS OF AILD LESIONS

To detect the cell lineage and clonal T cell and/or B cell proliferating in AILD lesions more directly, Southern blot analysis with probes for T cell receptor (TCR) and Ig genes were carried out.[16] As summarized in Table 30-5, clonal rearrangement of TCRβ genes were observed in 10 of 16 AILD lesions; 3 of 8 AILD cases and 7 of 8 AILD-T cases showed the TCRβ rearrangement. AILD-T cases had a higher tendency to show TCRβ gene rearrangement than AILD cases. One AILD-T case (Case G.N.) with a rearranged TCRβ gene exhibited clonal IgH and IgK gene rearrangement as well (Fig. 30-2), although no other cases, showed clonal rearrangements of IgH genes. Detailed serologic analysis was, however, not conducted in this case. Thus, the question whether the presence of two clones in a single tumor or a single clone with both IgK and TCRβ gene rearrangement was not solved. It is likely that the lineage specificity of the rearrangements of either Ig or TCR is not absolute.

In another case (Case 3), malignant lymphoma of T-cell type developed 2 years later. This lymphoma specimen exhibited the same size clonal rearrangement band as that ob-

TABLE 30-5
Clonal Rearrangements of TCR and Ig Genes in AILD and AILD-T Lesions

	No. of cases	No. of cases with gene rearrangements	
		TCR (%)	Ig (%)
AILD*	8	3 (38)	0 (0)
AILD-T	8	7 (88)	1 (13)

* AILD; angioimmunoblastic lymphadenopathy with dysproteinemia, without histologic manifestation of malignancy, AILD-T; AILD lesion with histologic manifestations of malignancy.

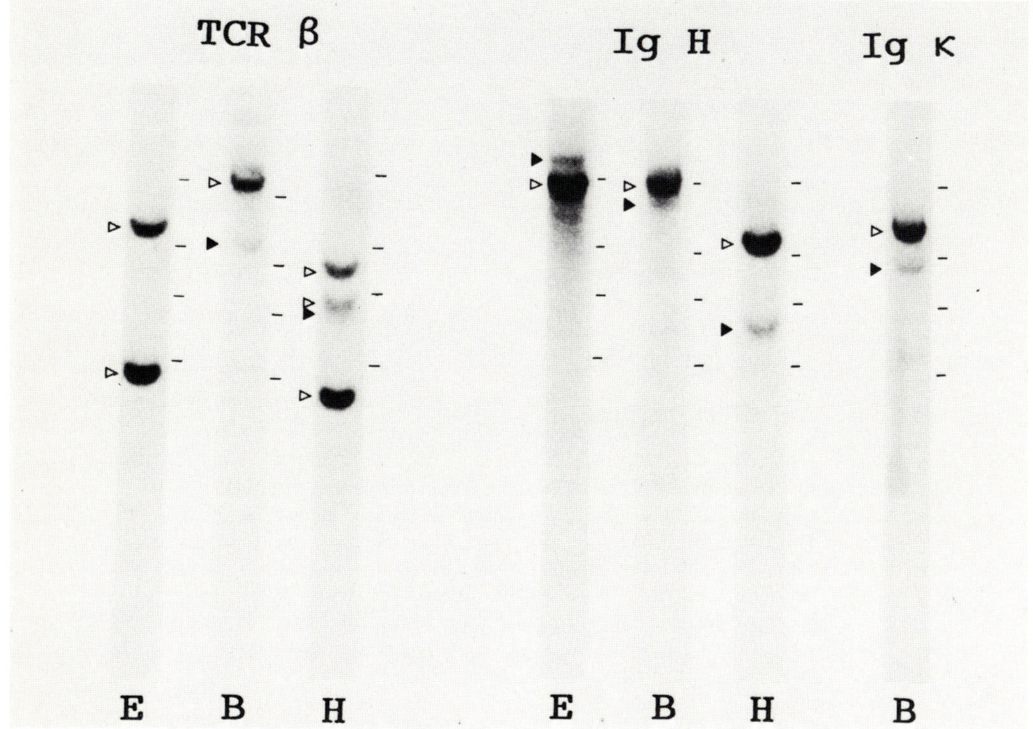

Fig. 30-2. Rearrangements of both TCR and Ig genes in AILD lesion of case G.N. DNA was digested with either EcoRI (E), BamHI (B) or HindIII (H) and hybridized with $C_T\beta$, J_H or Cκ probes. Open and closed arrowheads indicate the germline band, and the rearrangement band, respectively. Dashes on the right side of each lane indicate the position of the size marker.

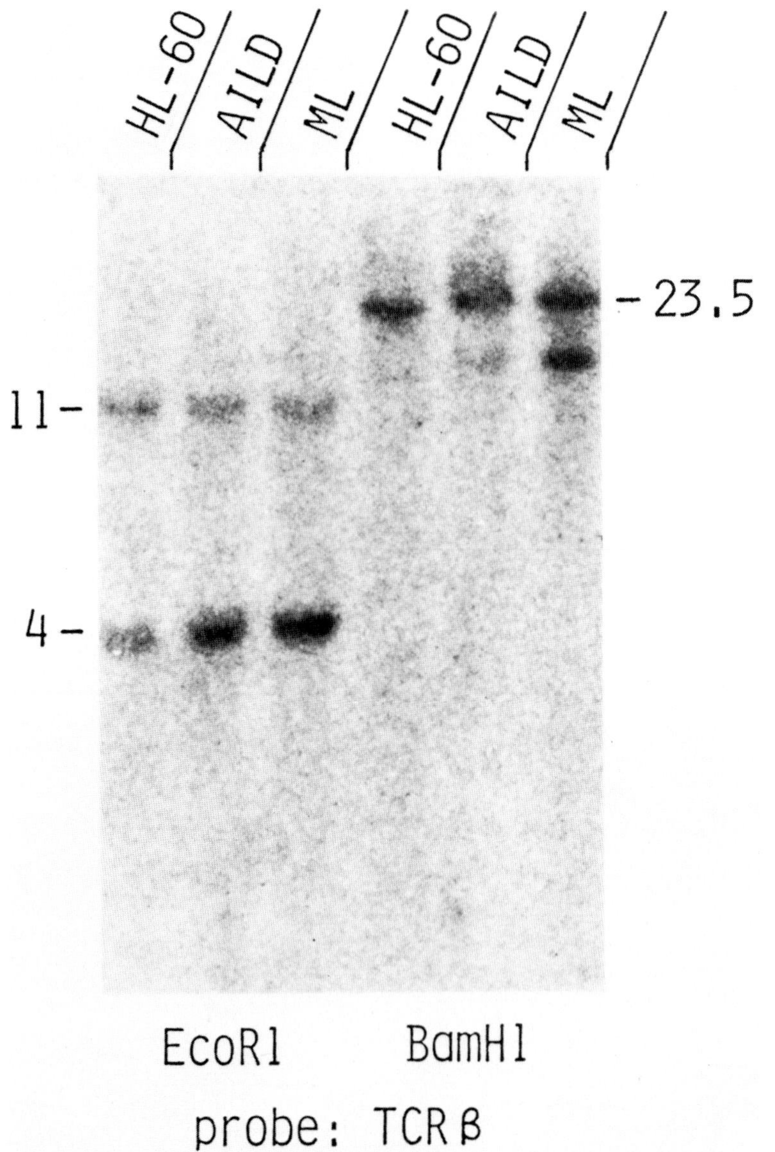

Fig. 30-3. Sequential analysis of TCRβ gene rearrangements in the primary AILD lesion and the malignant lymphoma (developed two year later) in case 3. DNA was digested with either EcoRI or BamHI, and hybridized with a $C_T\beta$ probe. The lane ''HL-60'' shows the results with HL-60 promyelocytic leukemia cell line. (As a control representing the germline pattern of TCRβ genes; 4 and 11 Kb in EcoRI digestion and 23.5 Kb in BamHI digestion.)

served in the previous AILD lesion with BamHI DNA digestion (Fig. 30-3). Expansion of the clonal T cell population was clearly shown by the increase in intensity of the rearranged band. This case suggested that the AILD lesion with clonal rearrangements might be T-cell lymphoma in early stage.

SUMMARY AND CONCLUSIONS

1. Double immunoenzymatic staining technique was established to determine the surface phenotype of proliferating lymphocytes with monoclonal antibodies against DNA polymerase α and lymphocyte membrane antigens.
2. Cell composition analysis was shown to have limited value for analysis of AILD lesions, because it failed to demonstrate a clonal T-cell population.
3. The proliferating lymphocytes of AILD lesion were peripheral T cells of either CD4-positive helper or CD8-positive suppressor phenotype.
4. No major histologic difference were recognized between CD4- and CD8- positive cases.
5. Clonal rearrangements of TCRβ gene were observed in 10 out of 16 AILD lesions by Southern blot analysis. AILD-T cases showed a higher frequency of TCRβ rearrangements than AILD cases.
6. Most AILD lesions are neoplastic disease originating from mature T cells as determined by combined analysis with double immunoenzymatic staining and Southern blotting.

ACKNOWLEDGMENTS

This work was supported in part by a Grant-in-Aid for the Comprehensive Ten-Year Strategy for Cancer Control from the Ministry of Health and Welfare; Grants-in-Aid for Cancer Research from the Ministries of Education, Science and Culture, and Health and Welfare in Japan; by a grant from the Cancer Research Institute Inc., New York, USA; and by a grant from the Foundation for Promotion of Cancer Research, Tokyo, Japan.

REFERENCES

1. Frizzera G, Moran EM, Rappaport H: Angioimmunoblastic lymphadenopathy with dysproteinemia. Lancet 1:1070–1073, 1974
2. Frizzera G, Moran EM, Rappaport H: Angioimmunoblastic lymphadenopathy. Diagnosis and clinical course. Am J Med 59:803–818, 1975
3. Lukes RJ, Tindle BH: Immunoblastic lymphadenoapthy; a hyperimmune entity resembling Hodgkin's disease. N Engl J Med 292:1–8, 1975
4. Radaszkiewics T, Lennert K: Lymphogranulomatosis X. Klinisches Bild, Therapie und Prognose. Dtsch Med Wochenschr 100:1157–1163, 1975
5. Nathwani BN, Rappaport H, Moran EM, et al: Malignant lymphoma arising in angioimmunoblastic lymphadenopathy. Cancer 41:578–606, 1978
6. Shimoyama M, Minato K, Saito H, et al: Immuno blastic lymphadenopathy (IBL)-like T cell-lymphoma. Jpn J Clin Oncol 9 (Suppl): 347–356, 1979
7. Watanabe S, Sato Y, Shimoyama M, et al: Immunoblastic lymphadenopathy, angioimmunoblastic lymphadenopathy, and IBL-like T-cell lymphoma. Cancer 58:2224–2232, 1986
8. Weiss LM, Strickler JG, Dorfman RF, et al: Clonal T-cell populations in angioimmunoblastic lymphadenopathy and angioimmunoblastic lymphadenopathy-like lymphoma. Am J Pathol 122:392–397, 1986
9. Griesser H, Feller A, Lennert K, et al: Rearrangement of the β chain of the T cell antigen receptor and immunoglobulin genes in lymphoproliferative disorders. J Clin Invest 78:1179–1184, 1986
10. O'Connor NTJ, Crick JA, Wainscoat JS, et al: Evidence for monoclonal T lymphocyte proliferation in angioimmunoblastic lymphadenopathy. J Clin Pathol 39:1229–1232, 1986
11. Namikawa R, Ueda R, Suchi T, et al: Double immunoenzymatic detection of surface phenotype of proliferating lymphocytes in situ with monoclonal antibodies against DNA polymerase α and lymphocyte membrane antigens. Am J Clin Pathol 87:725–731, 1987
12. Bensch KG, Tanaka S, Hu SZ, et al: Intercellular localization of human DNA polymerase α with monoclonal antibodies. J Biol Chem 275:8391–8396
13. Non-Hodgkin's Lymphoma Pathologic Classification Project. National Cancer Institute sponsored study of classification of non-Hodgkin's lymphoma: Summary and description of a working formulation for clinical usage. Cancer 49:2112–2135, 1982
14. Kadin ME, Berard CW, Nanba K, Wakasa H: Proceedings of the United States–Japan seminar. Hum Pathol 14:745–772, 1983
15. Namikawa R, Suchi T, Ueda R et al: Phenotyping of proliferating lymphocytes in angioimmunoblastic lymphadenopathy and related lesions by double immunoenzymatic staining technique. Am J Pathol 127:279–287, 1987
16. Suzuki H, Namikawa R, Ueda R, et al: Clonal T cell population in angioimmunoblastic lymphadenopathy and related lesions. Jpn J Cancer Res (Gann), 78:701–702, 1987

Index

Numerals in *italics* indicate a figure, "t" following a page number indicates tabular matter.